OBSTETRICS
by Ten Teachers

First published in 1917 as 'Midwifery', *Obstetrics by Ten Teachers* is well established as a concise, yet comprehensive, guide within its field. The 21st Edition has been thoroughly updated by its latest team of 'teachers', integrating clinical material with the latest scientific developments that underpin patient care.

Each chapter is highly structured, with learning objectives, definitions, aetiology, clinical features, investigations, treatments and key point summaries and additional reading where appropriate. A key theme for this edition is 'professionalism' and information specific to this is threaded throughout the text.

Along with its companion *Gynaecology by Ten Teachers*, 21st Edition, the books continue to provide an accessible 'one stop shop' in obstetrics and gynaecology for a new generation of doctors.

21st EDITION

OBSTETRICS
by Ten Teachers

Edited by

Louise C Kenny
Professor and Executive Pro-Vice Chancellor
Faculty of Health and Life Sciences
University of Liverpool, UK

Fergus McCarthy
Senior Lecturer
University College Cork
Consultant Obstetrician & Gynaecologist and
Maternal Fetal Medicine Subspecialist
Cork University Maternity Hospital
Cork, Ireland

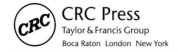

CRC Press
Taylor & Francis Group
Boca Raton London New York

CRC Press is an imprint of the
Taylor & Francis Group, an **informa** business

Designed cover image: From FatCamera via Getty Images

Twenty-first edition published 2024
by CRC Press
2385 NW Executive Center Drive, Suite 320, Boca Raton FL 33431

and by CRC Press
4 Park Square, Milton Park, Abingdon, Oxon, OX14 4RN

CRC Press is an imprint of Taylor & Francis Group, LLC

© 2024 Louise C Kenny and Fergus McCarthy

ISBN: 978-1-032-05120-8 (hbk)
ISBN: 978-1-032-05116-1 (pbk)
ISBN: 978-1-003-19611-2 (ebk)

DOI: 10.1201/9781003196112

Typeset in Palatino LT Std
by Evolution Design & Digital Ltd (Kent)

Access the Instructor and Student Resources: www.routledge.com/cw/mccarthy

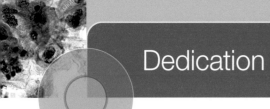

Dedication

This book is dedicated to Elaine, Vivienne, Alannah, Matthew and Evan (FMC)
And to my Mum (LCK)

Contents

Additional resources for students and lecturers to accompany this textbook are available online.

Visit www.routledge.com/cw/mccarthy for interactive SBAs and EMQs, videos and figure slides.

Preface

Obstetrics by Ten Teachers, first published in 1917, is now in its 21st Edition. An iconic text, it remains the oldest and one of the most respected and popular English-language texts in the discipline.

The 21st Edition builds on the solid foundations of over a century of previous editions but reflects recent advances in the field as well as the evolution of medical education. It contains new material, extensive online resources and additional tools for self-assessment, written by a new generation of 'Ten Teachers'. They are all leading clinicians, renowned in their fields, and all are intimately involved in the delivery of both undergraduate and postgraduate training in the UK and Ireland, allowing the book to reflect the current undergraduate curriculum. This volume has been carefully edited to ensure consistency of structure, style and content in common with its sister text, *Gynaecology by Ten Teachers*. The books can therefore be used together or independently as required.

It has been an honour and a privilege to edit a textbook that we once read as students and we fully appreciate the responsibility of revisiting a much-loved classic, particularly at this critical juncture for women's health. After almost a century of improvement, maternal mortality rates in some high-resource settings are increasing, largely driven by inequalities and disadvantage. Moreover, conditions that affect women more than men garner less research funding. Women have, for example, been historically under-represented in clinical trials and, despite work to rectify this bias, women are not necessarily included in proportions that match the prevalence or burden of disease. Consequently, effective cures for diseases that have been known about since the time of Hippocrates, such as pre-eclampsia, remain elusive. We therefore hope that the latest edition of *Obstetrics by Ten Teachers* inspires the next generation of doctors to follow the authors and editors into this discipline. There remains much to be done to make pregnancy and childbirth safe, fulfilling and equitable, everywhere and for everyone.

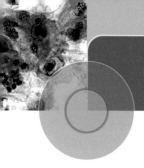

Contributors

Anna L David
Professor and Consultant
Obstetrics and Maternal Fetal Medicine
University College London Hospital
Director
Elizabeth Garrett Anderson Institute for Women's
 Health
University College London

Eugene Dempsey
Professor and Horgan Chair in Neonatology
Department of Paediatrics and Child Health
Infant Research Centre
University College Cork

Louise C Kenny
Professor and Executive Pro-Vice Chancellor
Faculty of Health and Life Sciences
University of Liverpool

Asma Khalil
Fetal Medicine Unit
St George's Hospital
St George's University of London
Fetal Medicine Unit
Liverpool Women's Hospital
University of Liverpool

David Lissauer
NIHR Professor
Global Maternal and Fetal Health
Women's & Children's Health
University of Liverpool
Queen Elizabeth Central Hospital
Blantyre, Malawi

Philippa J Marsden
Consultant in Obstetrics and Maternal Medicine
Head of Obstetrics
Honorary Reader in Medical Education
Royal Victoria Infirmary, Newcastle upon Tyne

Fergus McCarthy
Senior Lecturer
University College Cork
Consultant Obstetrician & Gynaecologist and
Maternal Fetal Medicine Subspecialist
Cork University Maternity Hospital

Deirdre J Murphy
Chair of Obstetrics
Professor and Consultant Obstetrician
Trinity College Dublin
Coombe Hospital Dublin

Surabhi Nanda
Consultant in Maternal Fetal Medicine
Liverpool Women's NHS Foundation Trust

Andrew D Weeks
Consultant Obstetrician
Professor of International Maternal Health
Department of Women's and Children's Health
University of Liverpool
Liverpool Women's Hospital

Abbreviations

2D	two-dimensional
3D	three-dimensional
4D	four-dimensional
AA	arterioarterial
AC	abdominal circumference
ACE	angiotensin-converting enzyme
A:Cr	albumin to creatinine
AED	anti-epileptic drug
AFI	amniotic fluid index
AFP	alpha-fetoprotein
AIDS	acquired immunodeficiency syndrome
ALARA	as low as reasonably achievable
AP	anterior–posterior
APH	antepartum haemorrhage
APS	antiphospholipid syndrome
ARM	artificial rupture of membranes
ART	antiretroviral therapy
AS	aortic stenosis
AV	arteriovenous
BAPM	British Association of Perinatal Medicine
BMI	body mass index
BNF	British National Formulary
BPD	biparietal diameter/bronchopulmonary dysplasia
bpm	beats per minute
BPP	biophysical profile
CF	cystic fibrosis
cffDNA	cell-free fetal deoxyribonucleic acid
CI	confidence interval
CMA	chromosomal microarray analysis
CMV	cytomegalovirus
CNS	central nervous system
COVID-19	coronavirus disease 2019
CPAP	continuous positive airway pressure
CPD	cephalopelvic disproportion
CPR	cardiopulmonary resuscitation
CRL	crown–rump length
CRM	clinical risk management
CT	computed tomography
CTG	cardiotocograph(y)
CVS	chorionic villus sampling

DDH	developmental dysplasia of the hip
DMD	Duchenne muscular dystrophy
DNA	deoxyribonucleic acid
DOHaD	Developmental Origins of Health and Disease
DV	ductus venosus
DVT	deep vein thrombosis
DWI	diffusion weighted imaging
ECG	electrocardiogram
ECV	external cephalic version
EDD	estimated date of delivery
(a)EEG	(amplitude integrated) electroencephalography
EFM	electronic fetal monitoring
EFW	estimated fetal weight
EIA	enzyme immunoassay
EMQ	extended matching question
ERCS	elective repeat caesarean section
ESBL	extended spectrum β-lactamase
FBC	full blood count
FBM	fetal breathing movement
FEV_1	forced expiratory volume in 1 second
fFN	fetal fibronectin
FGF(R)	fibroblast growth factor (receptor)
FGM	female genital mutilation
FGR	fetal growth restriction
FHR	fetal heart rate
FL	femur length
FOQ	family origin questionnaire
FVS	fetal varicella syndrome
GBS	group B *Streptococcus*
GCS	Glasgow Coma Score
GDM	gestational diabetes mellitus
GP	general practitioner
GUM	genitourinary medicine
Hb	haemoglobin
HbA	adult haemoglobin
HbAC	haemoglobin C trait
HbAS	sickle cell trait
HbA1c	glycated haemoglobin
HBcAb	hepatitis B core antibody
HbF	fetal haemoglobin
HBsAb	hepatitis B surface antibody
HBsAg	hepatitis B surface antigen
HbSC	sickle cell/haemoglobin C disease
HbSS	sickle cell disease
HBV	hepatitis B virus
HC	head circumference
(β)hCG	(beta-)human chorionic gonadotrophin

HCV	hepatitis C virus
HDFN	haemolytic disease of the fetus and newborn
HELLP	haemolysis, elevated liver enzymes and low platelets
HG	hyperemesis gravidarum
HIE	hypoxic-ischaemic encephalopathy
HIV	human immunodeficiency virus
HMO	human milk oligosaccharide
HSV	herpes simplex virus
IBD	inflammatory bowel disease
Ig	immunoglobulin
IM	intramuscular
iNO	inhaled nitric oxide
IOL	induction of labour
IQ	intelligence quotient
ISUOG	International Society of Ultrasound in Obstetrics and Gynecology
IUT	intrauterine transfusion
IV	intravenous
IVF	in vitro fertilization
IVH	intraventricular haemorrhage
LLETZ	large loop excision of the transformation zone
LMP	last menstrual period
LMWH	low-molecular-weight heparin
MBRRACE-UK	Mothers and Babies, Reducing Risk through Audits and Confidential Enquiries across the UK
MCA	middle cerebral artery
MCMA	monochorionic monoamniotic
M, C & S	microscopy, culture and sensitivity
MDT	multidisciplinary team
MEOWS	Modified Early Obstetric Warning System
MI	myocardial infarction
MMR	mumps, measles, rubella
MoM	multiples of median
MRI	magnetic resonance imaging
MRSA	methicillin-resistant *Staphylococcus aureus*
MS	multiple sclerosis
MSAF	meconium staining of amniotic fluid
MSU	midstream urine specimen
NEC	necrotizing enterocolitis
NICE	National Institute for Health and Care Excellence
NICU	neonatal intensive care unit
NIPT	non-invasive prenatal testing
NLS	Newborn Life Support
NRP	Newborn Resuscitation Program
NSAID	non-steroidal anti-inflammatory drug
NT	nuchal translucency
OA	occipito-anterior
OASI	obstetric anal sphincter injury

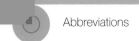
OGTT	oral glucose tolerance test
OP	occipito-posterior
OR	odds ratio
OT	occipito-transverse
OT(R)(-A)	oxytocin (receptor) (antagonist)
PAPP-A	pregnancy-associated plasma protein-A
PCR	polymerase chain reaction
P:Cr	protein to creatinine ratio
PDA	patent ductus arteriosus
PE	pulmonary embolism
PG	prostaglandin
PH	pulmonary hypertension
PlGF	placental growth factor
PPH	postpartum haemorrhage
PPHN	persistent pulmonary hypertension of the newborn
PPROM	pre-labour/prolonged premature rupture of membranes
PROM	preterm rupture of membranes
PSV	peak systolic velocity
PTL	preterm labour
RA	rheumatoid arthritis
RCM	Royal College of Midwives
RCOG	Royal College of Obstetricians and Gynaecologists
RDS	respiratory distress syndrome
REM	rapid eye movement
RhD	rhesus factor D
RNA	ribonucleic acid
ROP	retinopathy of prematurity
RR	relative risk
SBA	single best answer
SCBU	special care baby unit
SCD	sickle cell disease
SFH	symphysis–fundal height
sFlt-1	soluble fms-like tyrosine kinase
SGA	small for gestational age
SLE	systemic lupus erythematosus
SROM	spontaneous rupture of the membranes
SSRI	selective serotonin reuptake inhibitor
SUDEP	sudden unexpected death in epilepsy
(f)T3	(free) triiodothyronine
(f)T4	(free) thyroxine
TAPS	twin anaemia–polycythaemia sequence
TENS	transcutaneous electrical nerve stimulation
TH	therapeutic hypothermia
TRAP	twin reversed arterial perfusion
TSH	thyroid-stimulating hormone
TTTS	twin-to-twin transfusion syndrome
uE3	unconjugated oestriol

UKOSS	UK Obstetric Surveillance Survey
UTI	urinary tract infection
VBAC	vaginal birth after caesarean
VDRL	venereal diseases research laboratory
VEGF	vascular endothelial growth factor
VTE	venous thromboembolism
VWF	von Willebrand factor
VZIG	varicella zoster immunoglobulin
VZV	varicella zoster virus
WHO	World Health Organization

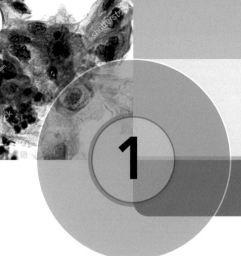

Obstetric history and examination

PHILIPPA J MARSDEN

1

Learning Objectives
- Understand the concept of preconceptual counselling and the opportunity that it provides.
- Understand the principles of taking an obstetric history.
- Understand the key components of an obstetric examination.
- Be able to perform an appropriate obstetric examination.

INTRODUCTION

Taking an obstetric history and performing an obstetric examination differs from a history and examination in other specialities in that the patient is often healthy and simply undergoing a normal life event. Antenatal care is designed to support the normal physiological process and to detect early signs of complications. For patients with a more complicated history, a detailed history and risk assessment offers a personalised approach with the opportunity to plan antenatal care carefully. The types of questions asked during the history change with gestation, as does the purpose and nature of the examination, and questioning and examination must always be undertaken with care and sensitivity.

PRECONCEPTUAL COUNSELLING

Pregnancy is increasingly being achieved in those of an advanced age, who frequently have one or more pre-existing medical conditions. As more patients with chronic illness look to conceive, who often have high levels of insight into their conditions, obstetricians are increasingly having the opportunity to meet with patients prior to conception to discuss their medical conditions and provide advice on optimizing their pregnancy and maximizing their chances of a healthy uncomplicated pregnancy. This often occurs via a preconceptual clinic.

The main purposes of preconceptual counselling are as follows:

- optimize maternal health before embarking on a pregnancy
  - recognise issues
  - amend lifestyle
  - address social issues
- reduce maternal and perinatal morbidity and mortality
- address chronic medical conditions
- address medications used (are they pregnancy friendly?)
- discuss the impact of the disease process on pregnancy versus the impact of pregnancy on the disease process

10.1201/9781003196112-1

- address challenges to falling pregnant – fertility issues
- plan antenatal follow-up and any screening needed for when pregnancy occurs
- discuss mode of delivery
- address breastfeeding – which medications are suitable
- plan postnatal follow-up and contraception

OBSTETRIC HISTORY

INTRODUCTION

When meeting a patient for the first time, introduce yourself and tell the patient why you have come to see them. Make sure that the patient is seated comfortably. Some patients may want another person to be present and this wish should be respected. A qualified interpreter (or interpreting service) should be used if appropriate.

The questions asked must be tailored to the purpose of the visit. At the booking visit, the history must be thorough and meticulously recorded. Once this baseline information is established, there is no need to go over this information at every visit. Everyone should attend for routine antenatal visits, usually performed by the midwife, and occasionally some attend for a specific reason or because a complication has developed.

Some areas of the obstetric history cover subjects that are intensely private. It is vital to maintain confidentiality and to be aware of and be sensitive to each individual situation.

DATING THE PREGNANCY

Pregnancy was historically dated from the last menstrual period (LMP), because the LMP was considered more reliable than the date of conception. The median duration from the first day of the LMP to birth is 40 weeks, and this can be used to work out the estimated date of delivery (EDD). This explains why, although a human pregnancy is approximately 38 weeks, we refer to the length of pregnancy as 40 weeks in duration. However, the National Institute for Health and Care Excellence (NICE) guideline on antenatal care recommends that pregnancy dates are set by ultrasound using the crown–rump

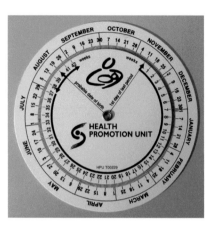

Figure 1.1 Gestation calendar wheel.

measurement between 11 weeks and 2 days and 14 weeks and 1 day. Almost everyone undergoing antenatal care in the UK will have an ultrasound scan late in the first trimester or early in the second trimester, and the EDD is determined at this point. Accurate dating early in pregnancy is important for assessing fetal growth in later pregnancy and reduces the risk of premature planned deliveries, such as induction of labour for postmature pregnancies (>41 weeks' gestation) and elective caesarean sections.

In the first trimester, there are pregnancy calculators (wheels) (**Figure 1.1**) available and pregnancy calculator apps for smartphones that can work out the EDD for you (**Figure 1.2**), which are useful before the dating scan.

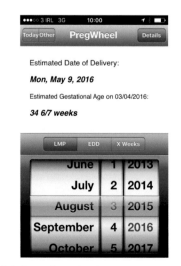

Figure 1.2 Gestation calendar app on a smartphone. (Courtesy of Dr Andrew Yu, Yale University.)

SOCIAL HISTORY

The social history is an important part of the obstetric history, as social circumstances can have a dramatic influence on pregnancy outcome, and requires considerable sensitivity. Mothers and Babies, Reducing Risk through Audits and Confidential Enquiries across the UK (MBRRACE-UK) has consistently reported that maternal mortality is highest among those who are older and those living in the most deprived areas. Recent reports highlighted that a quarter of those who died, whose birthplace was known, were born outside the UK and almost 1 in 10 had severe and multiple disadvantages including substance misuse, domestic abuse and mental health issues. Of those that died, 20% were known to social services and to child protection services.

Women from Black, Asian and minority ethnic groups have a much higher chance of dying during pregnancy or after birth and, although they have more health problems and are more affected by social and economic problems, systemic racism and racial bias may also affect their care. This is extremely important to remember when taking a history at any point in pregnancy, as there is evidence from Black, Asian and minority ethnic groups that they are treated differently, receive less empathy from health professionals, are not listened to, are not taken seriously and are less likely to disclose worries (**Figure 1.3**).

Women who are experiencing domestic abuse are at higher risk of abuse during pregnancy and of adverse pregnancy outcomes; because they may be prevented from attending antenatal appointments, they may be concerned that disclosure of their abuse may worsen their situation and they may be anxious about the reaction of health professionals. One-third of those who experience domestic abuse do so for the first time while pregnant, and pregnancy and the post-partum period is a risk factor for domestic abuse leading to homicide, with one in seven maternal deaths occurring in those who have told their health professional they are in an abusive relationship. This is why it is important to ask about domestic abuse in every pregnancy.

Enquiring about domestic abuse is difficult. It is recommended that everyone who is pregnant is seen on their own at least once during their pregnancy, so that they can discuss this, if needed, away from an abusive partner. If you happen to be the person with whom this information is shared, you must ensure that it is passed on to the relevant team, as this may be the only opportunity that the patient has to disclose it. It is a good idea to practise with your peers asking about domestic abuse sensitively, demonstrating empathy and compassion and signposting to support.

Smoking, alcohol and drug intake also form part of the social history. Smoking causes placental dysfunction and thus increases the risk of miscarriage,

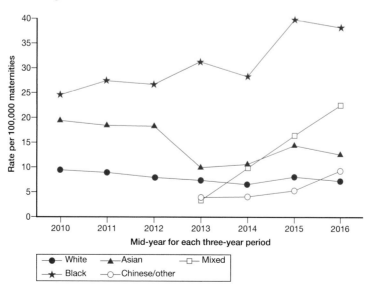

Figure 1.3 Maternal mortality rates from 2009 to 2017 among people from different ethnic groups in the UK.

stillbirth and neonatal death. There are interventions that can be offered to those who are still smoking in pregnancy (see **Chapters 3** and **6**).

Complete abstinence from alcohol is advised, as the safety of alcohol is not proven. However, alcohol is probably not harmful in small amounts (less than one drink per day). Binge drinking is particularly harmful and can lead to a constellation of features in the baby known as fetal alcohol syndrome (see **Chapters 3** and **6**).

Enquiring about recreational drug taking is more difficult. Approximately 0.5–1% of women continue to take recreational drugs during pregnancy. Be careful not to make assumptions. During the booking visit, the midwife should enquire directly about drug taking. If it is seen as part of the long list of routine questions asked at this visit, it is perceived as less threatening. However, sometimes this information comes to light at other times. Cocaine and crack cocaine are the most harmful of the recreational drugs taken, but all have some effects on the pregnancy, and all have financial implications (see **Chapter 6**).

The following are important aspects of the social history:

- whether the patient is single or in a relationship and what support they have at home
- what sort of housing the patient lives in (e.g. a flat with lots of stairs and no lift may be problematic)
- whether the patient works and, if so, for how long they are planning to work during the pregnancy
- whether the patient smokes/drinks or uses recreational drugs

PREVIOUS OBSTETRIC HISTORY

Past obstetric history is one of the most important areas for establishing risk in the current pregnancy. It is helpful to list the pregnancies in date order and to discover what the outcome was in each pregnancy.

The features that are likely to have impact on future pregnancies include:

- preterm delivery (increased risk of preterm birth)
- pre-eclampsia (increased risk of pre-eclampsia/fetal growth restriction)

- abruption (increased risk of recurrence)
- congenital abnormality (recurrence risk depends on type of abnormality)
- macrosomic baby (may be related to gestational diabetes)
- fetal growth restriction (increased recurrence)
- unexplained stillbirth (increased risk of gestational diabetes)

The method of delivery for any previous births must be recorded, as this can have implications for planning in the current pregnancy, particularly if there has been a previous caesarean section, difficult vaginal birth, postpartum haemorrhage or significant perineal trauma.

The shorthand for describing the number of previous pregnancies can be confusing:

- *gravidity* is the total number of pregnancies, regardless of how they ended
- *parity* is the number of live births or stillbirths, after 24 weeks. Note that miscarriages are denoted as a + (see below) and twins count as 2

Therefore, someone who has had six miscarriages with only one live baby born at 32 weeks and is pregnant again will be gravida 8, para 1 + 6.

In practice, when presenting a history, it is much easier to describe exactly what has happened; for example, 'JA is in their eighth pregnancy. They have had six miscarriages at gestations of 8–12 weeks and one spontaneous delivery of a live baby boy at 32 weeks. Baby Tom is now 2 years old and healthy.'

PAST GYNAECOLOGICAL HISTORY

EARLY PREGNANCY

In the first trimester, taking a detailed gynaecological history is important, particularly if scanning is not available and the LMP is being used to date the pregnancy. People with polycystic ovary syndrome can have very long menstrual cycles and may have ovulated much later in the cycle. Contraceptive history can also be relevant if conception has occurred soon after stopping the combined oral contraceptive pill or depot progesterone preparations, as, again, this makes dating by LMP more difficult. Also, some people will conceive with an intrauterine device still in situ. This carries an increased risk of miscarriage.

Previous episodes of pelvic inflammatory disease increase the risk of ectopic pregnancy. This is only of relevance in early pregnancy. However, it is important to establish that any infections have been adequately treated and that the partner was also treated. Chlamydia infection is common in teenagers and can cause problems if the baby if untreated.

Previous ectopic pregnancy increases the risk of recurrence from 1 in 100 pregnancies to 18 in 100. Those who have had an ectopic pregnancy should be offered an early ultrasound scan to establish the site of any future pregnancies.

RISK FACTORS FOR LATER PREGNANCY

The date of the last cervical smear should be noted. Every year, a small number of people are diagnosed as having cervical cancer in pregnancy. It is important that smears are not deferred in anyone at increased risk of cervical disease (e.g. previous cervical smear abnormality or very overdue smear). Gently taking a smear in the first trimester does not cause miscarriage and expectant parents should be reassured about this. If there has been irregular bleeding, the cervix should at least be examined to ensure that there are no obvious lesions present.

If someone has undergone treatment for cervical changes, this should be noted. Treatment to the cervix by knife cone biopsy or large loop excision of the transformation zone (LLETZ) can be associated with an increased risk of preterm birth, and depending on the depth of biopsy, measuring the cervical length in the second trimester may be recommended.

Recurrent miscarriage may be associated with a number of problems. Antiphospholipid syndrome increases the risk of further pregnancy loss, fetal growth restriction, pre-eclampsia and venous thromboembolism and patients need a great deal of support during pregnancy if they have experienced recurrent pregnancy losses.

Termination of pregnancy is a sensitive subject and, as first trimester terminations of pregnancy are not usually relevant to the pregnancy, information about such terminations must be sensitively requested and recorded. Some people do not wish this to be recorded in their hand-held notes. However, second-trimester terminations and terminations for congenital abnormalities may be relevant, and a sensitive way to ask is 'Have you had any other pregnancies?' allowing for disclosure of previous pregnancies.

Previous gynaecological surgery should be asked about, especially if it involved the uterus, and the presence of pelvic masses such as ovarian cysts and fibroids should also be noted, as both of these issues may also pose problems during pregnancy and may have an impact on delivery. A history of endometriosis is also important to be aware of, because of the adhesions and scarring associated with that disease, which can make a caesarean section complicated.

Having a history of subfertility and fertility treatment may increase anxiety about pregnancy and birth and therefore should be noted if the couple wish. However, legally, you should only write down in notes that a pregnancy is conceived by in vitro fertilization (IVF) or donor egg or sperm if you have written permission from the parent. Generally, if the patient has told you themselves that the pregnancy was an assisted conception, it is reasonable to state that in your presentation.

MEDICAL AND SURGICAL HISTORY

All pre-existing medical disease should be carefully noted and any associated drug history also recorded. The major pre-existing diseases that have an impact on pregnancy and their potential effects are covered in **Chapter 10**.

Previous surgery should be noted. Occasionally, surgery has been performed for conditions that may continue to be a problem during pregnancy and at delivery, such as Crohn disease.

A history of mental health illness is important to record. These enquiries should be made in a sensitive way at the antenatal booking visit and should include the severity of the illness and whether they received consultant care. If someone has had children before, it is important to ask whether they had problems with depression or 'the blues' after the births of any of them. People with significant mental illness in pregnancy should be cared for by a multidisciplinary perinatal mental health team, including the midwife, general practitioner, hospital consultant and psychiatric team.

- Diabetes mellitus
- Hypertension
- Cardiac disease
- Epilepsy
- Renal disease
- Connective tissue diseases (e.g. systemic lupus erythematosus)
- Venous thromboembolic disease: increased risk during pregnancy
- Human immunodeficiency virus (HIV) infection

Table 1.1 Organizations that offer advice on medicines during pregnancy and when breastfeeding

Type of information	Organization(s)
Evidence-based safety information about medication, vaccines, and chemical and radiological exposures in pregnancy	UK Teratology Information Service (UKTIS): https://uktis.org/ Best Use of Medicines in Pregnancy (BUMPS): https://www.medicinesinpregnancy.org/
Information about drugs/products and breastfeeding	UK Drugs in Lactation Advisory Service: http://www.midlandsmedicines.nhs.uk/content.asp?section=6&subsection=17&pageIdx=1

DRUG HISTORY

It is vital to establish what drugs have been taken, for which condition and for what duration during pregnancy. This includes over-the-counter medication and homeopathic/herbal remedies.

Pre-pregnancy counselling is advised for those with significant medical conditions and those who are taking potentially harmful drugs. In some cases, medication needs to be changed before pregnancy, if that is possible (e.g. anyone taking sodium valproate for epilepsy should be seen by a neurologist and counselled about changing to an alternative). Some people also need to know that they must continue their medication if they find out they are pregnant; for example, people with epilepsy often reduce or stop their medication for fear of potential fetal effects, with detriment to their own health. There are many instances in which there needs to be a discussion as to the pros and cons of taking medication in pregnancy; for example, someone with significant mental illness may be advised to continue medication, whereas someone with milder mental health issues may choose to stop medication pre-pregnancy after careful counselling.

The most important aspect here is that, once you have ascertained the drug history, you should give advice about the medication only if you have the knowledge and expertise to do so. The British National Formulary (BNF) does not give enough information to allow people to make an informed choice about the medication they take, but there are national organizations and websites that have much more information or are happy to be contacted for queries about medication in pregnancy and when breastfeeding. No one must ever be told to stop medication or not breastfeed without checking the full facts. **Table 1.1** sets out organizations that offer advice on medicines during pregnancy and when breastfeeding.

FAMILY HISTORY

Family history is important if it can have:

- an impact on the health of the parent in pregnancy or afterwards
- implications for the fetus or baby

A family history of certain conditions is particularly significant, namely a maternal history of a first-degree relative (sibling or parent) with:

- diabetes (increased risk of gestational diabetes)
- thromboembolic disease (increased risk of thrombophilia, thrombosis)
- pre-eclampsia (increased risk of pre-eclampsia)
- serious mental health illness (increased risk of puerperal psychosis)

For both parents, it is important to know about any family history of babies with congenital abnormality and any potential genetic problems, such as haemoglobinopathies.

Finally, any known allergies should be recorded. If someone gives a history of allergy, it is important to ask about how this was diagnosed and what sort of problems it causes.

OBSTETRIC EXAMINATION

In any clinical setting, attention to infection control is paramount. Arms should be bare from the elbow down and hands should always be washed or gel should be used before and after any patient contact. Before moving on to examine the patient, it is important to be aware of the clinical context. The examination should be directed at the presenting problem, if any, and the gestation. For instance, it is generally unnecessary to spend time defining the presentation at 24 weeks' gestation unless the presenting problem is threatened preterm labour.

MATERNAL WEIGHT AND HEIGHT

The measurement of weight and height at the initial examination is important, to identify people who are significantly underweight or overweight. Those with a body mass index (BMI: weight [kg]/height [m^2]) of <20 are at higher risk of fetal growth restriction and increased perinatal mortality. In the obese (BMI >30), the risks of gestational diabetes, venous thromboembolism and pre-eclampsia are increased. Additionally, fetal assessment, by both palpation and ultrasound, is more difficult. Obesity is also associated with increased birthweight and a higher perinatal mortality rate. Those with morbid obesity require referral to specialized clinics, which include antenatal anaesthetic assessments to plan the possible use of regional anaesthesia.

In those of normal weight at booking and in whom nutrition is of no concern, there is no need to repeat weight measurement in pregnancy.

BLOOD PRESSURE MEASUREMENT

Blood pressure measurement is an important aspect of antenatal care. The first recording of blood pressure should be made as early as possible in pregnancy and thereafter it should be performed at every visit.

Hypertension diagnosed for the first time in early pregnancy (blood pressure >140/90 mmHg on two separate occasions at least 4 hours apart) should prompt a search for underlying causes (e.g. renal or endocrine). Although 90% of cases will be due to chronic hypertension, this is a diagnosis of exclusion and can be confidently made only when other secondary causes have been excluded (see **Chapter 9**).

> **BOX 1.2: How to measure blood pressure in pregnancy**
>
> - Measure the blood pressure in a seated or semi-recumbent position.
> - Use an appropriately sized cuff. Using one too small will overestimate blood pressure.
> - If using an automated device, check it has been validated for use in pregnancy.
> - Ensure that manual devices have been recently calibrated.
> - Convention is to use Korotkoff V (i.e. disappearance of sounds), as this is more reproducible than Korotkoff IV.
> - Deflate the cuff slowly so that you can record the blood pressure to the nearest 2 mmHg.
> - Do not round up or down.

URINARY EXAMINATION

Early in pregnancy, all patients should be offered routine screening for asymptomatic bacteriuria by midstream urine culture. Identification and treatment of asymptomatic bacteriuria reduces the risk of pyelonephritis. The risk of ascending urinary tract infection in pregnancy is much higher than in the non-pregnant state. Acute pyelonephritis increases the risk of pregnancy loss/premature labour and is associated with considerable maternal morbidity.

At repeat visits, urinalysis using automated reagent strip readers should be performed. If there is proteinuria after 20 weeks, a thorough evaluation with regard to a diagnosis of pre-eclampsia should be undertaken.

GENERAL MEDICAL EXAMINATION

In those who are fit and healthy presenting for a routine visit, there is little benefit in a full formal physical examination. However, if a patient presents with a problem or is in certain at-risk groups, there may be a need to undertake a much more thorough physical examination.

CARDIOVASCULAR EXAMINATION

Routine auscultation for maternal heart sounds in those who are asymptomatic with no cardiac history is unnecessary. However, if someone has previously lived in an area where rheumatic heart disease is prevalent and/or has a known history of heart murmur or heart disease, a cardiovascular examination during pregnancy is indicated.

BREAST EXAMINATION

Formal breast examination is not necessary. Everyone should, however, be encouraged to perform self-examination at regular intervals.

EXAMINATION OF THE PREGNANT ABDOMEN

Always have a chaperone with you to perform this examination and, before starting, ask about pain and areas of tenderness.

In pregnancy, the abdomen should be examined in a semi-recumbent position to avoid aortocaval compression. The abdomen should be exposed from just below the breasts to the symphysis fundus.

Inspection

- Assess the shape of the uterus and note any asymmetry.
- Look for fetal movements.
- Note any signs of pregnancy such as striae gravidarum (stretch marks) or linea nigra (the faint brown line running from the umbilicus to the symphysis pubis).
- Look for scars. The common areas to find scars are:
  - suprapubic (caesarean section, laparotomy for ectopic pregnancy or ovarian masses)
  - sub-umbilical (laparoscopy)
  - right iliac fossa (appendicectomy)
  - right upper quadrant (cholecystectomy)

Palpation

The purpose of palpating the pregnant abdomen is to assess:

- the number of babies
- the size of the baby
- the lie of the baby
- the presentation of the baby
- whether the baby presenting part is engaged

Symphysis–fundal height measurement

Symphysis–fundal height (SFH) should be measured and recorded at each antenatal appointment from 24 weeks' gestation. Most UK hospitals now use customized SFH charts, which are generated at the first antenatal visit and are customized to each individual, taking into account the height, weight, ethnicity and parity (**Figure 1.4**). Using two standard deviations of the mean, it is possible to define the 10th and 90th centile values and these are normally marked on the chart.

Feel carefully for the top of the fundus and for the upper border of the symphysis pubis. The recommended method is using a tape measure with the centimetre marks face down, to place the tape measure at the top of the fundus and measure to the symphysis pubis (i.e. from the variable point to the fixed point). Turn the tape measure over and read the measurement. The fundal height approximates with the gestation so that, at 36 weeks, the fundal height should be approximately 36 cm ± 3 cm. However, customized growth charts are more sensitive and specific and serial measurements are of greater value in detecting growth trends than one-off measurements. It is therefore recommended that the measurement is plotted on a customized growth chart.

A large SFH raises the possibility of:

- a multiple pregnancy
- macrosomia
- polyhydramnios

A small SFH raises the possibility of:

- fetal growth restriction
- oligohydramnios

Fetal lie, presentation and engagement

After measuring the SFH, next palpate to count the number of fetal poles (**Figure 1.5**). A pole is a head or a bottom. If you can feel one or two, it is likely to be a singleton pregnancy. If you can feel three or four, a twin pregnancy is likely. Sometimes, large fibroids can mimic a fetal pole; remember this if there is a history of fibroids.

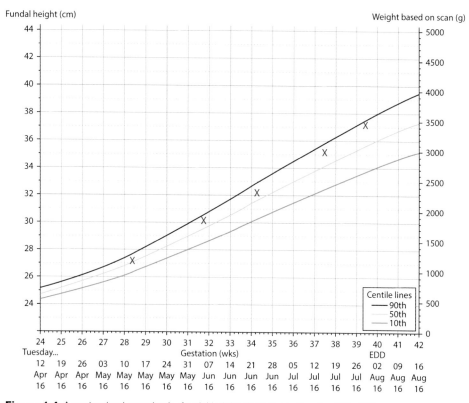

Fundal height (cm)
Weight based on scan (g)

| 24 | 25 | 26 | 27 | 28 | 29 | 30 | 31 | 32 | 33 | 34 | 35 | 36 | 37 | 38 | 39 | 40 | 41 | 42 |
Tuesday...
Gestation (wks)
EDD

12	19	26	03	10	17	24	31	07	14	21	28	05	12	19	26	02	09	16
Apr	Apr	Apr	May	May	May	May	May	Jun	Jun	Jun	Jun	Jul	Jul	Jul	Jul	Aug	Aug	Aug
16	16	16	16	16	16	16	16	16	16	16	16	16	16	16	16	16	16	16

Centile lines
— 90th
— 50th
— 10th

Figure 1.4 A customized symphysis–fundal height chart illustrating the 10th, 50th and 90th centiles and normal fetal growth. (Courtesy of Perinatal Institute.)

Determination of the fetal lie and presentation is of most importance in late pregnancy, as the likelihood of labour increases (i.e. after 36 weeks in an uncomplicated pregnancy). In addition, it is at this point in pregnancy that it is important to diagnose a breech presentation.

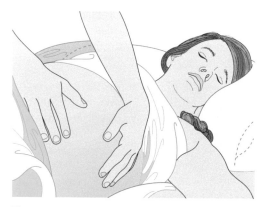

Figure 1.5 Palpation of the gravid abdomen.

If there is a pole over the pelvis, the lie is longitudinal regardless of whether the other pole is lying more to the left or right. An oblique lie is where the leading pole does not lie over the pelvis, but just to one side; a transverse lie is where the fetus lies directly across the abdomen.

Presentation can be either cephalic or breech. Using a two-handed approach and watching the face for pain or discomfort, gently feel for the presenting part. The head is generally much firmer than the bottom, although even in experienced hands it can sometimes be very difficult to tell. At the same time as feeling for the presenting part, assess whether it is engaged or not. If the whole head is palpable and it is easily movable, the head is likely to be 'free'. This equates to five-fifths palpable and is recorded as 5/5. As the head descends into the pelvis, less can be felt. When the head is no longer movable, it has 'engaged' and only one- or two-fifths will be palpable (**Figure 1.6**). You will see

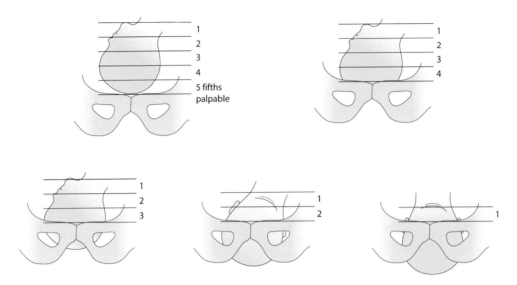

Figure 1.6 Palpation of the fetal head to assess engagement.

different methods from midwives and obstetricians of palpating the baby's head. There is no evidence that one technique is better or more uncomfortable than another and the most important aspect is to be considerate and watch for pain or discomfort while you are palpating.

Gentle palpation of the abdomen may reveal where the baby's back is (i.e. the side that feels fuller and smoother), as this will make auscultating the fetal heart beat easier, but don't worry if you can't. It takes a lot of experience.

Auscultation

If the fetus has been active during your examination and the mother reports that the baby is active, it is not necessary to auscultate the fetal heart. However, parents often like to hear their baby's heartbeat and nowadays most midwives and obstetricians use a hand-held Doppler device, which allows them to hear their baby's heartbeat. However, you may also see a Pinard stethoscope being used, particularly by community midwives. With both, place the device over where the fetal shoulder is likely to be (i.e. in a cephalic presentation, that would be halfway between the umbilicus and the anterior superior ischial spine on the side of the back). Hearing the heart sounds with a Pinard takes a lot of practise. If you cannot hear the fetal heart, never say that you cannot detect a heartbeat; instead, ask for help.

With twins, it is likely that a Doppler on a cardiotocograph (CTG) machine is necessary to be confident that both fetal hearts have been heard.

PELVIC EXAMINATION

Routine pelvic examination during antenatal visits is not necessary. However, there are circumstances in which a vaginal examination is necessary (in most cases, a speculum examination is all that is needed). These include:

- excessive or offensive discharge
- vaginal bleeding (in the known absence of a placenta praevia)
- to perform a cervical smear
- to confirm potential rupture of membranes
- to confirm and assess the extent of female genital mutilation (FGM) in those who have been subjected to this

Before commencing the examination, consent must be sought and a chaperone (nurse, midwife, etc.; never a relative) must be present (regardless of the gender of the examiner).

Assemble everything you will need (swabs, etc.) and ensure the light source works. Position the patient semi-recumbent with knees drawn up and ankles together. Ensure that the patient is adequately covered. If performing a speculum examination, a

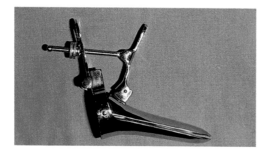

Figure 1.7 A Cusco speculum.

Cusco speculum is usually used (**Figure 1.7**). Select an appropriate size. Proceed as follows:

1. Wash your hands and put on a pair of gloves.
2. Use a plastic speculum.
3. Apply sterile lubricating gel or cream to the blades of the speculum. Do not use antiseptic cream if taking swabs for bacteriology.
4. Gently part the labia.
5. Introduce the speculum with the blades in the vertical plane.
6. As the speculum is gently introduced, aiming towards the sacral promontory (i.e. slightly downwards), rotate the speculum so that it comes to lie in the horizontal plane with the ratchet uppermost.
7. The blades can then slowly be opened until the cervix is visualized. Sometimes minor adjustments need to be made at this stage.
8. Assess the cervix and take any necessary samples.
9. Gently close the blades and remove the speculum, reversing the manoeuvres needed to insert it. Take care not to catch the vaginal epithelium when removing the speculum.

A digital examination may be performed when an assessment of the cervix is required. This can provide information about the consistency and effacement of the cervix that is not obtainable from a speculum examination.

The contraindications to digital examination are:

- known placenta praevia or vaginal bleeding when the placental site is unknown and the presenting part unengaged
- pre-labour rupture of the membranes (increased risk of ascending infection)

The patient should be positioned as before. Examining from the patient's right, two fingers of the gloved right hand are gently introduced into the vagina and advanced until the cervix is palpated. Prior to induction of labour, a full assessment of the Bishop's score can be made (see **Chapter 12**).

OTHER ASPECTS OF THE EXAMINATION

In anyone with suspected pre-eclampsia, the reflexes should be assessed. These are most easily checked at the ankle. The presence of more than three beats of clonus is pathological (see **Chapter 9**).

Oedema of the extremities affects 80% of term pregnancies and is not a good indicator for pre-eclampsia as it is so common. However, the presence of non-dependent oedema such as facial oedema should be noted.

KEY LEARNING POINTS

- Always introduce yourself and say who you are.
- Make sure you are wearing your identity badge.
- Wash your hands or use alcohol gel.
- Be courteous and gentle.
- Always ensure the patient is comfortable and warm.
- Always have a chaperone present when you examine patients.
- Explain what you are going to do and as you go along.
- Ask the patient to let you know if there is any discomfort.
- Tailor your history and examination to find the key information you need.
- Adapt to new findings as you go along.
- Present in a clear way.
- Be aware of giving sensitive information in a public setting.

PRESENTATION SKILLS

Part of the art of taking a history and performing an examination is being able to pass this information on to others in a clear and concise format. It is not necessary to give a full list of negative findings;

it is enough to summarize negatives, such as there is no important medical, surgical or family history of note. Adapt your style of presentation to meet the situation. A very concise presentation is needed for a busy ward round. In an examination, a full and thorough presentation may be required. Be very aware of giving sensitive information in a ward setting where other patients may be within hearing distance. The following template will prove useful for ensuring that you capture all the relevant history.

HISTORY TEMPLATE

DEMOGRAPHIC DETAILS

- Name
- Age
- Occupation
- Make a note of ethnic background

PREGNANCY SUMMARY

- Gestation and dates as calculated from ultrasound
- Gravidity/parity
- Whether singleton/multiple
- Presenting complaint or reason for attending

PRESENTING COMPLAINT

- Details of the presenting problem (if any) or reason for attendance (such as problems in a previous pregnancy).
- What action has been taken?
- Is there a plan for the rest of the pregnancy?
- What are the plans for birth, mode of birth and timing?
- What are the patient's main concerns?

CURRENT PREGNANCY

- Any other problems so far?
- Are they under consultant care? Ask why?
- Have they had additional tests?
- Have they been admitted to hospital for anything?

ULTRASOUND

- What scans have been performed? Were any problems identified?

PAST OBSTETRIC HISTORY

- List the previous pregnancies and their outcomes in order, including date, timing and mode of birth, and any complications for mum or baby

GYNAECOLOGICAL HISTORY

- Any gynaecological problems in the past?
- When was the last cervical smear? Was it normal? Have there ever been any that were abnormal? If yes, what treatment has been undertaken?
- Previous gynaecological surgery

PAST MEDICAL AND SURGICAL HISTORY

- Relevant medical problems
- Any previous operations: type of anaesthetic used, any complications

PSYCHIATRIC HISTORY

- Post-partum blues or depression
- Depression unrelated to pregnancy
- Major psychiatric illness

FAMILY HISTORY

- Diabetes, hypertension, genetic problems, psychiatric problems, etc.

SOCIAL HISTORY

- Smoking/alcohol/drugs
- Marital status
- Occupation, partner's occupation
- Who is available to help at home?
- Are there any housing problems?

DRUGS

- All medication including over-the-counter medication
- Folate supplementation

ALLERGIES

- To what?
- What problems do they cause?

FURTHER READING

NICE (2012). *Antenatal Care*. Quality standard [QS22]. Last updated 14 February 2023. http://www.nice.org.uk/guidance/qs22.

MBRRACE-UK. *Saving Lives, Improving Mothers' Care and Lessons Learned to Inform Maternity Care from the UK and Ireland*. https://www.npeu.ox.ac.uk/mbrrace-uk/reports.

SELF-ASSESSMENT

For interactive SBAs and EMQs relating to this chapter, visit www.routledge.com/cw/mccarthy.

CASE HISTORY 1

Preconceptual counselling is an increasingly important part of obstetric care, as it provides obstetricians an opportunity to review patients prior to getting pregnant and provide advice on maximizing the chance of a successful pregnancy outcome.

Mrs Singh is originally from Pakistan and attends your preconceptual clinic, as she intends to conceive. She gives her history with the following key points:

A 10-year history of systemic lupus erythematosus
B previously on mycophenolate mofetil and cyclophosphamide
C last lupus flare was 1 month ago
D switched to azathioprine 1 month ago
E on an angiotensin-converting enzyme inhibitor
F creatinine 246 μmol/L, protein creatinine ratio 174 mg/mmol
G not using any contraceptives

Address each of these points by identifying the key risk and what influence this may have on pregnancy. Suggest an action point to potentially improve the outcome or address the issue.

ANSWERS

A Systemic lupus erythematosus is an autoimmune condition associated with increased risks of adverse pregnancy outcome including miscarriage, pre-eclampsia, growth restriction and stillbirth. The patient should be counselled regarding this.
Pregnancy increases the risk of flare-ups by 40–60%.
B Mycophenolate mofetil and cyclophosphamide are teratogenic and are contraindicated in pregnancy. If they have been used recently, appropriate time should be given to allow 'wash out'.
C The best chance of a good pregnancy outcome is related to stable/quiescent disease. Ideally, medical conditions should be stable for 6 months prior to conception with no changes to medications in this period.
D Azathioprine is safe to use in pregnancy, as the fetal liver lacks the enzyme that converts azathioprine to its active metabolites.
E Angiotensin-converting enzyme inhibitor is contraindicated in pregnancy and an alternative agent must be used. Consultation with a renal physician should occur.
F These levels indicate significant renal impairment, which increases the possibility of an adverse pregnancy outcome. Consultation with a renal physician should occur and optimization of medicine and renal function should occur prior to conception.
G Until optimal control of the systemic lupus erythematosus occurs, the patient should be advised not to become pregnant. All efforts should focus on making the systemic lupus erythematosus as stable as possible and improving the patient's renal function. This will maximize their chances of having as healthy a pregnancy as possible with minimal risks to their baby.

CASE HISTORY 2

Mrs O'Shea, a 41-year-old single woman from Ireland, attends your clinic for a booking visit. This is her second pregnancy and her first child is in foster care. She gives a history of alcohol and drug use and smokes 30 cigarettes daily. She also reports having an abusive partner.

Identify the key issues raised and prepare a plan for management during the pregnancy.

ANSWER

Mrs O'Shea is a very high-risk pregnancy with significant concerns for both herself and her baby's health. Firstly, a social work review should occur with the inclusion of child protection services. This should also address Mrs O'Shea's own safety due to her abusive partner. She should be counselled regarding drug and smoking cessation and offered support to assist her with this. She should be managed within a perinatal medicine high-risk clinic with a multidisciplinary input.

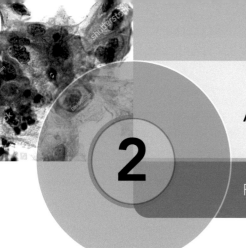

Antenatal care

2

FERGUS McCARTHY

Learning Objectives
- Understand the principles of routine antenatal care.
- Be aware of the rationale for, and purpose of, clinical investigations during each trimester.
- Differentiate normal pregnancy symptoms from potential underlying pathology.

INTRODUCTION

Every year in England and Wales, approximately 700,000 babies are delivered. The majority of pregnancies occur in those who are healthy and low risk with no pre-existing medical problems and result in spontaneous vaginal deliveries. A minority will have pre-existing medical conditions that may be affected by pregnancy or may affect the course of pregnancy and require specialist input. The purpose of antenatal care is to optimize pregnancy outcomes by providing support and reassurance to those who are low risk and, by stratifying care, allowing those at high risk of adverse pregnancy events to receive specialized care in a timely manner.

This chapter provides information on best practice for baseline care of all pregnancies and comprehensive information on the antenatal care in the case of the uncomplicated singleton pregnancy. It provides evidence-based information on baseline investigations that are performed and indications for referral to specialist care.

DEVELOPMENT OF ANTENATAL CARE

Modern maternity care has evolved over more than 100 years. Many of the changes have been driven by political and consumer pressure and a recognition of the need to align appropriate care to optimal outcomes. Antenatal care continues to evolve with the ongoing publication of good-quality research aimed at optimizing perinatal outcomes, but the scope and delivery of antenatal care varies widely across the globe, with maternal mortality rates varying substantially between low- and high-income countries. According to the World Health Organization (WHO), in 2020, globally there were approximately 800 maternal deaths a day from preventable causes

10.1201/9781003196112-2

related to pregnancy and childbirth, meaning that someone dies as a result of pregnancy around every 2 minutes; 99% of all these maternal deaths occur in low-income countries.

HISTORY OF MATERNITY CARE IN THE UK

In 1929, the government in the UK released a document that set out a minimum standard for antenatal care that was so prescriptive in its recommendations that, until very recently, it was practised in many regions, despite the lack of research to demonstrate its effectiveness. The National Health Service Act 1946 came into effect on 5 July 1948 and created the NHS in England and Wales. The introduction of the NHS allowed maternity services to be available to all without cost. As part of these arrangements, a specified fee was paid to the general practitioner (GP) depending on whether they were on the obstetric list (undertaking pregnancy care). This encouraged a large number of GPs to take an interest in maternity care, reversing the previous trend to leave this work to midwives.

Antenatal care became perceived as beneficial, acceptable and available for all. This was reinforced by the finding that the perinatal death rate seemed to be inversely proportional to the number of antenatal visits. In 1963, the first perinatal mortality study showed that the perinatal mortality rate was lowest for those who attended between 10 and 24 times in pregnancy. This failed to take into account prematurity and poor education as reasons for decreased visits and increased mortality. However, antenatal care became established, and with increased professional contact came the drive to continue to improve outcomes, with an emphasis on decreasing maternal and perinatal mortality.

The development and introduction of ultrasound to antenatal care late in the 1960s had a considerable influence on antenatal care, initially limited to confirming multifetal pregnancies, but later being used increasingly for the detection of fetal anomalies. This new intervention became quickly established, but limited evidence exists supporting its routine regular use. The move towards hospital deliveries began in the early 1950s. At this time, with limited hospital maternity facilities, one in three were planned home deliveries. The Cranbrook Report in 1959 recommended that there be sufficient hospital maternity beds for 70% of all deliveries to take place in hospital, and the subsequent Peel Report (1970) recommended that a bed should be available for every woman to deliver in hospital if she so wished.

Obstetricians were not alone in the movement towards hospital deliveries. Parents themselves were pushing to at least be allowed the choice to deliver in hospital. By 1972, only 1 in 10 deliveries were planned for home, and the publication of the Short Report (1980) from the Social Services Committee led to further centralization of hospital delivery. It made a number of recommendations. Among these were the following:

- An increasing number of births should occur in large units; assessment of pregnancy should be improved for smaller consultant units and isolated GP units and home deliveries should be phased out further.
- It should be mandatory that all those who are pregnant should be seen at least twice by a consultant obstetrician – preferably as soon as possible after the first visit to the GP in early pregnancy and again in late pregnancy.

This and subsequent reports – including UK government reports in 1982, 1984 and 1985, *Birth to Five* (Department of Health, 2005) and the *2012/13 Choice Framework* (Department of Health, 2012) – led to a policy of increasing centralization of units for delivery and, consequently, maternity care.

The gradual decline in maternal and perinatal mortality was thought to be due in greater part to hospital deliveries, although proof of this was lacking. Indeed, the decline in perinatal mortality was least in those years when hospitalization increased the most. As other new interventions became available and were increasingly used, such as continuous fetal monitoring and induction of labour, a change in practice began to establish these as the norm for most births, without robust evaluation of their impact through randomized controlled trials or other high-quality research methodology. In England and Wales between 1966 and 1974, the induction rate rose from 12.7% to 38.9%. During the 1980s, with increasing consumer awareness, the unquestioning acceptance of unproven technologies was challenged. Groups such as the National Childbirth Trust began to question not only the need for any intervention but also the need to come to the hospital at all. The professional bodies also began to question the effectiveness of antenatal care.

The government set up an expert committee to review policy on maternity care and to make recommendations. This committee published the report *Changing Childbirth* (Department of Health, Report of the Expert Maternity Group, 1993), which provided purchasers and providers with a number of action points aiming to improve choice, information and continuity of care for everyone during pregnancy. It outlined a number of indicators of success to be achieved within 5 years:

- the carriage of hand-held notes in pregnancy
- midwifery-led care in 30% of pregnancies
- a known midwife at delivery in 75% of cases
- a reduction in the number of antenatal visits for those with low-risk pregnancies

This landmark report provided a new impetus to examine the provision of maternity care in the UK and enshrined choice as a concept in maternity care.

More recently, government publications on maternity care such as *Maternity Matters* (2007) have aimed to address inequalities in maternity care provision and uptake; this publication enables commissioners to assess maternity care in their area and to ensure that safe and effective care is available to all pregnant women. Antenatal and postnatal care now centres on increased choice and empowerment of couples, including birth at home or in a stand-alone midwifery unit. The most recent *National Maternity Review* report (2016) led to the introduction of the Maternity Transformation Programme, which emphasizes the following principles:

- personalized woman-centred care
- continuity of carer
- better postnatal and perinatal mental health care
- a fairer payment system for different types of care
- safer care, with multi-professional working and training, and measurement of performance using routinely collected data

Despite the call for safer, personalized care, in 2017 the discovery of a large series of adverse outcomes at one NHS Trust in England led to bereaved parents to call for a public inquiry. The final report of the Ockenden review, commissioned by the Secretary of State of Health, was published in 2022. One of the main findings was that patient safety was often overlooked in the pursuit of a vaginal birth and that the affected hospital failed to learn from repeated adverse outcomes. The report also included wide-ranging recommendations for maternity services across England, including standards around workforce planning, staffing, multidisciplinary training and learning from adverse outcomes.

OVERVIEW OF ANTENATAL CARE

The aims of antenatal care are to:

- optimize pregnancy outcomes for parents and babies
- prevent, detect and manage those factors that adversely affect the health of the pregnant woman and baby
- provide advice, reassurance, education and support for the pregnant woman and their family
- deal with the 'minor ailments' of pregnancy
- provide general health screening

Antenatal care aims to make the pregnant woman the focus. They should be treated with kindness and dignity at all times, and due respect given to personal, cultural and religious beliefs. Services should be readily accessible and there should be continuity of care. There is a need for high-quality, culturally appropriate, verbal and written information on which women can base their choices through a truly informed decision-making process that is led by them.

In the UK and many countries worldwide, maternity care is provided by a community-based team of midwives and family practitioners (such as GPs), a hospital consultant team or a combination of the two. In the case of a complex pregnancy, a hospital-based obstetric team leads the antenatal care and this is known as consultant care. Those with low-risk pregnancies with no overtly complicating factors usually have community-based care and are said to be under midwifery care. A further group have risk factors identified at booking, for example previous caesarean section, which mandate clinical input by obstetricians, but the majority of routine care can still be provided by the community team. This is referred to as shared care.

ADVICE, REASSURANCE AND EDUCATION

Pregnancy is a time of great uncertainty and stress and this is compounded by the many physical changes experienced during pregnancy. Common symptoms include nausea, heartburn, constipation, shortness of breath, dizziness, swelling, backache, abdominal discomfort and headaches. Generally, these reflect physiological adaptations to pregnancy but may become extremely debilitating. Occasionally they will represent the first presentation of a more serious problem.

Information regarding smoking, alcohol consumption and the use of drugs (both legal and illegal) during pregnancy is extremely important. In some populations, almost one-third of pregnant women smoke during pregnancy, despite its association with fetal growth restriction, preterm labour, placental abruption and intrauterine fetal death. A major role of antenatal care is to help limit these harmful behaviours during pregnancy, for example by inclusion in smoking cessation programmes. Alcohol or illegal substance misuse may require more specialized skills from support services, including perinatal mental health teams. The information given should be of high quality and evidence based. It should be provided in a culturally appropriate manner and in different formats (e.g. written information) where appropriate and possible.

Parentcraft education is the term often used to describe formal group discussion of issues relating to pregnancy, labour and delivery, and care of the newborn. These sessions offer an opportunity for couples to meet others in the same situation and help to establish a network of social contacts that may be useful after the delivery. They may include a tour of the maternity department, the aim of which is to lessen anxiety and increase the sense of maternal control surrounding delivery.

FIRST TRIMESTER

When someone becomes pregnant, one of the first interactions with the health services is known as the booking visit. At this point, or shortly afterwards, a midwife will take a detailed history and, with consent, perform an examination and a series of routine investigations so that appropriate care can be offered. If risk factors are identified that may potentially have an impact on the pregnancy outcome, the midwife will access specialized services on behalf of the pregnant individual. This may mean referral to a hospital consultant obstetric clinic or other specialist services as appropriate. Medical or psychosocial issues raised at the booking visit may need to be explored in some depth.

BODY MASS INDEX AND WEIGHT ASSESSMENT

Height and weight should be measured at the booking visit and body mass index (BMI) calculated and assessed. If the BMI is more than 35 kg/m^2, review is recommended by an obstetric consultant or another healthcare professional who can provide appropriate advice on the increased pregnancy risks (**Table 2.1**) and interventions to minimize excessive gestational weight gain. The Institute of Medicine has guidelines on recommended weight increase in pregnancy. For those of normal weight (BMI 18.5–24.9 kg/m^2), the recommended total weight gain in pregnancy is 11–16 kg (25–35 lb); for those who are overweight (BMI 25–29.9 kg/m^2), it is 7–11 kg (15–25 lb); and, for those who enter pregnancy in the obese range (BMI ≥30 kg/m^2), it is 5–9 kg (11–20 lb).

Anyone with raised BMI should be counselled regarding appropriate weight in pregnancy and the risks. In general, the risks increase as BMI rises.

GENERAL PREGNANCY DIETARY ADVICE

The Royal College of Obstetricians and Gynaecologists (RCOG) provides the following dietary advice for optimal weight control in pregnancy:

- Do not eat for two; maintain your normal portion size and try and avoid snacks.
- Eat fibre-rich foods such as oats, beans, lentils, grains, seeds, fruit and vegetables as well as wholegrain bread, brown rice and wholewheat pasta.
- Base your meals on starchy foods such as potatoes, bread, rice and pasta, choosing wholegrain options where possible.
- Restrict intake of fried food, drinks and items of confectionery that are high in added sugars, and other foods high in fat and sugar.
- Eat at least five portions of a variety of fruit and vegetables each day.

- Dieting in pregnancy is not recommended but controlling weight gain in pregnancy is advocated.

It may be difficult to make these dietary changes for the first time during pregnancy, and further work is needed to determine how best to facilitate adherence to this guidance.

GENERAL EXERCISE ADVICE

Aerobic and strength conditioning exercise in pregnancy is considered safe and beneficial. It may help recovery following delivery, reduce back and

Table 2.1 Maternal and neonatal complications associated with high BMI in pregnancy

Maternal	Fetal
Antenatal	
Difficulty accurately assessing growth and anatomy of fetus	Increased congenital malformations; if BMI is >40 kg/m², risk of neural tube defects is three times that if BMI is <30 kg/m². If BMI is >30 kg/m², high-dose folic acid (5 mg once daily) is recommended pre-pregnancy and for the first 12 weeks' gestation
Increased risk of GDM: three times more likely to develop GDM than those with BMI <30 kg/m²	Macrosomia and associated complications
Hypertensive disorders of pregnancy: increased risk of chronic hypertension, gestational hypertension and pre-eclampsia	Fetal growth restriction and associated complications
Increased risk of VTE	Miscarriage; overall miscarriage risk is 20%, which increases to 1 in 4 (25%) if BMI is >30 kg/m²
	Stillbirth: doubling of stillbirth risk from 0.5% to 1 in 100 (1%)
Intrapartum	
Difficulty with analgesia (epidurals and spinal) and general anaesthesia if needed	Macrosomia and shoulder dystocia: risk of macrosomia (neonatal weight >4 kg) increases from 7% to 14% compared with those with a BMI of between 20 and 30 kg/m²
Difficulty with monitoring in labour	
Increased instrumental delivery rate	
Increased caesarean section rate	
Postnatal	
VTE risk	Increased risk of childhood obesity and diabetes in later life
Wound breakdown and infection	
Postnatal depression	

BMI, body mass index; GDM, gestational diabetes mellitus; VTE, venous thromboembolism.

pelvic pain during pregnancy and contribute to overall wellness. The aim of exercise during pregnancy is to stay fit, rather than to reach peak fitness. Contact sports should be avoided and a more tailored exercise programme may be needed for those with pre-existing medical conditions. However, there are very few people for whom some exercise is not appropriate and healthcare professionals can encourage walking, swimming and other forms of non-contact exercise in pregnancy. Pelvic floor exercises during pregnancy and immediately after birth may reduce the risk of urinary and faecal incontinence in the future. Following delivery, it is generally safe to resume exercise gradually as soon the individual feels ready.

The RCOG provides modified heart rate target zones for exercise in pregnancy. These are age dependent and are as follows:

- <20 years of age: target range 140–155 beats per minute (bpm)
- 20–29 years of age: 135–150 bpm
- 30–39 years of age: 130–145 bpm
- >40 years of age: 125–140 bpm

BREASTFEEDING EDUCATION

Breastfeeding protects against diarrhoea and common childhood illnesses such as pneumonia and may also have longer term health benefits for the breastfeeding parent and child, such as reducing the risk of obesity later in life. Breastfeeding has also been associated with a higher intelligence quotient (IQ) in children, although it is not clear whether this is a result of confounding. The WHO recommends initiation of breastfeeding within an hour of birth, exclusive breastfeeding for the first 6 months of life and continued breastfeeding beyond 6 months and at least up to 2 years of age. Although evidence for interventions to promote breastfeeding are limited, a recent systematic review demonstrated that the greatest improvements in initiation and continuation of breastfeeding were seen when education was provided concurrently across the various settings including in the home, the community and the health system. Baby-friendly hospital support in the health system was the most effective intervention to improve rates of any breastfeeding. As a result, early education in pregnancy about breastfeeding is advocated to improve uptake and engage pregnant parents with breastfeeding services to allow them to be fully prepared.

OPTIONS FOR PREGNANCY CARE

Provided that there are no contraindications to midwifery-led care (such as medical comorbidities or previous obstetric complications that may warrant consultant-led care), the options available for delivery include the following:

- *Home birth*: according to the Birthplace Study published in 2011, in England and Wales approximately 2% of pregnant women opt to deliver at home, cared for by a midwife. The advantages of home birth include familiar surroundings, no interruption of labour to go to hospital, no separation from other children or the birth partner during or after birth, continuity of care and reduced interventions. The disadvantages are that 45–50% of first pregnancies (and 10–12% of second and subsequent pregnancies) planned for home birth are transferred to hospital and there is a poor perinatal outcome in approximately twice as many first-time home births than in those occurring in hospital (9.3 versus 5.3 adverse perinatal events per 1,000 births, respectively; adjusted odds ratio 1.75, 95% confidence interval 1.07–2.86). Other disadvantages include limited analgesic options (e.g. no epidurals are available).
- *Midwifery units or birth centres*: these may be stand-alone units located on a separate site to hospital birth centres or may be adjacent to hospitals ('co-located') with access to obstetric, neonatal and anaesthetic care. Advantages of midwifery units may include continuity of care, fewer interventions and convenience of location. Disadvantages include transfer out to a hospital birth centre (40% of first births and 10% of second and subsequent births) and limited access to certain analgesic options. No difference was found in the risk of adverse perinatal outcomes between midwifery units and hospital units (4.5 adverse perinatal events/1,000 births in free-standing midwifery

units; 4.7 events/1,000 births in alongside midwifery units; and 5.3 events/1,000 births in obstetric units).

- *Hospital birth centre*: in hospital birth centres, midwives continue to provide care during labour but doctors are available should the need arise. There is direct access to obstetricians, anaesthetists and neonatologists. Disadvantages include a lack of continuity of care and a greater likelihood of intervention (compared with midwifery units and home births).

ANTENATAL URINE TESTS

Asymptomatic bacteriuria is associated with increased risk of preterm delivery and the development of pyelonephritis during pregnancy. A mid-stream specimen of urine (MSU) should be sent for culture and sensitivity at the booking visit to screen for asymptomatic bacteriuria. Urinalysis is performed every antenatal visit. Urine is screened for protein (to detect renal disease or pre-eclampsia), persistent glycosuria (to detect pre-existing diabetes or gestational diabetes mellitus [GDM]) and nitrites (to detect urinary tract infections). If nitrites are detected on urine dipstick testing, an MSU is sent for microscopy, culture and sensitivity to detect asymptomatic bacteria and appropriate treatment initiated if a positive culture is identified.

BLOOD PRESSURE ASSESSMENT

Blood pressure falls by a small amount (a few mmHg) in the first trimester and increases to prepregnancy levels by the end of the second trimester. First-trimester blood pressure assessment also allows the detection of previously unrecognized chronic hypertension; this enables early initiation of treatment including antihypertensive agents (to reduce episodes of severe hypertension) and lowdose aspirin (which reduces the risk of pre-eclampsia and decreases perinatal mortality).

BOOKING TESTS IN PREGNANCY

Table 2.2 lists the booking tests often performed at the booking visit.

Table 2.2 Summary of booking investigations

Investigation	Indication
FBC	Haemoglobin, platelet count, mean cell volume
MSU	Asymptomatic bacteriuria
Blood group and antibody screen	Rhesus status and atypical antibodies
cffDNA	Fetal rhesus status in rhesus-negative pregnancies
Haemoglobinopathy screening	Screening is based on the FOQ and blood test results
Infection screen	Hepatitis B, syphilis, HIV (and rubella status)
Dating scan and first-trimester screening	Accurate pregnancy dating with provision of risk assessment for trisomy 21, 18 and 13 and identification of major congenital anomalies

cffDNA, cell-free fetal deoxyribonucleic acid; FBC, full blood count; FOQ, family origin questionnaire; HIV, human immunodeficiency virus; MSU, mid-stream specimen of urine.

FULL BLOOD COUNT

Full blood count (FBC) measurement allows identification of anaemia, to allow early initiation of treatment. Anaemia in pregnancy is defined as a haemoglobin (Hb) level of <110 g/L in the first trimester, <105 g/L in the second and third trimesters and <100 g/L in the post-partum period. The detection of anaemia should prompt examination of the mean cell volume to identify likely iron deficiency anaemia (microcytic anaemia) or folate or vitamin B12 deficiency (macrocytic anaemia). Further investigations may include B12, folate or iron (ferritin) studies. Appropriate treatment should be initiated.

In accordance with the recommendations of the British Society for Haematology, a trial of oral iron should be considered as the first-line management option for anaemia in pregnancy, with an increment demonstrated at 2 weeks confirming a positive response. Those with known haemoglobinopathy should have serum ferritin checked and should be offered oral supplements if their ferritin level is <30 µg/L.

An FBC also allows the identification of low platelets, which may rarely represent de novo immune thrombocytopaenic purpura. Gestational thrombocy-topaenia (a fall in platelet count in pregnancy) rarely presents in the first trimester and is more commonly detected beyond 28 weeks' gestation. Therefore, a low platelet count in the first trimester warrants further investigation and haematological input; in many settings, the threshold for referral is $<100 \times 10^9/l$, but individual maternity units may set their own criteria. A baseline platelet count is also useful later in pregnancy if there are concerns regarding conditions such as pre-eclampsia or haemolysis, elevated liver enzymes and low platelets (HELLP) syndrome, which may present with thrombocytopaenia.

BLOOD GROUP

Blood group is checked at booking to identify those who are rhesus D-negative so that they may be informed of the risks of rhesus isoimmunization and sensitization from a rhesus D-positive fetus. Anti-D is administered to rhesus D-negative pregnant women in instances of potential sensitizing events such as post-chorionic villus sampling, amniocentesis or trauma to the abdomen.

The British Committee for Standards in Haematology recommends that following potentially sensitizing events, anti-D immunoglobulin should be administered as soon as possible and always within 72 hours of the event. In pregnancies less than 12 weeks' gestation, anti-D immunoglobulin prophylaxis is indicated only following ectopic pregnancy, molar pregnancy and therapeutic termination of pregnancy and in cases of uterine bleeding where this is repeated, heavy or associated with abdominal pain. The minimum dose of anti-D should be 250 IU and a test for feto-maternal haemorrhage is not required. For potentially sensitizing events between 12 and 20 weeks' gestation, a minimum dose of 250 IU should be administered within 72 hours of the event and a test for feto-maternal haemorrhage is not required. Pregnant women who are rhesus D-negative are now offered prophylactic anti-D administration at 28 weeks' gestation. Antenatal anti-D immuno-globulin prophylaxis using either a single large dose at 28 weeks' gestation or two doses given at 28 and 34 weeks' gestation achieves a significant reduction in the incidence of sensitization to rhesus D due to occult sensitizing events. Following birth, rhesus D-negative individuals also receive anti-D post-partum once a baby is confirmed as being rhesus D-positive on testing of a cord blood sample.

Assessment of blood group in all pregnant women at 28 weeks' gestation also identifies those with other atypical antibodies so that appropriate monitoring can be put in place.

Newer techniques such as non-invasive prenatal testing of maternal blood for fetal rhesus status (determined by analysis of cell-free fetal deoxyribo-nucleic acid [cffDNA]) may limit the need for anti-D prophylaxis in pregnancies where the fetus is known to be rhesus D-positive, and this is widely used in many countries and is >99% sensitive and specific for the prediction of fetal rhesus status. Knowing the fetal rhesus status allows for targeted anti-D administration only in pregnancies with rhesus-positive babies. For further details, see **Chapter 6**.

GESTATIONAL DIABETES

Pregnant women who have had previous GDM should be offered a glucose tolerance test or random blood glucose in the first trimester, with the aim of detecting pre-existing diabetes that may have developed since a preceding pregnancy.

THALASSAEMIA

Thalassaemia is a group of inherited blood disorders in which the Hb is abnormal as a result of mutations in genes that code Hb. They are inherited in an autosomal recessive pattern. Although the thalassaemias can occur worldwide, the carrier rate is particularly common in people from Southeast Asia, and also affects those of Mediterranean, North African, Middle Eastern, Indian and Asian origin. A mutation that affects the alpha chain causes alpha-thalassaemia, while beta-thalassaemia occurs as a result of a mutation in the beta chain. The alpha chains are produced by four genes, two on each chromosome 16, inherited as pairs. The severity of the condition depends on how many of those genes have been altered. If one gene is mutated, individuals are asymptomatic. If someone carries two mutations (alpha-thalassaemia trait) they may have mild anaemia. Haemoglobin H disease occurs when an individual carries three mutated genes, and this leads to chronic anaemia that requires regular blood transfusion. Alpha-thalassaemia major occurs when all four genes are mutated and is almost uniformly fatal in utero without intervention.

There are only two beta genes, one each on chromosome 11. The beta-thalassaemia phenotype can range from moderate to severe. Beta-thalassaemia major occurs when both beta genes are affected, and affected individuals will require blood transfusions for the rest of their lives. Beta-thalassaemia intermedia is the milder form of the condition and is non-transfusion dependent. Screening for thalassaemia in the UK is offered to all pregnant women at the booking visit using the family origin questionnaire (FOQ) and/or FBC results; those at high risk of having an affected fetus should then be referred to a fetal medicine unit to discuss the option of invasive confirmatory testing.

SICKLE CELL SCREEN

Similar to the other haemoglobinopathies, certain ethnic groups are at a higher risk of carrying sickle cell trait. The carrier rate for sickle cell trait (HbAS) is approximately 1 in 10 among Afro-Caribbean people, but as high as 1 in 4 in people from West Africa. The carrier frequency for haemoglobin C trait (HbAC) is approximately 1 in 30, but up to 1 in 6 in some groups (e.g. Ghanaians). Homozygous sickle cell disease (HbSS) is the most serious form of the disease and these individuals have chronic haemolytic anaemia and suffer from sickle cell crisis, which may be precipitated by infection. It is also possible to have a combination of HbS (sickle haemoglobin) and another beta-globin variant such as sickle cell/haemoglobin C disease (HbSC). These individuals have slightly milder features than seen in HbSS but are still at risk of sickle cell crises. Partners of pregnant women with sickle cell disease or trait are offered screening early in pregnancy, with the option of invasive testing to detect an affected fetus if both parents are carriers.

FIRST-TRIMESTER INFECTION SCREEN

Rubella

For many years, immunity to rubella has been tested at booking visits in most countries. Public Health England has recently stopped routine testing for rubella (from April 2016) on the grounds that rubella infection levels in the UK are so low that they are defined as eliminated by the WHO. Rubella infection in pregnancy is now very rare; the mumps, measles, rubella (MMR) immunization programme has demonstrated that over 90% of children aged up to 2 years had received at least one mumps, measles and rubella vaccination. As the screening test used can potentially give inaccurate results and cause unnecessary stress, the screening programme has been stopped.

The majority of pregnant women are rubella immune and no further action is required. When an individual is found not to be immune in pregnancy, they are advised to avoid contact with individuals known to be currently infected and are offered the combined MMR vaccination following delivery (see **Chapter 11**).

Syphilis

Syphilis is a sexually transmitted disease caused by transmission of *Treponema pallidum*, a spirochaete bacterium. In pregnancy, it may cause miscarriage or stillbirth and can cause active disease in newborn infants if contracted antenatally. Between 2011 and 2012, there were 2,978 cases of syphilis diagnosed in the UK. Although diagnosis is rare in pregnancy, due to the increasing incidence of the disease and the fact that it may be safely treated with penicillin in pregnancy, screening for syphilis in pregnancy is still routinely performed (see **Chapter 11**).

Hepatitis B

Hepatitis screening is performed in pregnancy to reduce infant infection. Without preventative measures, 90% of babies born to pregnant women with hepatitis B will contract the virus and develop chronic infection, which is associated with liver failure, cirrhosis and hepatocellular carcinoma. A baby born following a pregnancy known to be affected by active hepatitis B should receive hepatitis B vaccine and one dose of hepatitis B immune globulin within the first 12 hours of life. This confers over 95% protection against chronic hepatitis B infection. The infant will need additional doses of hepatitis B vaccine at 1 and 6 months of age. The test for screening for hepatitis B involves detection of hepatitis B surface antibody (HBsAb or anti-HBs). Detection of the antibody implies immunity to hepatitis B. Hepatitis

B surface antigen (HBsAg) indicates the presence of hepatitis B in the blood. Hepatitis B core antibody (HBcAb or anti-HBc) indicates that a person may have been exposed to the hepatitis B virus (see **Chapter 11**).

Hepatitis C

The National Institute for Health and Care Excellence (NICE) currently recommends that pregnant women should not be offered routine screening for hepatitis C virus because there is insufficient evidence to support its clinical and cost-effectiveness. Screening for hepatitis C may be offered to those individuals considered to be at high risk, including those with current or previous intravenous drug use and hepatitis B and/or human immunodeficiency virus (HIV) infection. The risk of vertical transmission in pregnancy is approximately 5%, but this increases significantly to 36% if there is coinfection with HIV. Screening is performed by examining for hepatitis C virus immunoglobulin (Ig) G antibodies (see **Chapter 11**).

Human immunodeficiency virus

The estimated HIV prevalence among pregnant women in the UK is 2 per 1,000. With appropriate interventions, the risk of transmission to the neonate is as low as 0.1%. Interventions to minimize vertical transmission include initiation of antiretroviral therapy (ART) by 24 weeks' gestation if naive to ART, planned elective caesarean section for those with a viral load ≥400 HIV ribonucleic acid (RNA) copies/mL at 36 weeks' gestation and exclusive formula feeding from birth regardless of viral load and ART use. It is recommended that pregnant women who decline initial screening should be offered screening again at 28 weeks' gestation.

ULTRASOUND FOR FIRST-TRIMESTER DATING AND SCREENING

Accurate dating through first-trimester ultrasound is key to avoiding issues later in pregnancy, such as incorrect identification of growth restriction and inadvertent induction of labour for post-term pregnancy. First-trimester ultrasound also enables early identification of multifetal pregnancies, screening for trisomies and examination of the fetus for gross anomalies such as anencephaly and cystic hygromas. The dating scan and first trimester screening is best performed between 11 + 3 and 13 + 6 weeks' gestation, when the crown–rump length (CRL) measures between 45 and 84 mm. From 14 and 20 weeks' gestation, the head circumference is used to date the pregnancy.

Beyond 20 weeks' gestation, the impact of genes and environmental factors can cause variability in fetal size. Dating a pregnancy by ultrasound scan therefore becomes progressively less accurate as the gestation advances. This is just one of the potential problems of 'late booking'.

First-trimester screening currently involves:

- Measurement of nuchal translucency (NT). The median and 95th centile for NT is 1.2 mm and 2.1 mm with a CRL of 45 mm, and 1.9 mm and 2.7 mm for a CRL of 84 mm.
- Measurement of maternal free beta-human chorionic gonadotrophin (βhCG) and pregnancy-associated plasma protein-A (PAPP-A). In trisomy 21 pregnancies, the concentration of free βhCG is higher (around two multiples of median [MoM]) and the concentration of PAPP-A is lower (approximately 0.5 MoM).
- The pregnant woman's age.

Using an algorithm based on the above criteria, the detection rate for trisomy 21 is approximately 90%. The false-positive rate can be reduced to 3% by additionally examining the nasal bone, ductus venosus flow and tricuspid flow, and this gives a detection rate of approximately 95%. Screening may also be performed in the second trimester between 14 and 20 weeks' gestation and consists exclusively of risk prediction using maternal biomarkers. The quadruple test measures maternal alpha-fetoprotein (AFP), hCG, unconjugated oestriol (uE3) and inhibin A and has an 80% detection rate with a 5% false-positive rate. Newer technologies including non-invasive prenatal testing are now available with reported sensitivities for detection of Down syndrome of more than 99% with a screen-positive rate of <0.2%. These are being used increasingly throughout the UK and Europe and are discussed further in **Chapter 5**.

IDENTIFICATION OF HIGH-RISK PREGNANCIES

PREGNANCIES AT HIGH RISK OF DEVELOPING PRE-ECLAMPSIA

NICE currently recommends that pregnant women who are considered to be at high risk of pre-eclampsia should have low-dose aspirin (75–150 mg) treatment initiated early in pregnancy until delivery. Individuals considered to be at high risk include those with:

- hypertensive disease during a previous pregnancy
- chronic kidney disease
- autoimmune disease such as systemic lupus erythematosus or antiphospholipid syndrome
- type 1 or type 2 diabetes
- chronic hypertension

Furthermore, pregnant women with two or more moderate risk factors for pre-eclampsia are also recommended to commence aspirin early in pregnancy until delivery. Moderate risk factors for the development of pre-eclampsia include:

- primiparity
- advanced age (>40 years)
- pregnancy interval of more than 10 years
- BMI ≥35 kg/m^2 at booking visit
- family history of pre-eclampsia
- multifetal pregnancy

All pregnant women should be screened at every antenatal visit for pre-eclampsia by measurement of blood pressure and urinalysis for protein.

PREGNANCIES AT HIGH RISK OF PRETERM BIRTH

Pregnant women considered to be at high risk of preterm birth include those with previous preterm birth, late miscarriage, multifetal pregnancies and cervical surgery such as previous cone biopsy. These individuals may be offered serial cervical length screening with or without the use of fetal fibronectin to detect increased risk of preterm birth.

FETAL GROWTH RESTRICTION

NICE guidelines recommend that symphysis–fundal height (SFH) measurements should be performed at every antenatal appointment from 24 weeks' gestation. Concerns that fetal growth may be slow, or has stopped altogether, should prompt ultrasound scanning. There is no consensus on the recommended 'routine' use of ultrasound in pregnancy. The majority of units offer dating scans (at end of first trimester) and anomaly scans (at around 20–22 weeks' gestation) but no further growth assessment unless clinically indicated. Some units offer an additional third-trimester growth scan but this is still being evaluated in research studies.

VITAMIN D DEFICIENCY

The RCOG advises that there are no data to support routine screening for vitamin D deficiency in pregnancy in terms of health benefits or cost-effectiveness. Individuals thought to be at increased risk of vitamin D deficiency on the basis of skin colour or coverage, obesity, risk of pre-eclampsia or gastroenterological conditions limiting fat absorption may be screened, but this testing is expensive. Daily vitamin D supplementation with oral cholecalciferol or ergocalciferol is safe in pregnancy. NICE guidance states that all pregnant and breastfeeding women should be advised to take 10 µg of vitamin D supplements daily. Severe vitamin D deficiency in pregnancy results in increased risk of neonatal rickets.

SECOND-TRIMESTER CARE

ANOMALY SCAN

Between 20 and 22 weeks' gestation, it is recommended that fetal anatomy be assessed. This is a detailed structural scan aimed at detecting conditions such as spina bifida, major congenital anomalies, diaphragmatic hernia and renal agenesis. Prenatal diagnosis is covered in detail in **Chapter 5**.

GESTATIONAL DIABETES MELLITUS

Universal screening for GDM is available in some countries, including the USA and Australia. However,

NICE advocates risk-based screening in the UK. GDM is diagnosed if the fasting plasma glucose level is 5.6 mmol/L or above, or a 2-hour plasma glucose level is 7.8 mmol/L or above.

Risk factors for the development of GDM include previous gestational diabetes, previous macrosomia (≥4.5 kg), raised BMI (≥30 kg/m^2), a first-degree relative with diabetes or being of Asian, black Caribbean or Middle Eastern origin. If risk factors are present, 2-hour 75 g oral glucose tolerance test (OGTT) should be offered at 24–28 weeks' gestation. Pregnant women with a previous history of GDM should have an OGTT at 16–18 weeks' gestation. The test should be repeated at 24–28 weeks of pregnancy.

GOVERNANCE OF MATERNITY CARE

Many clinical, political and consumer bodies now contribute to optimizing care in pregnancy. These include the following.

NATIONAL INSTITUTE FOR HEALTH AND CARE EXCELLENCE

NICE has evaluated maternity care in great detail and continues to publish many important guidelines relating to different aspects of pregnancy, covering antenatal, intrapartum and postnatal care. These provide the benchmark by which NHS Trusts are judged on their ability to provide care. The process of guideline development is rigorous, and stakeholders are consulted at each stage of development. The guidelines are available through the NICE website (www.nice.org.uk) and provide the framework for standards of care within England and Wales.

NATIONAL SCREENING COMMITTEE

Screening has formed a part of antenatal care since its inception. The National Screening Committee is responsible for developing standards and strategies for the implementation of these. The National Screening Committee has unified and progressed standards for all aspects of antenatal screening across the UK. The provision of national standards means that new tests are critically evaluated before being offered to populations. Conditions for which screening is currently not recommended, such as group B streptococcus carriage, are regularly reviewed against current evidence. The National Screening Committee recently recommended the cessation of testing for rubella immunity.

ROYAL COLLEGE OF OBSTETRICIANS AND GYNAECOLOGISTS

The RCOG has many roles. These include developing national guidelines (not covered by the previously mentioned bodies), setting standards for the provision of care, training and revalidation, audit and research. The RCOG publishes a large number of guidelines pertinent to pregnancy, with patient information leaflets to accompany many of these. These guidelines are reviewed 3-yearly and are accessible to all on the RCOG website (www.rcog.org.uk). The RCOG works in partnership with other colleges such as the Royal College of Midwives (RCM) to set standards for maternity care. These standards provide important drivers to organizations, such as the Clinical Negligence Scheme for Trusts, in setting standards for levels of care and performance by hospitals.

CONSUMER GROUPS

As well as providing support and advice for pregnant women, often at times of great need, consumer

⊙━ KEY LEARNING POINTS

- Antenatal care improves pregnancy outcomes, and a variety of models exist.
- There are key visits during the pregnancy when essential investigations or decisions are taken regarding antenatal care and delivery.
- Antenatal care should be seen as an opportunity for education, reassurance and screening for potential problems.
- Continued efforts should be made to improve access to antenatal care for disadvantaged and minority groups.

groups allow them to have a louder voice in the planning and provision of maternity care. National consumer groups such as the National Childbirth Trust have representatives on many influential panels, such as the National Screening Committee and RCOG working groups. At local level, each hospital should have a maternity services liaison committee. When these committees work well, they can provide essential consumer input into service delivery at local level.

FURTHER READING

Qureshi H, Massey E, Kirwan D, Davies T, Robson S, White J, Jones J, Allard S (2014). BCSH guideline for the use of anti-D immunoglobulin for the prevention of haemolytic disease of the fetus and newborn. *Transfusion Medicine*, 24(1): 8–20.

British HIV Association (2014). British HIV Association guidelines for the management of HIV infection. *HIV Medicine*, 15(Suppl. 4): 1–77. https://www.bhiva.org/file/FCUcXrfVgWsYl/BHIVA-Pregnancy-guidelines-update-2014.pdf.

NHS England (2023). Fetal anomaly screening programme handbook: Guidance – Overview. https://www.gov.uk/government/publications/fetal-anomaly-screening-programme-handbook/overview.

Public Health England (2015). Infectious Diseases in Pregnancy Screening (IDPS). https://assets.publishing.service.gov.uk/government/uploads/system/uploads/attachment_data/file/439996/Infectious_Disease_in_Pregnancy_Screening__IDPS_.pdf.

NICE (2012). *Antenatal Care*. Quality standard [QS22]. Last updated: 14 February 2023. http://www.nice.org.uk/guidance/qs22.

RCOG guidance: https://www.rcog.org.uk/guidelines.

SELF-ASSESSMENT

For interactive SBAs and EMQs relating to this chapter, visit www.routledge.com/cw/mccarthy.

CASE HISTORY 1

Mrs Singh, a 39-year-old woman originally from Pakistan, is approximately 8 weeks' gestation and attends a booking visit with her community midwife, who fills out her client-held records. This is Mrs Singh's fourth pregnancy, having had two normal deliveries and then a caesarean section for a transverse lie. The previous babies' weights were 2.30 kg, 2.40 kg and 2.35 kg, all born at 39 weeks' gestation. Mrs Singh's booking blood pressure is 140/95 mmHg and her BMI is 37.

Identify the key issues raised and prepare a plan for management during the pregnancy.

ANSWER

Mrs Singh is originally from Pakistan, although she has been a UK citizen for many years. This makes a language problem less likely. However, there is no record that a thalassaemia screen has ever been performed. This is important because thalassaemia trait (carrier status) might contribute to maternal anaemia. Furthermore, if the father of this baby is also a carrier, the child will have a one in four chance of having thalassaemia. It is reassuring that all the children are fit and well, but this does not exclude the possibility that they are both carriers.

Mrs Singh is 39 years old. This slightly increases the risks of pregnancy complications including pre-eclampsia, but, more significantly, it is associated with an increase in the risk of certain fetal chromosomal abnormalities, principally Down syndrome. The decision to undergo screening and invasive testing is a personal one, often influenced by cultural and religious beliefs, but an offer of screening should be made to all pregnant women.

Mrs Singh likely has chronic hypertension (possibly related to her body weight) but is not currently on medication. Mrs Singh should be commenced on 75–150 mg aspirin once daily to reduce the risk of pre-eclampsia. She should also be assessed further for consideration of starting an antihypertensive agent.

Mrs Singh's children have all been of low birthweight. It is difficult to determine whether they were constitutionally (genetically) small but healthy or whether they were pathologically small (i.e. growth restricted). Serial ultrasound scans should be performed as surveillance for fetal growth restriction.

(Contd.)

(Contd.)

Mrs Singh has a raised BMI; this increases her risks of anaesthetic complications (such as failure to intubate or successfully site a spinal anaesthetic) and also her risks of developing GDM. An OGTT will be recommended at 24–28 weeks' gestation to screen for this.

Finally, the mode of delivery after a previous caesarean section requires discussion. The transverse lie was probably secondary to uterine laxity, but this would need to be confirmed by obtaining the previous pregnancy notes. The options for mode of delivery (vaginal birth after caesarean versus elective repeat caesarean section) will need to be discussed. Malpresentation at term may occur again.

In conclusion, Mrs Singh has a number of factors that increase the risk of complications in this pregnancy. Shared care under a hospital consultant would be the appropriate form of antenatal care.

CASE HISTORY 2

Mrs Murphy, a 43-year-old woman from Ireland, attends your clinic for a booking visit. This is her second pregnancy. The first resulted in severe preterm pre-eclampsia resulting in emergency caesarean section at 27 weeks' gestation of a baby boy, John, weighing 550 g. John is 3 years old and has significant developmental issues. This is an egg donation pregnancy. Her blood pressure is 150/100 mmHg and her BMI is 45.

Identify the key issues raised and prepare a plan for management during the pregnancy.

ANSWER

Mrs Murphy is at very high risk of recurrence of preterm pre-eclampsia. She is obese and likely has underlying chronic hypertension that is poorly controlled. She is of advanced maternal age and this is an egg donation pregnancy, both of which are additional risk factors for pre-eclampsia. Mrs Murphy requires treatment with an appropriate antihypertensive agent such as labetolol with the aim of getting her blood pressure to <135/85 mmHg, commencement of aspirin 75–150 mg aspirin once daily until 36 weeks' gestation and referral to a dietician and to a high-risk perinatal medicine clinic. Mrs Murphy will require serial growth scans and regularly (likely fortnightly) assessment for monitoring of blood pressure and signs and symptoms of pre-eclampsia.

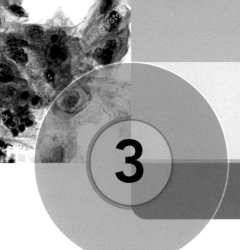

3

Normal fetal development and growth

ANNA L DAVID

Learning Objectives

- Understand that fetal growth and birthweight are important determinants of immediate neonatal health and long-term adult health.
- Appreciate the fetal, maternal and placental factors that affect fetal growth and development.
- Be familiar with fetal circulation and the specific shunts that prioritize delivery of oxygenated blood from the placenta to the fetal brain, and appreciate how fetal circulation transitions at birth to adult circulation.
- Be aware of normal fetal organ development during pregnancy, how fetal structural abnormalities arise and how they can affect the fetus and neonate.
- Recognize the importance of normal amniotic fluid physiology to fetal growth and development.

INTRODUCTION

Knowledge of normal development, growth and maturation is important for understanding the complications that may arise in pregnancy and for the neonate. For example, an understanding of normal lung development will explain why preterm infants are at higher risk of respiratory distress syndrome than term infants, and why bowel protruding into the umbilical cord at 10 weeks' gestation is normal and is not diagnosed as an omphalocele (exomphalos).

This chapter provides an overview of the development, growth and maturation of the main body organs and systems in the human fetus and the implications of disordered growth.

FETAL GROWTH

Fetal growth and the eventual weight of the fetus at birth are important, not only for the immediate health of the neonate but also for long-term adult health and even into the next generation. The Developmental Origins of Health and Disease (DOHaD) hypothesis describes that reduced fetal growth is strongly associated with a number of chronic conditions later in life. This increased susceptibility results from adaptations made by the fetus in an environment with limited nutrient supply. These chronic conditions include coronary heart disease, stroke, diabetes and hypertension.

Fetal size can be assessed antenatally in two ways. The symphysis–fundal height (SFH) measurement is

29

taken externally by using a tape measure to assess the uterine size from the superior edge of the pubic symphysis to the uterine fundus. Second, ultrasound can be used to measure the dimensions of specific fetal parts, and the estimated fetal weight (EFW) is then calculated using equations such as those described by Hadlock (see **Chapter 4**). Fetal size is described in terms of the fetus's size for gestational age and is presented on centile charts. Centile charts can be designed for a population or can be personalized based on maternal factors.

Figure 3.1 shows the EFW centile chart for two fetuses. Fetus A has an EFW that is growing normally along the 75th centile. Fetus B is small and has suboptimal fetal growth; the EFW starts below the 5th centile and moves progressively further away from the normal centiles as gestation advances.

Customized centile charts (**Figure 1.2**, **Chapter 1**) take into consideration factors that are known to affect fetal growth such as maternal height, weight, parity, ethnicity and fetal sex.

A fetus that is less than the 10th centile is described as being small for gestational age (SGA) (**Figure 3.1,** Fetus B). This is a statistical concept designed to categorize on size but not necessarily on neonatal outcome. An SGA fetus may be constitutionally small; in other words, their growth potential was reached and they were destined to be that small. Many fetuses that are SGA, however, have failed to reach their full growth potential, a condition called fetal growth restriction (FGR). FGR is associated with a significant increased risk of perinatal morbidity and mortality. Growth-restricted fetuses are more likely to suffer intrauterine hypoxia/asphyxia and, as a consequence, be stillborn or demonstrate signs and symptoms of hypoxic-ischaemic encephalopathy, including seizures and multi-organ damage or failure in the neonatal period. Other complications to which these growth-restricted babies are more prone include neonatal hypothermia, hypoglycaemia, infection and necrotizing enterocolitis. In the medium term, cerebral palsy is more prevalent. It is now recognized from large epidemiological studies that low birthweight infants (defined as EFW <2,500 g) and SGA babies are more likely to develop hypertension, cardiovascular disease (ischaemic heart disease and stroke) and diabetes in adult life, indicating that the impact of FGR is long lasting.

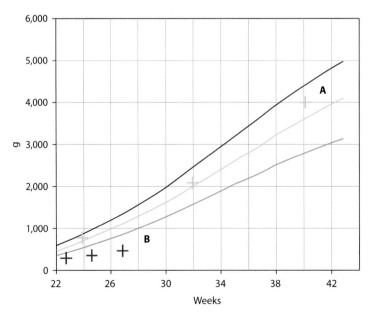

Figure 3.1 Population centile chart for estimated fetal weight by ultrasound measurements. Fetus **A** has normal growth (green crosses); fetus **B** has suboptimal growth (red crosses).

Recognizing the small fetus and distinguishing the 'small but healthy' SGA baby from those that are 'small and unhealthy' is a major obstetric challenge. Interventions such as the induction of labour or caesarean section to deliver the growth-restricted SGA fetus early from the intrauterine environment may improve outcome. Not all growth-restricted fetuses, however, are SGA: although a baby's birthweight is within the normal range for gestation (above the 10th centile), they may have failed to reach their full growth potential. Detecting these fetuses is even more difficult than identifying the small growth-restricted fetus.

DETERMINANTS OF FETAL GROWTH AND BIRTHWEIGHT

Determinants of fetal growth and birthweight are multifactorial. They include the influence of the natural growth potential of the fetus, which is dictated largely by the fetal genome and epigenome, but also the intrauterine environment, which is influenced by both maternal and placental factors. The birthweight is therefore the result of the interaction between the fetus and the maternal uterine environment. Fetal growth is dependent on adequate delivery to, and transfer of nutrients and oxygen across, the placenta, which relies on appropriate maternal nutrition and placental perfusion. Factors affecting these are discussed here and in **Chapter 9**. Other factors are important in determining fetal growth and include fetal hormones that affect the metabolic rate, the growth of tissues and the maturation of individual organs. In particular, insulin-like growth factors coordinate a precise and orderly increase in growth throughout late gestation. Insulin and thyroxine (T4) are required through late gestation to ensure appropriate growth in normal and adverse nutritional circumstances. Fetal hyperinsulinaemia, which occurs in association with maternal diabetes mellitus when maternal glycaemic control is suboptimal, results in fetal macrosomia with, in particular, excessive fat deposition. This leads to complications such as late stillbirth, shoulder dystocia and neonatal hypoglycaemia. Other factors related to fetal, maternal and placental influences are discussed in **Chapter 9**.

FETAL INFLUENCES
GENETIC

The fetal genome plays a significant role in determining fetal size. Early-onset and sometimes severe FGR is seen in fetuses with chromosomal defects such as the trisomies, particularly of chromosomes 13 (Patau syndrome) and 18 (Edwards syndrome), as well as triploidy. FGR is also common in trisomy 21 (Down syndrome). The other genetic influence is fetal sex, with slightly greater birthweights in males.

EPIGENETIC

Epigenetic changes play a role in determining fetal size. Epigenetic changes are modifications of deoxyribonucleic acid (DNA), which occur without any alteration in the underlying DNA sequence, and can control whether a gene is turned on or off and how much of a particular message is made. In genomic imprinting, the epigenetic process silences one parental allele, resulting in monoallelic expression. Genes that are paternally expressed tend to promote fetal growth, whereas maternally expressed genes suppress growth.

INFECTION

Although relatively uncommon in the UK, infection has been implicated in FGR, particularly rubella, cytomegalovirus, *Toxoplasma* and syphilis (discussed in further detail in **Chapter 11**). When a fetus is found to be very small on ultrasound measurement (for example EFW less than the 5th centile for gestational age), it is common to test the maternal blood for antibodies (immunoglobulin (Ig)G and IgM) to these infections. The results are then compared with samples taken at booking (see **Chapter 2**) to determine if the mother has evidence of seroconversion during pregnancy, which would suggest an acute infection.

MATERNAL INFLUENCES
PHYSIOLOGICAL INFLUENCES

In normal pregnancy, maternal physiological influences on birthweight include height, pre-pregnancy weight, age and ethnic group. Heavier and taller mothers tend to have bigger babies, and certain ethnic groups have lighter babies (e.g. South Asian and Afro-Caribbean ethnicities). Parity also has an influence, with increasing parity being associated with increased birthweight. Age influences are related to the association of age with parity (i.e. older mothers are more likely to be parous). In older pregnant women, however, there is an increased risk of chromosomal abnormalities and acquired maternal disease, for example hypertension, which lead to lower birthweights. Teenage pregnancy is also associated with FGR.

BEHAVIOURAL INFLUENCES

Maternal behavioural influences are also important, with smoking, alcohol and recreational drug use all associated with reduced fetal growth and birthweight. Mothers who smoke during pregnancy deliver babies up to 300 g lighter than non-smoking mothers. This effect may be through toxins, for example carbon monoxide, or vascular effects on uteroplacental circulation. Stopping smoking, even part way through pregnancy, is associated with higher birthweight. Alcohol crosses the placenta, and a dose-related effect has been noted, with up to a 500 g reduction in birthweight, along with other anomalies such as developmental delay occurring in those individuals who drink heavily (two drinks per day). Recreational drug use is often associated with smoking and alcohol use. Heroin use is independently associated with a reduction in birthweight. Cocaine use is associated with spontaneous preterm birth, low birthweight and small head circumference. Placental abruption is associated with cigarette smoking and the use of recreational drugs such as cocaine.

CHRONIC DISEASE

Chronic maternal disease may restrict fetal growth. Such diseases are largely those that affect placental function or result in maternal hypoxia, and include hypertension (essential or secondary to renal disease) and lung or cardiac conditions (cystic fibrosis, cyanotic heart disease). Hypertension can lead to placental infarction that impairs placental function. Maternal thrombophilia can also result in placental thrombosis and infarction.

PLACENTAL INFLUENCES

Normal placental development and function from early pregnancy is key to ensuring that the fetus receives adequate oxygen and nutrients from the mother. Placental insufficiency occurs when there is inadequate transfer of nutrients and oxygen across the placenta to the fetus. It can be due to poor maternal uterine artery blood flow, a thicker placental trophoblast barrier and/or abnormal fetus villous development. Placental infarction secondary to the maternal chronic conditions discussed previously or acute premature separation like in placental abruption can impair nutrient and oxygen transfer and hence reduce fetal growth. Recurrent bleeding from the placenta (antepartum haemorrhage) can, over time, compromise placental function, leading to poor fetal growth in the latter part of pregnancy. FGR is discussed further in **Chapter 9**.

FETAL DEVELOPMENT

CARDIOVASCULAR SYSTEM AND FETAL CIRCULATION

Fetal circulation is quite different from that of an adult (**Figure 3.2**). Fetal circulation is characterized by four shunts that ensure that the oxygenated blood from the placenta is prioritized for delivery to the fetal brain. These shunts are the:

- umbilical circulation
- ductus venosus
- foramen ovale
- ductus arteriosus

The umbilical circulation carries fetal blood to and from the placenta for gas and nutrient exchange. The umbilical arteries arise from the caudal end of the dorsal fetal aorta and carry deoxygenated blood from the fetus to the placenta. Normally, two umbilical arteries are present, but a single umbilical artery is relatively common (approximately 0.5% of fetuses) and can be associated with reduced fetal growth velocity and some congenital anomalies. Oxygenated blood is returned to the fetus via the umbilical vein to the fetal liver. A small proportion of blood oxygenates the liver, but the bulk passes

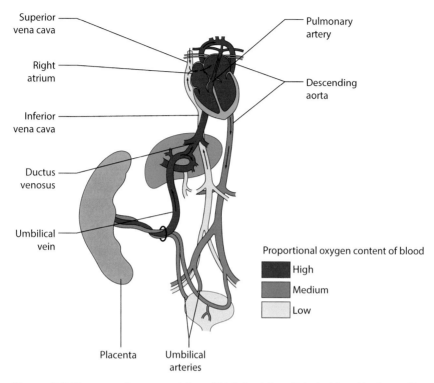

Figure 3.2 Diagrammatic representation of fetal circulation. (Adapted from Harrington K, Campbell S (1995). *A Colour Atlas of Doppler Ultrasonography in Obstetrics*. Arnold.)

through the ductus venosus, bypassing the liver, and joins the inferior vena cava as it enters the right atrium. The ductus venosus is a narrow vessel, and high blood velocities are generated within it. This streaming of the ductus venosus blood, together with a membranous valve in the right atrium (the crista dividens), prevents mixing of the well-oxygenated blood from the ductus venosus with the desaturated blood of the inferior vena cava. The ductus venosus stream passes across the right atrium through a physiological defect in the atrial septum called the foramen ovale to the left atrium. From here, the blood passes through the mitral valve to the left ventricle and hence to the aorta. About 50% of the blood goes to the head and upper extremities, providing high levels of oxygen to supply the fetal heart, upper thorax and brain; the remainder passes down the aorta to mix with blood of reduced oxygen saturation from the right ventricle. Deoxygenated blood returning from the fetal head and lower body flows through the right atrium and ventricle and into the pulmonary artery, after which it bypasses

the lungs to enter the descending aorta via the ductus arteriosus that connects the two vessels. Only a small portion of blood from the right ventricle passes to the fetal lungs, as they are not functional before birth. By this means, the desaturated blood from the right ventricle passes down the aorta to enter the umbilical arterial circulation where it is returned to the placenta for reoxygenation.

Prior to birth, the ductus arteriosus remains patent due to the production of prostaglandin E2 and prostacyclin, which act as local vasodilators. Premature closure of the ductus arteriosus has been reported with maternal administration of cyclooxygenase inhibitors before birth. At birth, the cessation of umbilical blood flow causes cessation of flow in the ductus venosus, a fall in pressure in the right atrium and closure of the foramen ovale. Ventilation of the lungs opens the pulmonary circulation, with a rapid fall in pulmonary vascular resistance, which dramatically increases the pulmonary circulation. The ductus arteriosus closes functionally within a few days of birth.

Occasionally, this transition from fetal to adult circulation is delayed, usually because the pulmonary vascular resistance fails to fall despite adequate breathing. This delay, termed persistent fetal circulation, results in left-to-right shunting of blood from the aorta through the ductus arteriosus to the lungs. The baby remains cyanosed and can suffer from life-threatening hypoxia. This delay in closure of the ductus arteriosus is most commonly seen in infants born preterm (<37 weeks' gestation). It results in congestion in the pulmonary circulation and a reduction in blood flow to the gastrointestinal tract and brain, and is implicated in the pathogenesis of necrotizing enterocolitis and intraventricular haemorrhage, both of which are complications associated with preterm birth.

CENTRAL NERVOUS SYSTEM

Neural development is one of the earliest systems to begin and one of the last to be completed during pregnancy, generating the most complex structure within the fetus. The early central nervous system begins as a simple neural plate that folds to form a groove, then a tube, open initially at each end. Failure of these openings to close contributes to a major class of neural abnormalities called neural tube defects (see **Chapter 5**). Later development of the fetal brain involves elaborate folding of the neurocortex, which occurs in the second half of pregnancy. There is a rapid increase in total grey matter in the last trimester, which is mainly due to a fourfold increase in cortical grey matter.

RESPIRATORY SYSTEM

The lung first appears as an outgrowth from the primitive foregut at about 3–4 weeks post-conception and, by 4–7 weeks, epithelial tube branches and vascular connections are forming. By 20 weeks, the conductive airway tree and parallel vascular tree is well developed. By 26 weeks, with further development of the airway and vascular tree, type I and II epithelial cells are beginning to differentiate. Pulmonary surfactant, a complex mixture of phospholipids and proteins that reduces surface tension at the air–liquid interface of the alveolus, is produced by the type II cells starting from about 30 weeks.

Dilatation of the gas-exchanging airspaces, alveolar formation and maturation of the surfactant system continues between this time and delivery at term. The fetal lungs are filled with fluid, the production of which starts in early gestation and ends in the early stages of labour. At birth, the production of this fluid ceases and the fluid present is absorbed. Adrenaline, to which the pulmonary epithelium becomes increasingly sensitive towards term, appears to play a major role in this process. With the clearance of the fluid and with the onset of breathing, the resistance in the vascular bed falls and results in an increase in pulmonary blood flow. A consequent increased pressure in the left atrium leads to closure of the foramen ovale.

Pulmonary surfactant prevents the collapse of small alveoli during expiration by lowering surface tension. The predominant phospholipid in surfactant (80% of the total) is phosphatidylcholine (lecithin), the production of which is enhanced by cortisol, growth restriction and prolonged rupture of the membranes, and is delayed in maternal diabetes mellitus. Inadequate amounts of surfactant result in poor lung expansion and poor gas exchange. In infants delivering preterm, prior to the maturation of the surfactant system, this results in a condition known as respiratory distress syndrome (RDS). It typically presents within the first few hours of life with signs of respiratory distress, including tachypnoea and cyanosis. It occurs in more than 80% of infants born between 23 and 27 weeks, falling to 10% of infants born between 34 and 36 weeks. Acute complications include hypoxia and asphyxia, intraventricular haemorrhage and necrotizing enterocolitis. The incidence and severity of RDS can be reduced by administering steroids antenatally to mothers 12–24 hours before they deliver preterm. The steroids cross the placenta and stimulate the premature release of stored fetal pulmonary surfactant in the fetal alveoli.

Numerous, but intermittent, fetal breathing movements (FBMs) occur in utero, especially during rapid eye movement (REM) sleep. By opposing lung recoil, FBM helps to maintain the high level of lung expansion that is essential for normal growth and structural maturation of the fetal lungs. During 'apnoeic' periods between successive episodes of FBM, active laryngeal constriction has the effect of opposing lung recoil by resisting the escape of lung

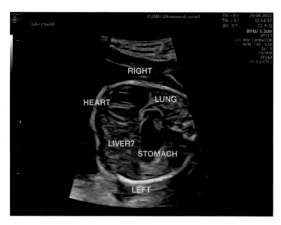

Figure 3.3 Ultrasound images of a fetus with a severe left-sided congenital diaphragmatic hernia. There is a herniated fetal liver, stomach and bowel in the left side of the thorax, compressing the heart to the right side of the thorax (right-sided mediastinal shift).

liquid via the trachea. The prolonged absence or impairment of FBM is likely to result in a reduced mean level of lung expansion that can lead to hypoplasia of the lungs. An adequate amniotic fluid volume is also necessary for normal lung maturation. Oligohydramnios (reduced amniotic fluid volume), decreased intrathoracic space (e.g. congenital diaphragmatic hernia) or chest wall deformities can result in pulmonary hypoplasia, which leads to progressive respiratory failure from birth.

BOX 3.1: Causes of pulmonary hypoplasia

Reduced or absent FBMs
- Inherited neuromuscular disorders (e.g. myotonic dystrophy)

Reduced (oligohydramnios) or absent (anhydramnios) amniotic fluid
- Preterm prelabour rupture of the membranes <24 weeks' gestation
- Bilateral congenital renal agenesis (Potter syndrome)
- Lower urinary tract obstruction

Decreased intrathoracic space
- Congenital diaphragmatic hernia
- Congenital cystic adenomatoid malformation of the lung
- Skeletal dysplasia (e.g. thanatophoric dysplasia)

ALIMENTARY SYSTEM

The primitive gut is present by the end of the fourth week, having been formed by folding of the embryo in both craniocaudal and lateral directions, with the resulting inclusion of the dorsal aspect of the yolk sac into the intraembryonic coelom. The primitive gut consists of three parts – the foregut, midgut and hindgut – and is suspended by a mesentery through which the blood supply, lymphatics and nerves reach the gut parenchyma. The foregut endoderm gives rise to the oesophagus, stomach, proximal half of the duodenum, liver and pancreas. The midgut endoderm gives rise to the distal half of the duodenum, jejunum, ileum, caecum, appendix, ascending colon and transverse colon. The hindgut endoderm develops into the descending colon, sigmoid colon and rectum.

Between 5 and 6 weeks, probably due to the lack of space in the abdominal cavity as a consequence of the rapidly enlarging liver and elongation of the intestine, the midgut is extruded into the umbilical cord as a physiological hernia. The gut undergoes a 270° anticlockwise rotation prior to re-entering the abdominal cavity by 12 weeks' gestation. Failure of the gut to re-enter the abdominal cavity results in the development of an omphalocele (otherwise called an exomphalos) and this condition is associated with chromosomal anomalies (**Figure 3.4**).

Other malformations include those that result from failure of the normal rotation of the gut, fistulae and atresias. Malrotation anomalies can result in

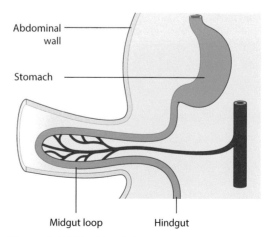

Figure 3.4 Midgut herniation.

volvulus and bowel obstruction. Atresias exist when there is a segment of bowel in which the lumen is not patent and most commonly occur in the upper gastrointestinal tract (i.e. the oesophagus or duodenum). As the fetus continually swallows amniotic fluid, any obstruction that prevents fetal swallowing or passage of amniotic fluid along the gut will result in the development of polyhydramnios (excess amniotic fluid). Gastrointestinal fistulae can also occur, the most common being a tracheo-oesophageal fistula (**Figure 3.5**), in which a connection exists between the distal end of the oesophagus and the trachea. Without surgical intervention, the neonate can develop complications after birth, as breathing causes air to pass from the trachea to the oesophagus and stomach, and feeding results in swallowed milk and stomach acid passing into the lungs. Some babies with tracheo-oesophageal fistula also have other congenital anomalies. This is known as VACTERL (vertebral, anal, cardiac, tracheal, (o)esophageal, renal and limb anomalies).

Peristalsis in the intestine occurs from the second trimester. The large bowel is filled with meconium at term. Defaecation in utero, and hence meconium in the amniotic fluid, is associated with post-term pregnancies and fetal hypoxia. Aspiration of meconium-stained liquor by the fetus at birth can result in meconium aspiration syndrome and respiratory distress.

In the last trimester of pregnancy, while body water content gradually diminishes, glycogen and fat stores increase about fivefold. Preterm infants have a reduced ability to withstand starvation and are at risk of hypoglycaemia, as they have virtually no fat. This is aggravated by an incompletely developed alimentary system and may manifest in a poor and unsustained suck, uncoordinated swallowing mechanism, delayed gastric emptying and poor absorption of carbohydrates, fat and other nutrients. Growth-restricted fetuses also have reduced glycogen stores and are therefore more prone to hypoglycaemia within the early neonatal period.

LIVER, PANCREAS AND GALL BLADDER

The pancreas, liver and epithelial lining of the biliary tree derive from the endoderm of the foregut. The liver and biliary tree appear late in the third week or early in the fourth week as the hepatic diverticulum, which is an outgrowth of the ventral wall of the distal foregut. The larger portion of this diverticulum gives rise to the parenchymal cells (hepatocytes) and the hepatic ducts, while the smaller portion gives rise to the gall bladder. By the sixth week, the fetal liver performs haematopoiesis. This peaks at 12–16 weeks and continues until approximately 36 weeks.

In utero, the normal metabolic functions of the liver are performed by the placenta. For example, unconjugated bilirubin from haemoglobin breakdown is actively transported from the fetus to the mother, with only a small proportion being conjugated in the liver and secreted in the bile (the mechanism after birth). The fetal liver also differs from the adult organ in many processes; for example, the fetal liver has a reduced ability to conjugate bilirubin because of relative deficiencies in the necessary enzymes such as glucuronyl transferase. After birth, the loss of the placental route of excretion of unconjugated bilirubin, in the presence of reduced conjugation, particularly in the premature infant, may result in transient unconjugated hyperbilirubinaemia or physiological jaundice of the newborn.

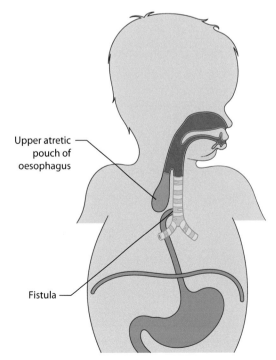

Upper atretic pouch of oesophagus

Fistula

Figure 3.5 Tracheo-oesophageal fistula.

Glycogen is stored within the liver in small quantities from the first trimester, but storage is maximal in the third trimester, with abundant stores being present at term. Growth-restricted and premature infants have deficient glycogen stores; this renders them prone to neonatal hypoglycaemia.

KIDNEY AND URINARY TRACT

The kidney, recognized in its permanent final form (metanephric kidney), is preceded by the development and subsequent regression of two primitive forms: the pronephros and the mesonephros. The pronephros originates at about 3 weeks in a ridge that forms on either side of the midline in the embryo, known as the nephrogenic ridge. In this region, epithelial cells arrange themselves in a series of tubules and join laterally with the pronephric duct. The pronephros is non-functional in mammals. Each pronephric duct grows towards the tail of the embryo. As it does so, it induces intermediate mesoderm in the thoracolumbar area to become epithelial tubules called mesonephric tubules. The pronephros degenerates while the mesonephric (Wolffian) duct extends towards the most caudal end of the embryo, ultimately attaching to the cloaca.

During the fifth week of gestation, the ureteric bud develops as an out-pouching from the Wolffian duct. This bud grows towards the head of the embryo and into the intermediate mesoderm and, as it does so, it branches to form the collecting duct system (ureter, pelvis, calyces and collecting ducts) of the kidney and induces the formation of the renal secretory system (glomeruli, convoluted tubes, loops of Henle). Subsequently, the lower portions of the nephric duct will migrate caudally (downwards) and connect with the bladder, thereby forming the ureters. As the fetus develops, the torso elongates and the kidneys rotate and migrate upwards within the abdomen, which causes the length of the ureters to increase.

Failure of the normal migration of the kidney upwards can result in a pelvic kidney, where it remains in the pelvic area (**Figure 3.6**). Abnormal development of the collecting duct system can result in duplications such as duplex kidneys (**Figure 3.6**).

The most common sites of congenital urinary tract obstructive uropathies are at the pyeloureteric

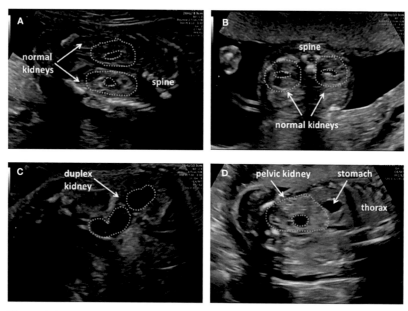

Figure 3.6 Normal kidneys in coronal view (**A**) and transverse view (**B**). The kidneys are outlined with blue dots and the renal pelvis in each kidney is outlined in green dots. (**C**) A duplex kidney with two separate dilated renal pelvises (green dots). (**D**) A pelvic kidney with a normal size renal pelvis (green dots outline the renal pelvis; blue dots outline the renal cortex).

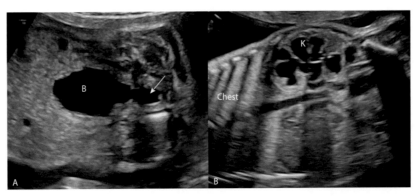

Figure 3.7 Posterior urethral valves. (**A**) The typical 'keyhole' sign in the fetal bladder (labelled 'B'), where the dilated upper posterior urethra is indicated (white arrow). (**B**) Dilatation of the collecting system of the fetal kidney (labelled 'K').

junction, at the vesicoureteric junction or as a consequence of posterior urethral valves, an obstructing membrane in the posterior male urethra (**Figure 3.7**). Severe obstruction in utero can lead to hydronephrosis and renal interstitial fibrosis, with postnatal renal failure.

In humans, all of the branches of the ureteric bud and the nephronic units have been formed by 32–36 weeks' gestation. However, these structures are not yet mature, and the maturation of the excretory and concentrating ability of the fetal kidneys is gradual and continues after birth. In the preterm infant, this may lead to abnormal water, glucose, sodium or acid–base homeostasis.

As fetal urine forms much of the amniotic fluid, renal agenesis will result in a severe reduction in (oligohydramnios) or the absence of amniotic fluid (anhydramios). Babies born with bilateral renal agenesis (Potter syndrome), which is associated with other features such as widely spaced eyes, small jaw and low set ears (results that are secondary to oligohydramnios), do not pass urine and usually die as a consequence of either 'renal failure' or pulmonary hypoplasia, again secondary to severe oligohydramnios.

SKIN AND HOMEOSTASIS

Fetal skin protects and facilitates homeostasis. The skin and its appendages (nails, hair) develop from the ectodermal and mesodermal germ layers. The epidermis develops from the surface ectoderm; the dermis and the hypodermis (the latter attaches the dermis of the skin to underlying tissues) both develop from mesenchymal cells in the mesoderm.

By the fourth week following conception, a single-cell layer of ectoderm surrounds the embryo. At about 6 weeks, this ectodermal layer differentiates into an outer periderm and an inner basal layer. The periderm eventually sloughs as the vernix, a creamy protective coat that covers the skin of the fetus. The basal layer produces the epidermis and the glands, nails and hair follicles.

Over the ensuing weeks, the epithelium becomes stratified and, by 16–20 weeks, all layers of the epidermis are developed and each layer assumes a structure characteristic of the adult. Preterm babies have no vernix and have thin skin; this allows a proportionately large amount of insensible water loss. Thermal control in cool, ambient temperatures is limited by a large surface-to-body weight ratio and poor thermal insulation. Heat may be conserved by peripheral vasoconstriction and can be generated by brown fat catabolism, but this is deficient in preterm or growth-restricted babies because of the small amount of subcutaneous fat and the immaturity of vascular tone regulation in the former. The response to warm ambient temperatures is also poor and can result in overheating of the infant.

Hair follicles begin to develop as hair buds between 12 and 16 weeks from the basal layer of the epidermis. By 24 weeks, the hair follicles produce delicate fetal hair called lanugo, first on the head and then on other parts of the body. This lanugo is usually shed before birth.

BLOOD AND IMMUNE SYSTEM

Red blood cells and immune effector cells are derived from pluripotent haematopoietic cells, first noted in the blood islands of the yolk sac. By 8 weeks, the yolk sac is replaced by the liver as the source of these cells and, by 20 weeks, almost all of these cells are produced by the bone marrow.

The development of the thymus and the secondary lymphoid organs is a highly ordered process that undergoes a rapid expansion in the first trimester of pregnancy and appears to be largely finished by the time of birth. T-cell precursors transit to the thymus by 9 weeks' gestation, and mature, naive and memory αβ T-cells are readily found by 12–14 weeks in spleen and lymph nodes; circulating mature T-cells are present by 16 weeks of gestation. In the second trimester, the fetal tissues have an increased frequency of regulatory T-cells, more than at any other time in fetal, neonatal or adult development, and this is important for the induction of specific tolerance. Complement proteins are present by the middle of the second trimester and reach 50% of adult levels at term. Lymphoid precursor cells develop into B-lymphocytes, detected in the fetal liver at 8 weeks of gestation, and appear in fetal blood circulation by 12 weeks of gestation. They undergo subsequent functional maturation in secondary lymphoid tissue (e.g. lymph nodes and spleen). Ig somatic hypermutation and class switch recombination already occur during intrauterine life, although much of the IgG in the fetus originates from the maternal circulation and crosses the placenta to provide passive immunity to the fetus and neonate. The fetus normally produces only small amounts of IgM and IgA, which do not cross the placenta. Detection of IgM/IgA in the newborn, without IgG, is indicative of fetal infection.

Most haemoglobin in the fetus is fetal haemoglobin (HbF), which has two gamma-chains (alpha-2, gamma-2). This differs from the adult haemoglobins HbA and HbA2, which have two beta-chains (alpha-2, beta-2) and two delta-chains (alpha-2, delta-2), respectively. Ninety percent of haemoglobin in the fetus is HbF between 10 and 28 weeks of gestation. From 28 to 34 weeks, a switch to HbA occurs and, at term, the ratio of HbF to HbA is 80:20; by 6 months of age, only 1% of haemoglobin is HbF. A key feature of HbF is a higher affinity for oxygen than HbA. This, in association with a higher haemoglobin concentration (at birth, the mean capillary haemoglobin is 18 g/dL), enhances transfer of oxygen across the placenta.

Abnormal haemoglobin production results in thalassaemia. The thalassaemias are a group of genetic haematological disorders characterized by reduced or absent production of one or more of the globin chains of haemoglobin. Beta-thalassaemia results from reduced or absent production of the beta-globin chains. As the switch from HbF to HbA occurs, the absent or insufficient beta-globin chains shorten red cell survival, with destruction of these cells within the bone marrow and spleen. Beta-thalassaemia major results from the inheritance of two abnormal beta genes; without treatment, this leads to severe anaemia, FGR, poor musculoskeletal development and skin pigmentation due to increased iron absorption. In the severest form of alpha-thalassaemia, in which no alpha-globin chains are produced, severe fetal anaemia occurs with cardiac failure, hepatosplenomegaly and generalized oedema. Abnormal fluid present in more than one cavity (for example fetal ascites, or pleural or pericardial effusion) is called fetal hydrops. The infants are stillborn or die shortly after birth.

ENDOCRINE SYSTEM

Major components of the hypothalamic–pituitary axis are in place by 12 weeks' gestation. Thyrotrophin-releasing hormone and gonadotrophin-releasing hormone have been identified in the fetal hypothalamus by the end of the first trimester. Testosterone produced by the interstitial cells of the testis is also synthesized in the first trimester of pregnancy and increases until 17–21 weeks, which mirrors the differentiation of the male urogenital tract. Growth hormone is similarly present from early pregnancy and is detectable in the circulation from 12 weeks. The thyroid gland produces T4 from 10 to 12 weeks. Growth-restricted fetuses exist in a state of relative hypothyroidism, which may be a compensatory measure to decrease metabolic rate and oxygen consumption.

BEHAVIOURAL STATES

From conception, the fetus follows a developmental path, with milestones that continue into childhood. The first activity is the beating of the fetal heart, followed by fetal movements at 7–8 weeks. These start as just discernible movements and graduate through startles to movements of arms and legs, breathing movements and, by 12 weeks, yawning, sucking and swallowing. This means that, in the first trimester of pregnancy, the fetus exhibits movements that are observed after birth. Further maturation does not add new movements but results in a change in terms of combinations of movements and activity that reflect fetal behavioural states. In the second trimester, for example, cycles of the absence or presence of movements change, meaning that periods over which body movements are absent increase.

Four fetal behavioural states have been described, annotated 1F–4F. 1F is quiescence, 2F is characterized by frequent and periodic gross body movements with eye movements, 3F is characterized by no gross body movements but eye movements and 4F is vigorous continual activity again with eye movements. 1F is similar to quiet or non-REM sleep in the neonate, 2F is REM sleep, 3F is quiet wakefulness and 4F is active wakefulness. An understanding of fetal behaviour can assist in assessing fetal condition and well-being.

AMNIOTIC FLUID

By 12 weeks' gestation, the amnion comes into contact with the inner surface of the chorion and the two membranes become adherent, but never intimately fuse. Neither the amnion nor the chorion contains vessels or nerves, but both do contain a significant quantity of phospholipids, as well as enzymes involved in phospholipid hydrolysis. Choriodecidual function is thought to play a pivotal role in the initiation of labour through the production of prostaglandins E2 and F2a.

The amniotic fluid is initially secreted by the amnion, but by the 10th week it is mainly a transudate of the fetal serum via the skin and umbilical cord. From 16 weeks' gestation, the fetal skin becomes impermeable to water and the net increase in amniotic fluid is through a small imbalance between the contributions of fluid through the kidneys and lung fluids and removal by fetal swallowing. The amniotic fluid contains growth factors and multipotent stem cells, the function of which at present is unknown. Amniotic fluid volume increases progressively (10 weeks, 30 mL; 20 weeks, 300 mL; 30 weeks, 600 mL; 38 weeks, 1,000 mL), but from term there is a rapid fall in volume (40 weeks, 800 mL; 42 weeks, 350 mL). The reason for the late reduction has not been explained. The amniotic fluid index is calculated as the total measurement of the deepest pool in the four quadrants of the uterus (**Figure 3.8**).

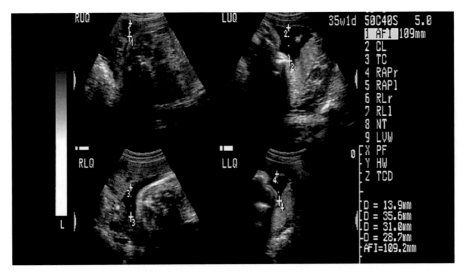

Figure 3.8 Amniotic fluid measurement and normal ranges.

KEY LEARNING POINTS

- Determinants of birthweight are multifactorial and include the influence of the natural growth potential of the fetus and the intrauterine environment.
- Fetal circulation is quite different from that of the adult. Its distinctive features are as follows:
  - Oxygenation occurs in the placenta, not the lungs.
  - The right and left ventricles work in parallel rather than in series.
  - The heart, brain and upper body receive blood from the left ventricle, while the placenta and lower body receive blood from both the right and the left ventricles.
- Surfactant prevents collapse of small alveoli in the newborn lung during expiration by lowering surface tension. Its production is maximal after 28 weeks.
- RDS is common in babies born prematurely and is associated with surfactant deficiency.
- The fetus requires an effective immune system to resist intrauterine and perinatal infections. Lymphocytes appear from 8 weeks and, by the middle of the second trimester, all phagocytic cells, T- and B-cells and complement are available to mount a response.
- Fetal skin protects and facilitates homeostasis.
- In utero, the normal metabolic functions of the liver are performed by the placenta. The loss of the placental route of excretion of unconjugated bilirubin, in the face of conjugating enzyme deficiencies, particularly in the premature infant, may result in transient unconjugated hyperbilirubinaemia or physiological jaundice of the newborn.
- Growth-restricted and premature infants have deficient glycogen stores; this renders them prone to neonatal hypoglycaemia.
- The function of the amniotic fluid is to:
  - protect the fetus from mechanical injury
  - permit movement of the fetus while preventing limb contracture
  - prevent adhesions between the fetus and amnion
  - permit fetal lung development in which there is two-way movement of fluid into the fetal bronchioles; absence of amniotic fluid in the second trimester is associated with pulmonary hypoplasia.

The function of the amniotic fluid is to:

- protect the fetus from mechanical injury
- permit movement of the fetus while preventing limb contracture
- prevent adhesions between the fetus and amnion
- permit fetal lung development in which there is two-way movement of fluid into the fetal bronchioles; absence of amniotic fluid in the second trimester is associated with pulmonary hypoplasia

Major alterations in amniotic fluid volume occur when there is reduced contribution of fluid into the amniotic sac in conditions such as renal agenesis, cystic kidneys or FGR; oligohydramnios results. Reduced removal of fluid in conditions such as congenital neuromuscular disorders, anencephaly and oesophageal/duodenal atresia, which prevent fetal swallowing, is associated with polyhydramnios.

FURTHER READING

Moore KL, Persaud TVN, Torchia MG (2015). *The Developing Human: Clinically Oriented Embryology*, 10th edn. Saunders.

SELF-ASSESSMENT

For interactive SBAs and EMQs relating to this chapter, visit www.routledge.com/cw/mccarthy.

CASE HISTORY 1

A 26 year old is admitted to the labour ward at 28 weeks' gestation. She gives a history suggestive of preterm prelabour rupture of the membranes and is experiencing uterine contractions. The mother receives an injection of dexamethasone corticosteroids to mature the fetal lungs and an infusion of magnesium sulphate is begun for fetal neuroprotection. On abdominal examination, the fetus is in cephalic presentation. On vaginal examination, there is clear liquor draining, the cervix is found to be 8 cm dilated and she rapidly goes on to have an uncomplicated vaginal delivery of a male infant weighing 1,250 g within an hour of presenting to hospital. At birth, he is intubated because of poor respiratory effort and is transferred to the neonatal intensive care unit.

As a premature infant, from which complications is he particularly at risk?

ANSWERS

Fetal growth
Deficient glycogen stores in the liver increase the risk of hypoglycaemia. This is compounded by the increased glucose requirements of premature infants.

Cardiovascular system
Patent ductus arteriosus may result in pulmonary congestion, worsening lung disease and decreased blood flow to the gastrointestinal tract and brain. The duct can be closed by administering prostaglandin synthetase inhibitors, for example indomethacin, or by surgical ligation.

Respiratory system
RDS and apnoea of prematurity may lead to hypoxia. The administration of antenatal steroids to the mother reduces the risk and severity of RDS. For maximal benefit to be gained, steroids need to be administered at least 24 hours before delivery. In this case, delivery occurred too rapidly for steroids to be administered. The severity of RDS can also be reduced by giving surfactant via the endotracheal tube used to ventilate the baby.

Fetal blood
Anaemia of prematurity is common because of low iron stores and red cell mass at birth, reduced erythropoiesis and decreased survival of red blood cells. Treatment is by blood transfusion, iron supplementation or, in some cases, the use of erythropoietin.

Immune system
Preterm babies have an increased susceptibility to infection due to impaired cell-mediated immunity and reduced levels of immunoglobulin. Suspected infection should be treated early with antibiotics because deterioration in these premature small infants can be rapid.

Skin and homeostasis
Hypothermia is common in preterm infants secondary to a relatively large body surface area, thin skin, a lack of subcutaneous fat and a lack of a keratinized epidermal layer of skin. High insensible water losses due to skin immaturity may aggravate dehydration and electrolyte problems secondary to immaturity in renal function (see the following section 'Kidney and urinary tract'). The environment can be controlled by nursing this type of infant in an incubator.

Alimentary system
Necrotizing enterocolitis is an inflammatory condition of the bowel leading to necrosis and is thought to be secondary to alterations in gut blood flow, hypotension, hypoxia, infection and feeding practices. Feeding problems are common in preterm infants because they have immature suck and swallowing reflexes and gut motility. Parenteral nutrition is usually required in these very premature infants, with gradually increasing volumes of milk given by nasogastric tube.

Liver and gall bladder
Jaundice (hyperbilirubinaemia) secondary to liver immaturity and a shorter half-life of red blood cells is common in premature infants. Treatment with phototherapy is required because premature infants are at greater risk of bilirubin encephalopathy.

Kidney and urinary tract
Immaturity of the kidneys can lead to a poor ability to concentrate or dilute urine. This can result in dehydration and electrolyte disturbances: hypernatraemia and hyponatraemia, hyperkalaemia and metabolic acidosis.

Central nervous system
Periventricular and intraventricular haemorrhages result from bleeding from the immature rich capillary bed of the germinal matrix lining the ventricles. Such haemorrhages are more likely in the presence of hypoxia. Major degrees of haemorrhage can result in hydrocephalus and neurological abnormalities such as cerebral palsy. Periventricular leukomalacia is ischaemic necrosis in the white matter surrounding the lateral ventricles and commonly leads to cerebral palsy. The administration of peripartum magnesium sulphate reduces the risk of cerebral palsy and is recommended for pregnant women between 24+0 and 29+6 weeks of pregnancy who are in established preterm labour or having a planned preterm birth.

CASE HISTORY 2

A 24-year-old nulliparous woman had a detailed fetal anomaly ultrasound scan at 20 weeks' gestation. This showed reduced amniotic fluid index (2 cm), an enlarged, thick-walled bladder and a dilated urethra with a 'keyhole' sign, bilateral hydroureteronephrosis (dilated ureter and renal pelvis) and bilateral echogenic kidneys. The fetus was a male. There were no other fetal structural abnormalities. The findings at the dating scan at 12 weeks had been apparently normal. She had no family or personal history of renal problems.

What is the likely diagnosis and what is the prognosis?

ANSWER

The likely diagnosis is posterior urethral valves, which is the most common congenital cause of bladder outflow obstruction in male neonates (sometimes called lower urinary tract obstruction). This occurs in 1 in 5,000 live male births and is caused by an obstructing membrane

in the posterior male urethra as a result of abnormal in utero development. The differential diagnosis includes urethral atresia and bilateral vesicoureteric reflux. The majority of cases are suspected prenatally and referred to specialist centres at birth.

Early prenatal diagnosis (before 24 weeks' gestation), ultrasound evidence of echogenic renal parenchyma and reduced amniotic fluid volume have been identified as predictors of a poor prognosis, as in this case. Prenatal interventions such as percutaneous ultrasound-guided vesicocentesis (drainage of the bladder) can be used to relieve the obstruction temporarily. Ultrasound-guided placement of a vesicoamniotic shunt (between the bladder and the amniotic cavity) seems to improve perinatal survival. Whether this treatment or conservative management is used, however, the surviving children have a high rate of end-stage renal failure requiring dialysis and transplantation. The condition accounts for 25–30% of paediatric renal transplantations in the UK.

CASE HISTORY 3

A 30-year-old multiparous woman is referred to the fetal medicine unit because the midwife is concerned about the size of the uterus during a routine antenatal check at 30 weeks' gestation. The SFH measures 38 cm. Down syndrome screening by the combined test gave a low risk (1 in 20,000). On ultrasound examination, the fetal measurements are on the 80th centile. There is increased amniotic fluid with a single deepest pool of 10 cm (normal range <8 cm) and an amniotic fluid index of 35 cm (normal range <25 cm). Fetal movements and fetal umbilical artery and middle cerebral artery Doppler measurements are normal. In the transverse fetal abdominal views, there was a double bubble seen on the left side of the abdomen (**Figure 3.9**). There were no other abnormalities detectable; in particular, the fetal face was normal. The placenta was anterior high and had a normal structural appearance.

What is the most likely diagnosis and what are the differential diagnoses? What is the optimum management for the rest of the pregnancy and at birth?

ANSWER

Polyhydramnios occurs in approximately 1–1.5% of pregnancies. This is a case of mild polyhydramnios (single deepest pool of liquor 8–11 cm). An underlying disease is only found in 17% of cases in mild polyhydramnios. In contrast, an underlying disease is detected in 91% of cases in moderate (12–15 cm) to severe polyhydramnios (>15 cm).

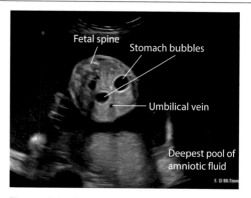

Figure 3.9 Ultrasound image showing the 'double bubble' appearance and polyhydramnios associated with duodenal atresia.

The most likely diagnosis is duodenal atresia, namely the congenital absence or complete closure of a portion of the lumen of the duodenum, which occurs in 1:2,500–5,000 live births. In 25–40% of cases, there is associated trisomy 21 (Down syndrome). The differential diagnosis includes:

- an obstructive structural malformation that prevents fetal swallowing (e.g. facial cleft or congenital high airways obstruction syndrome [CHAOS]) or prevents passage of amniotic fluid along the gut (e.g. oesophageal atresia)

(Contd.)

(Contd.)

- congenital problems that prevent normal swallowing function (e.g. neurological structural problems such as anencephaly or neuromuscular disorders such as myotonic dystrophy)
- fetal anaemia (e.g. due to rhesus incompatibility or virus infection such as with parvovirus B19); usually there are other associated findings such as pleural effusion or ascites
- multiple pregnancies, particularly those with a monochorionic placenta
- maternal diabetes

Management of a case of polyhydramnios includes a detailed fetal anomaly scan to observe fetal movements and structures, counselling about the risk of trisomy 21 and an offer of fetal karyotyping by amniocentesis, a glucose tolerance test for maternal diabetes and a maternal antibody blood test for virus infections.

In this case, the patient declined amniocentesis. She was seen antenatally by the paediatric surgeons to discuss surgical management postnatally. She was counselled about the risk of spontaneous preterm labour, preterm prelabour rupture of the membranes, abnormal fetal presentation and cord prolapse in labour. She was monitored by scan every 2 weeks; the amniotic fluid index remained the same and she had only mild uterine activity. She did not require amnioreduction (amniocentesis to drain off excessive fluid). She presented in labour at 36 weeks' gestation with the fetus in cephalic presentation and had a normal vaginal delivery. The neonate weighing 3.7 kg was born with good Apgar scores and he was transferred to the neonatal intensive care unit for monitoring. At 1 day of age, he underwent laparoscopic duodenostomy for duodenal atresia and had a good recovery. His karyotype performed postnatally was normal euploid.

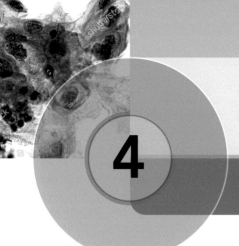

Assessment of fetal well-being

4

ANNA L DAVID

Learning Objectives
- Understand the principles of imaging in obstetrics and its safety and benefits for examining the fetus during gestation.
- Know how ultrasound is used in pregnancy to confirm gestational age, to detect fetal structural abnormalities, to monitor fetal growth and development, to study the placenta and to assess fetal well-being.
- Recognize the value of antenatal cardiotocography to assess fetal well-being and to screen for fetal hypoxia.
- Be aware of the role of Doppler ultrasound to monitor and guide the management of pregnancies at risk of adverse outcomes.

INTRODUCTION

Ultrasound is the principal imaging modality used in obstetrics. Indeed, diagnostic ultrasound is used to screen all pregnancies in most high- and middle-income countries. Ultrasound is used to date pregnancies, to monitor growth of the fetus and to identify congenital abnormalities. Colour and spectral Doppler are used to interrogate the uterine, placental and fetal blood vessels, providing information on uteroplacental function, fetal well-being and the fetal circulatory response to hypoxia and anaemia, for example.

Antenatal tests of fetal well-being are now principally based on ultrasound techniques and are designed to identify fetuses that are in the early or late stages of fetal hypoxia. Continuous wave Doppler ultrasound is employed in cardiotocography to provide continuous tracings of the fetal heart rate, the patterns of which alter when the fetus is hypoxic.

Three-dimensional (3D) ultrasound and increasingly magnetic resonance imaging (MRI) are used to provide further information when a fetal abnormality is suspected.

DIAGNOSTIC ULTRASOUND IN OBSTETRIC PRACTICE

In 1959, Professor Ian Donald, the Regius Chair of Midwifery at Glasgow University, noted that clear echoes could be obtained from the fetal head using

45

10.1201/9781003196112-4

ultrasound. Since the reporting of this initial discovery, the technique of ultrasound has developed into one that now plays an essential role in the care of pregnant women.

The ultrasound technique uses very high-frequency sound waves of between 3.5 and 7.0 MHz emitted from a transducer. Transducers can be placed and moved across the abdomen (transabdominal, **Figure 4.1**) or mounted on a probe that can be inserted into the vagina (transvaginal, **Figure 4.2**).

Transvaginal ultrasonography is useful in early pregnancy, for examining the cervix later in pregnancy and for identifying the lower edge of the placenta (to assess for placenta praevia). It is also useful in early pregnancy in individuals with significant amounts of abdominal adipose tissue through which abdominal ultrasound waves would need to travel, and hence be attenuated prior to reaching the uterus and its

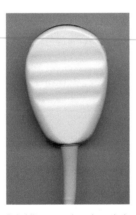

Figure 4.1 Ultrasound probe: abdominal.

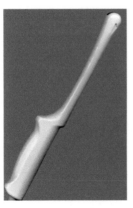

Figure 4.2 Ultrasound probe: transvaginal.

contents, making visualization difficult. In general, however, after 12 weeks' gestation, an abdominal transducer, which is a flat or curvilinear probe with a much wider array, is used. Crystals within the transducer emit a focused ultrasound beam in a series of pulses and then receive the reflected signals from within the uterus between the pulses. The strength of the reflected sound wave depends on the difference in 'acoustic impedance' between adjacent structures. The acoustic impedance of a tissue is related to its density; the greater the difference in acoustic impedance between two adjacent tissues the more reflective will be their boundary. The returning signals are transformed into visual signals and generate a continuous picture of the moving fetus. Movements such as fetal heartbeat and structures in the fetus can be assessed and measurements can be made accurately on the images displayed on the screen. Such measurements enable the assessment of gestational age, size and growth in the fetus. Ultrasound images obtained can also be processed with computer software to produce 3D images and even four-dimensional (4D, moving 3D images), which provide more detail on fetal anatomical structure and the identification of anomalies.

The use of Doppler ultrasound allows the assessment of the velocity of blood within fetal and placental vessels and provides indirect assessment of the fetal and placental condition. Doppler ultrasound makes use of the phenomenon of the Doppler frequency shift, that is, the reflected wave will be at a different frequency from the transmitted one if it interacts with moving structures, such as red blood cells flowing along a blood vessel, with the change in frequency being proportional to the velocity of the blood cells. If the red blood cells are moving towards the beam, the reflected signal will be at a higher frequency than the transmitted one and conversely the reflected beam will be at a lower signal if the flow is away from the beam. In this modality, signals from a particular vessel can be isolated and displayed in graphic form, with the velocity plotted against time. The significance of changes observed in waveform patterns obtained from placental and fetal vessels, and how these observations can be used in clinical practice, will be discussed in the section 'Doppler investigation' later in the chapter.

Ultrasound scanning is currently considered to be a safe, non-invasive, accurate and cost-effective investigation in the fetus. There are guidelines that cover the safe use of ultrasound in pregnancy. These include the as low as reasonably achievable (ALARA) principle, a practice mandate adhering to the principle of keeping radiation doses to patients and personnel as low as possible. Examination times are kept as short as is necessary to produce a useful diagnostic result, particularly before 10 weeks' gestation when the embryo may be more sensitive to the effects of thermal and mechanical injury. This chapter will consider the diagnostic use of these techniques in more detail.

The main uses of ultrasonography in pregnancy are in the areas discussed in the following sections.

DIAGNOSIS AND CONFIRMATION OF VIABILITY IN EARLY PREGNANCY

The gestational sac can be visualized from as early as 4–5 weeks' gestation and the yolk sac at about 5 weeks (**Figure 4.3**). The embryo can be observed and measured at 5–6 weeks' gestation. Beating of the fetal heart can be visualized by about 6 weeks.

Transvaginal ultrasound plays a key role in the diagnosis of disorders of early pregnancy, such as incomplete or missed miscarriage (anembryonic pregnancy or 'blighted ovum'), where no fetus is present (**Figure 4.4**) and ectopic pregnancy. In a missed miscarriage, for example, the fetus can be identified, but with an absent fetal heartbeat. In an anembryonic pregnancy, there is a gestation sac present but it is empty because the fetus has failed to develop. An ectopic pregnancy is suspected if, in the presence of a positive pregnancy test, an ultrasound

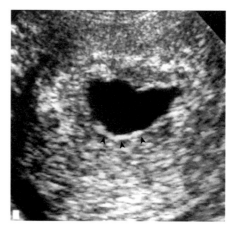

Figure 4.4 Ultrasound image showing an empty gestation sac (arrowheads) in a case of an anembryonic pregnancy.

scan does not identify a gestation sac within the uterus, there is an adnexal mass with or without a fetal pole or there is fluid in the pouch of Douglas.

DETERMINATION OF GESTATIONAL AGE AND ASSESSMENT OF FETAL SIZE AND GROWTH

Up to approximately 20 weeks' gestation, the range of values around the mean for measurements of fetal length, head size and long bone length is narrow and hence assessment of gestation based on these measures is accurate. The crown–rump length (CRL) is used up to 13 weeks + 6 days (see **Figure 5.3**) and the head circumference (HC) is used from 14 to 20 weeks' gestation. The biparietal diameter (BPD) (**Figure 4.5**)

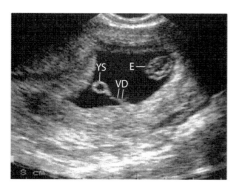

Figure 4.3 Ultrasound sac showing the yolk sac (YS) and embryo (E) with the vitelline duct (VD).

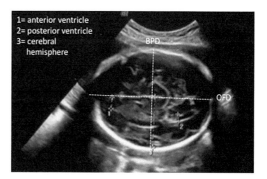

Figure 4.5 Biparietal diameter (BPD). (1, anterior ventricle; 2, posterior ventricle; 3, cerebral hemisphere. OFD, occipitofrontal diameter.)

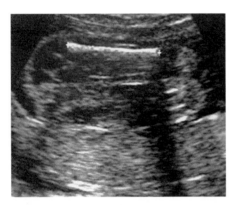

Figure 4.6 Femur length.

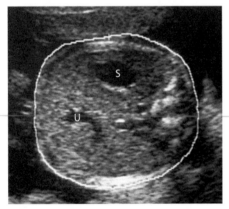

Figure 4.7 Abdominal circumference measurement demonstrating the correct section showing the stomach (S) and the umbilical vein (U).

and femur length (FL) (**Figure 4.6**) can also be used to determine gestational age. Essentially, the earlier the measurement is made, the more accurate the prediction, and measurements made from an early CRL (accuracy of prediction 6 ± 5 days) will be preferred to a BPD at 20 weeks (accuracy of prediction 6 ± 7 days).

In the latter part of pregnancy, measuring fetal abdominal circumference (AC) (**Figure 4.7**) and HC will allow assessment of the size and growth of the fetus and will assist in the diagnosis and management of fetal growth restriction (FGR). In addition to AC and HC, BPD and FL, when combined in an equation, provide a more accurate estimate of fetal weight (EFW) than any of the parameters taken singly.

In pregnancies at high risk of FGR, serial measurements are plotted on the normal reference range. Growth patterns are helpful in distinguishing between different types of growth restriction (symmetrical and asymmetrical). Asymmetry between head measures (BPD, HC) and AC can be identified in FGR, where a brain-sparing effect will result in a relatively large HC compared with the AC (**Figure 4.8**). The opposite would occur in a diabetic pregnancy, where the abdomen is disproportionately large due to the effects of insulin on the fetal liver and fat stores. Cessation of growth is an ominous sign of placental failure.

Gestational age cannot be accurately calculated by ultrasound after 20 weeks' gestation because of the wider range of normal values of AC and HC around the mean.

MULTIPLE PREGNANCY

Ultrasound is now the most common way in which multiple pregnancies are identified (**Figure 4.9**). In addition to identifying the presence of more than one fetus, it is used to determine the chorionicity of the pregnancy, which is important in stratifying the risk of particular pregnancy complications that occur in monochorionic multiple pregnancies.

Monochorionic twin pregnancies (i.e. those who 'share' a placenta) are associated with an increased risk of pregnancy complications such as twin-to-twin transfusion syndrome and a higher perinatal mortality rate than dichorionic twin pregnancies. It is therefore clinically useful to be able to determine chorionicity early in pregnancy (see **Chapter 7**).

The dividing membrane between monochorionic twins is formed by two layers of amnion and in dichorionic twins the dividing membrane consists of two layers of chorion and two of amnion. Dichorionic twin pregnancies therefore have a thicker dividing membrane than monochorionic twin pregnancies and this can be perceived qualitatively on ultrasound. Sonographically, dichorionic twin pregnancies in the first trimester of pregnancy have a thick inter-twin separating membrane (septum), flanked on either side by a very thin amnion. This is in contrast to a monochorionic twin pregnancy, which on two-dimensional (2D) ultrasound has a very thin inter-twin septum.

Another method of determining chorionicity in the first trimester uses the appearance of the septum at its origin from the placenta. On ultrasound, a tongue of placental tissue is seen within the base of dichorionic membranes and has been termed the

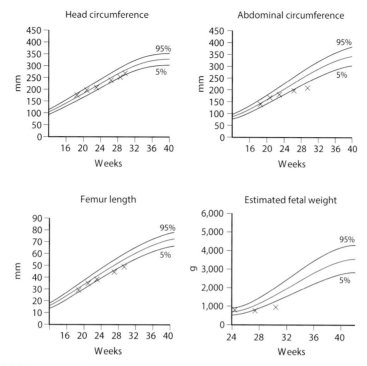

Figure 4.8 Ultrasound plots on reference range for head circumference, abdominal circumference, femur length and estimated fetal weight in a case of early-onset fetal growth restriction. Note that head circumference remains above the 5th centile, while the abdominal circumference falls below the 5th centile. This is a case of asymmetric fetal growth restriction with head sparing.

'twin peak' or 'lambda' sign (see **Figure 4.9**). The optimal gestation at which to perform such ultrasonic chorionicity determination is 9–10 weeks. Dichorionicity may also be confirmed by the identification of two placental masses and later in pregnancy by the presence of different-sex fetuses.

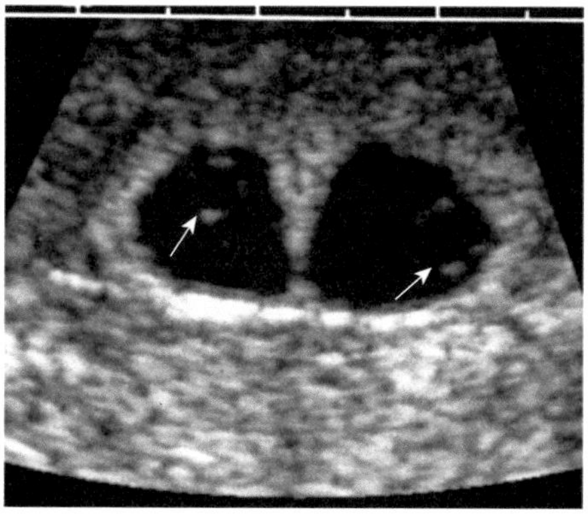

Ultrasound is also invaluable in the management of twin pregnancy in terms of confirming fetal presentations, which may be difficult on abdominal palpation, evidence of growth restriction, fetal anomaly and the presence of placenta praevia, all of which are more common in this type of pregnancy, and any suggestion of twin-to-twin transfusion syndrome.

DIAGNOSIS OF FETAL ABNORMALITY

Major fetal structural abnormalities occur in 2–3% of pregnancies and many can be diagnosed by an ultrasound scan at around or before 20 weeks' gestation. Increasingly, as ultrasound technology improves, these abnormalities are being detected at the first trimester 'dating' scan. Common examples include spina bifida and hydrocephalus (ventriculomegaly), skeletal abnormalities such as achondroplasia, abdominal wall defects such as exomphalos and gastroschisis, cleft lip/palate and congenital cardiac abnormalities (see **Chapter 3**).

Figure 4.9 Early twin dichorionic pregnancy (arrows); note the 'peaked' inter-twin membrane.

When a fetal structural abnormality is detected, a referral is normally made to a fetal medicine specialist for further advice about prognosis and management.

Detection rates of between 40% and 90% have been reported at the 20-week 'anomaly' scan. Through developments in ultrasound machine resolution and the application of specific fetal imaging views, for example the four-chamber view and the three-vessel trachea view (**Figure 4.10**), there have been improvements in the detection rates of cardiac anomalies in particular.

Parents, however, do need to be aware that a 'normal scan' is not a guarantee of a normal baby. A number of factors can influence the success of detecting an abnormality. Some are very difficult to visualize or to be absolutely certain about. Some conditions, for example hydrocephalus (ventriculomegaly), may not have been obvious at the time of early scans or even at the mid-pregnancy anomaly scan. Neuronal migration disorders that affect cerebral development may not manifest until the third trimester. Pregnant women should be informed of the limitations of routine ultrasound screening and that detection rates vary by the type of fetal anomaly, body mass index and the position of the unborn baby at the time of the scan. The position of the baby in the uterus will influence visualization of organs such as the heart, face and spine. Repeat scans are sometimes required if visualization is a problem in anticipation that the fetus will be in a more accessible position.

Some obstetric ultrasound findings are considered variants of normal but are noteworthy because they also increase the risk for underlying fetal aneuploidy such as Down syndrome. These findings are known as 'soft markers' and are considered distinct from fetal structural malformations. Detection of first trimester ultrasonic 'soft' markers for chromosomal abnormalities, such as an increased fetal nuchal translucency (NT) (the area at the back of the neck), are now in common use to enable detection of fetuses at risk of chromosomal anomalies such as Down syndrome (see **Chapter 5**). On the routine anomaly scan, detection of an increased nuchal fold (>6 mm), for example, should prompt referral to a fetal medicine specialist for advice.

PLACENTAL LOCALIZATION

Placenta praevia, a placenta that is inserted wholly or in part into the lower segment of the uterus, can cause life-threatening haemorrhage in pregnancy. Ultrasonography has become indispensable to localize the site of the placenta. Ultrasonographic identification of the lower edge of the placenta to exclude or confirm placenta praevia as a cause for antepartum haemorrhage is now a part of routine clinical practice. The transvaginal approach, undertaken with caution, can be helpful in clearly identifying the lower placental edge if it is not seen clearly with an abdominal probe.

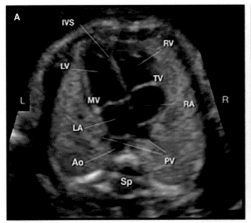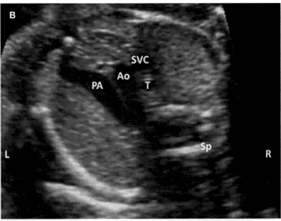

Figure 4.10 Ultrasound images of the fetal heart views used to screen for cardiac anomalies. (**A**) Four-chamber view. (**B**) Three-vessel trachea view. (Ao, aorta; IVS, interventricular septum; L, left; LA, left atrium; LV, left ventricle; MV, mitral valve; PA, pulmonary artery; PV, pulmonary veins; R, right; RA, right atrium; RV, right ventricle; Sp, spine; SVC, superior vena cava; T, trachea; TV, tricuspid valve.)

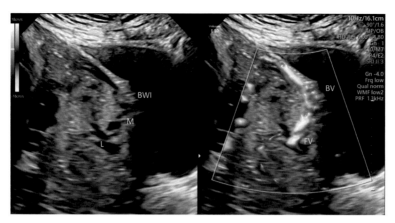

Figure 4.11 2D ultrasound images of placenta accreta spectrum illustrating the use of colour Doppler to improve the assessment of vascular perfusion in the right-hand image. The maternal bladder is kept full to better visualize the interface between the placenta and the bladder wall. (BV, bridging vessels; BWI, bladder wall interruption; FV, feeder vessels; L, large and irregular lacunae adjacent to the myometrium; M, myometrium indistinguishable from placenta.)

At the 20-week scan, it is customary to identify those pregnancies with a low-lying placenta. At this stage, the lower uterine segment has not yet formed and most low-lying placentas will appear to 'migrate' upwards as the lower segment stretches in the late second and third trimesters. About 15–20% of pregnancies are complicated by a low-lying placenta at 20 weeks, and only 10% of this group will eventually be shown to have a placenta praevia (for management, see **Chapter 14**).

Ultrasound is also used to identify whether there is placenta accreta spectrum, a disorder in which the placenta is abnormally attached to the myometrium (accreta) and may even attach to other pelvic organs such as the bladder, bowel and pelvic vessels (percreta). If undiagnosed, this can lead to catastrophic acute haemorrhage and maternal death. Sonographic markers include loss of the clear zone, a hypoechoic plane in the myometrium underneath the placental bed, placental bulge into surrounding organs such as the bladder on 2D ultrasound and placental hypervascularity using colour Doppler (**Figure 4.11**).

ASSESSMENT OF FETAL WELL-BEING

Ultrasound can be used to assess fetal well-being by evaluating the amniotic fluid, fetal movements, tone and breathing in the biophysical profile (BPP).

Doppler ultrasound can be used to assess placental function and identify evidence of blood flow redistribution in the fetus, which is a sign of hypoxia. These aspects of ultrasound use will be discussed in the section 'Doppler investigation' later in the chapter.

MEASUREMENT OF CERVICAL LENGTH

Evidence suggests that approximately 50% of pregnancies that result in birth before 34 weeks' gestation will be found to have a short cervix at the midtrimester of pregnancy. Cervical length is best measured using a transvaginal probe that allows accurate identification of the internal and external os (see **Chapter 8**). Current National Institute for Health and Care Excellence (NICE) guidance (NICE guideline [NG25]: *Preterm Labour and Birth*, 2015) recommends serial cervical length assessment from 16 weeks' gestation in anyone with a history of spontaneous preterm birth or midtrimester loss.

Ultrasonography is also of value in other obstetric conditions such as:

- confirmation of intrauterine death
- confirmation of fetal presentation in uncertain cases
- diagnosis of uterine and pelvic abnormalities during pregnancy, for example fibromyomata and ovarian cysts

ULTRASOUND SCHEDULE IN CLINICAL PRACTICE

NICE recommends that all pregnant women be offered scans at between 10 and 14 weeks' and 18 and 21 weeks' gestation (Clinical guideline [CG62]: *Antenatal Care for Uncomplicated Pregnancies*, 2015). The first trimester scan is principally to determine gestational age, to detect multiple pregnancies and to determine NT as part of screening for Down syndrome. The 18–21-week scan primarily screens for structural anomalies, giving couples reproductive choice (e.g. termination of pregnancy versus continuing with the pregnancy) and allowing antenatal care and delivery to be planned, including intrauterine therapy if available. Evidence suggests that routine ultrasound in early pregnancy appears to enable better gestational age assessment, earlier detection of multiple pregnancies and earlier detection of clinically unsuspected fetal malformation at a time when termination of pregnancy is possible. In uncomplicated pregnancies, scans are performed only after this stage in pregnancy if there is a clinical indication, such as concern about fetal growth or well-being, discussed in the section 'Ultrasound in the assessment of fetal well-being' later in the chapter. Additional ultrasound examinations, particularly for fetal growth and well-being, are offered to pregnant women who are identified as needing additional antenatal care (NICE guideline [NG201]: *Antenatal Care*, 2021), for example those who had problems during a previous pregnancy or who have pre-existing medical complications.

ULTRASOUND IN THE ASSESSMENT OF FETAL WELL-BEING

AMNIOTIC FLUID ASSESSMENT

Ultrasound can be used to identify both increased and decreased amniotic fluid volumes. The fetus has a role in the control of the volume of amniotic fluid. It swallows amniotic fluid, absorbs it in the gut and later excretes urine into the amniotic sac. Congenital abnormalities that either structurally or functionally impair the fetus's ability to swallow, for example oesophageal atresia or anencephaly, will result in an increase in amniotic fluid. Congenital abnormalities that result in a failure of urine production or passage, for example renal agenesis and posterior urethral valves, will result in reduced or absent amniotic fluid (**Chapter 3**).

The amount of amniotic fluid in the uterus is a guide to fetal well-being in the third trimester. A reduction in amniotic fluid volume is referred to as oligohydramnios and an excess is referred to as polyhydramnios. Definitions of oligohydramnios and polyhydramnios are based on sonographic criteria. Two ultrasound measurement approaches give an indication of amniotic fluid volume: the maximum vertical pool and the amniotic fluid index.

The maximum vertical pool is measured after a general survey of the uterine contents. Measurements of less than 2 cm suggest oligohydramnios, and measurements of greater than 8 cm suggest polyhydramnios.

The amniotic fluid index is measured by dividing the uterus into four 'ultrasound' quadrants (see **Figure 3.8**). A vertical measurement is taken of the deepest pool of fluid that is free of umbilical cord in each quadrant and the results are summated. The amniotic fluid index alters throughout gestation, but in the third trimester it should be between 10 and 25 cm; values below 10 cm indicate a reduced volume and those below 5 cm indicate oligohydramnios, while values above 25 cm indicate polyhydramnios.

Amniotic fluid volume is decreased in FGR as a consequence of redistribution of fetal blood away from the kidneys to vital structures such as the brain and heart, with a consequent reduction in renal perfusion and urine output.

CARDIOTOCOGRAPHY

A cardiotocograph (CTG) is a continuous tracing of the fetal heart rate used to assess fetal well-being, together with an assessment of uterine activity. Cardiotocography is sometimes called electronic fetal monitoring. The CTG recording is obtained with the patient positioned comfortably in a left lateral or semi-recumbent position to avoid compression of the maternal vena cava. Two external transducers are placed on the abdomen, each attached with a belt.

One transducer is a pressure-sensitive contraction tocodynometer (stretch gauge) that measures the pressure required to flatten a section of the abdominal wall. This correlates with the internal uterine pressure and indicates if there is any uterine activity (contractions). The second transducer uses ultrasound and the Doppler effect to detect motion of the fetal heart and measures the interval between successive beats, thereby allowing a continuous assessment of fetal heart rate. Recordings are then made for at least 30 minutes, with the output from the CTG machine producing two 'lines' traced onto a running piece of paper, one a tracing of fetal heart rate and a second a tracing of uterine activity. The pregnant woman may be given a button to press to record any fetal movements that they have felt. In addition, the CTG machine may record fetal movements detected via the tocodynometer.

IMPORTANT CARDIOTOCOGRAPH FEATURES

Fetal cardiac behaviour is regulated through the autonomic nervous system and by vasomotor, chemoceptor and baroreceptor mechanisms. Pathological events, such as fetal hypoxia, modify these signals and hence cardiac response, including variation in heart rate patterns, which can be detected and recorded in the CTG. Features that are reported from a CTG to define normality and identify abnormality and potential concern for fetal well-being include the:

- baseline rate
- baseline variability
- accelerations
- decelerations

Each of these is discussed in the following sections. Interpretation of the CTG must be in the context of any risk factors, for example suspected FGR or fetal anaemia, and all features must be considered in order to make a judgement about the likelihood of fetal compromise.

Baseline fetal heart rate

The normal fetal heart rate at term is 110–150 beats per minute (bpm). Higher rates are defined as fetal tachycardia and lower rates are defined as fetal

bradycardia. The baseline fetal heart rate falls with advancing gestational age as a result of maturing fetal parasympathetic tone and, prior to term, 160 bpm is taken as the upper limit of normal. The baseline rate is best determined over a period of 5–10 minutes. Fetal tachycardias can be associated with maternal or fetal infection, acute fetal hypoxia, fetal anaemia and drugs such as adrenoceptor agonists, for example ritodrine.

Baseline variability

Under normal physiological conditions, the interval between successive fetal heartbeats (beat-to-beat) varies. This is called short-term variability and increases with increasing gestational age. It is not visible on a standard CTG but can be measured with computer-assisted analysis (see the section 'Computerized cardiotocograph' later in this chapter). In addition to these beat-to-beat variations in heart rate, there are longer term fluctuations in heart rate occurring between two and six times per minute. This is known as 'baseline variability'. Normal baseline variability reflects a normal fetal autonomic nervous system. A normal CTG is shown in **Figure 4.12**.

Baseline variability is considered abnormal when it is variability of 5 bpm or less (**Figure 4.13**). As well as gestational age, baseline variability is modified by fetal sleep states and activity, and also by hypoxia, fetal infection and drugs suppressing the fetal central nervous system, such as opioids, and hypnotics (all of which reduce baseline variability). As fetuses display deep sleep cycles of 20–30 minutes at a time, baseline variability may be normally reduced for this length of time, but should be preceded and followed by a period of normal baseline variability on the CTG trace.

Fetal heart rate accelerations

Accelerations are increases in the baseline fetal heart rate of at least 15 bpm, lasting for at least 15 seconds. The presence of two or more accelerations on a 20–30-minute antepartum fetal CTG defines a reactive trace and is indicative of a non-hypoxic fetus (i.e. they are a positive sign of fetal health).

Fetal heart rate decelerations

Decelerations are transient reductions in fetal heart rate of 15 bpm or more, lasting for more than 15 seconds. Decelerations can be indicative of fetal hypoxia or umbilical cord compression. There is a higher

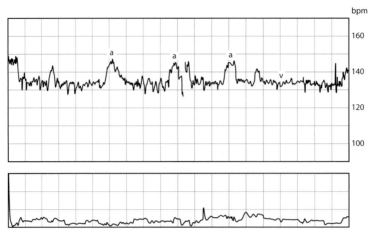

Figure 4.12 A normal fetal cardiotocograph showing a normal rate, normal variability (v) and the presence of several accelerations (a).

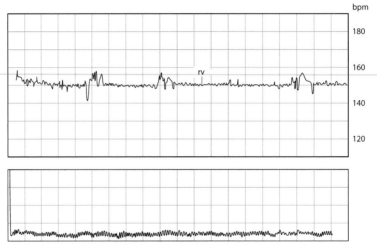

Figure 4.13 A fetal cardiotocograph showing a baseline of 150 bpm but with reduced variability (rv).

chance of fetal hypoxia being present if there are additional abnormal features such as reduced variability or baseline tachycardia (**Figure 4.14**).

From the preceding descriptions, a normal antepartum fetal CTG can therefore be defined as a baseline of 110–150 bpm, with baseline variability exceeding 10 bpm and with more than one acceleration being seen in a 20–30-minute tracing. Reduced baseline variability, an absence of accelerations and the presence of decelerations are all suspicious features. A suspicious CTG must be interpreted within the clinical context. If many antenatal risk factors have already been identified, a suspicious CTG may

warrant delivery of the baby, although when no risk factors exist, a repeated investigation later in the day may be more appropriate.

COMPUTERIZED CARDIOTOCOGRAPH

Standard CTG interpretation has high intra- and interobserver variability, as it is based on pattern recognition, and this leads to differences in interpretation among different clinicians. Computerized CTG interpretation is objective and more consistent than standard CTG interpretation, with normal ranges for computerized CTG parameters available throughout

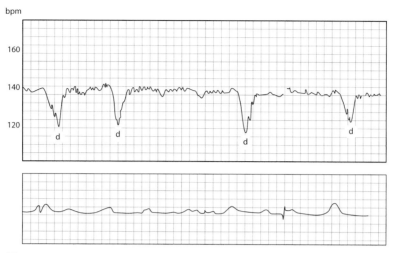

Figure 4.14 An admission cardiotocograph from a term pregnancy. Although the baseline fetal heart rate is normal, there is reduced variability, an absence of fetal heart rate accelerations and multiple decelerations (d). The decelerations were occurring after uterine tightening and are therefore termed 'late'.

gestation. Compared with standard CTG, a Cochrane review found that the use of computerized CTG was associated with a reduction in perinatal mortality.

Antenatal (pre-labour) computerized CTG uses Dawes Redman criteria, which take into account the standard features of visual assessment such as accelerations, decelerations and basal heart rate, as well as parameters that are difficult or impossible to measure visually, such as short-term variation, sinusoidal rhythm and the number of minutes of high variation.

Fetal heart rate variation is the most useful predictor of fetal well-being in small-for-gestational-age (SGA) fetuses, and a short-term variation of ≤3 ms (within 24 hours of delivery) has been associated with a higher rate of metabolic acidaemia and early neonatal death. The computer software assesses these parameters and can report a first normal result within 10 minutes (**Figure 4.15**). If the CTG is clearly abnormal or if criteria are not met by 60 minutes, further senior obstetric assessment of fetal well-being is recommended.

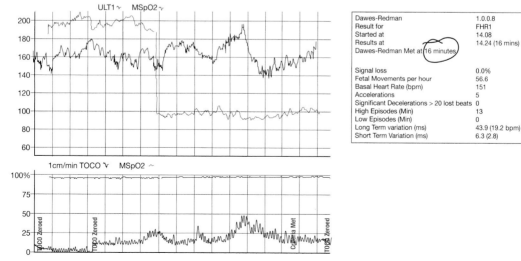

Figure 4.15 Computerized antenatal cardiotocograph showing Dawes Redman criteria have been met, indicating a normal fetus.

BIOPHYSICAL PROFILE

When the fetus is hypoxic, there may be reduced or absent fetal breathing movements (FBMs, movements of the fetal chest) and gross body movements, less flexor tone and fewer accelerations in fetal heart rate. The BPP (**Figure 4.16**) includes fetal variables: FBMs, fetal gross body movement, fetal tone, and CTG and amniotic fluid volume, assigning a score from 0 to 2 for each, with a total score out of 10. Low overall scores (0–4) are considered abnormal and indicate significant fetal compromise. A score of 6 is equivocal and requires a repeat profile within a reasonable timescale (hours) to exclude a period of fetal sleep as a cause.

A systematic review of the effectiveness of BPP as a surveillance tool in high-risk pregnancies (five studies, testing 2,974 fetuses) found that the use of BPP was not associated with a reduction in perinatal deaths or Apgar scores of <7 at 5 minutes. There are a number of problems with the BPP that limit its utility. BPPs can be time consuming. Fetuses spend approximately 30% of their time asleep, during which they are not very active and do not exhibit FBMs. It is therefore necessary to scan for at least 30 minutes to exclude this physiological cause of a poor score. Ultimately, however, by the time a fetus develops an abnormal BPP score prompting delivery, it is likely to already be severely hypoxic. While delivery may reduce the perinatal death rate (death in utero or within the first week of life), it may not increase long-term survival and, in particular, survival without significant mental and physical impairment. There is currently insufficient evidence from randomized trials to support the use of BPP as a test of fetal well-being in high-risk pregnancies.

DOPPLER INVESTIGATION

The principles of Doppler have already been discussed. Waveforms can be obtained from the umbilical and fetal vessels and the maternal uterine artery. Data obtained from the umbilical artery provide indirect information about placenta function, whereas data from the fetal vessels provide information on the fetal response to hypoxia. Doppler insonation of the uterine artery can be used to assess the degree of placental insufficiency (see **Chapter 3**).

UMBILICAL ARTERY

Waveforms obtained from the umbilical artery provide information on placental resistance to blood flow and hence, indirectly, placenta 'health' and function. An infarcted placenta secondary to maternal hypertension, for example, will have increased resistance to flow. A normal umbilical arterial waveform is shown in **Figure 4.17**. The plot is obtained using Doppler ultrasound of velocity of blood flow against time and demonstrates forward flow of blood throughout the whole cardiac cycle (i.e. both systole and diastole). A useful analogy to understand the concept of umbilical Doppler and placental resistance is to consider

Parameter	Score 2	Score 0
Non-stress cardiotocograph	Reactive	Fewer than two accelerations in 40 minutes
Fetal breathing movements	≥30 movements in 30 minutes	Fewer than 30 seconds of fetal breathing in 30 minutes
Fetal body movements	Three or more movements in 30 minutes	Two or fewer gross body movements in 30 minutes
Fetal tone	One episode of limb flexion	No evidence of fetal movement or flexion
Amniotic fluid volume	Large cord-free pocket of fluid over 1 cm	Less than 1 cm pocket of fluid

Figure 4.16 Biophysical profile scoring system.

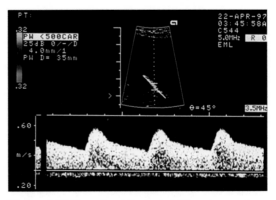

Figure 4.17 Normal umbilical arterial Doppler waveform.

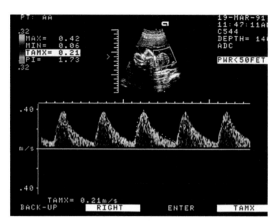

Figure 4.18 Reduced end-diastolic flow in umbilical artery compared with the normal waveform in Figure 4.17.

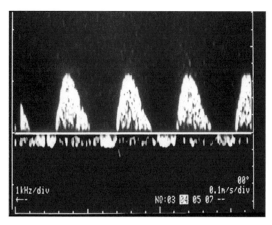

Figure 4.19 Reverse end-diastolic flow in the umbilical artery.

the umbilical artery as a hose carrying water towards a placenta, which in a healthy pregnancy will act like a sponge and in an infarcted placenta will act more like a brick wall. So, with a normal pregnancy, blood will flow through the placenta without difficulty like water from a hose directed at the sponge and will pass straight through the sponge. In a diseased placenta, the blood will reflect back from the high-resistance placenta like water from a hose being bounced back from the wall at which it is directed. In the normal pregnancy, the normal constant forward flow of blood in diastole will be seen, but, in the diseased placenta, flow during diastole may be reduced, absent or even reversed (**Figure 4.18**). Reversed end-diastolic flow effectively means that, during diastole, there is flow of fetal blood away from the placenta and back to the fetus.

Most studies investigating the value of using this technique in clinical practice have looked at resistance to flow, which is indicated by the diastolic component. A reduced amount of diastolic flow implies high resistance downstream to the vessel being studied and implies low perfusion (see **Figure 4.18**). An increased diastolic flow indicates low resistance downstream and implies high perfusion. Doppler indices such as the pulsatility index or the resistance index are useful, as they calculate the variability of blood velocity in a vessel, comparing the amount of diastolic flow relative to systolic flow. When these indices are high, there is high resistance to blood flow; when these indices are low, resistance to blood flow is low. Normally, diastolic flow in the

umbilical artery increases (i.e. placental resistance falls) throughout gestation. Absent or reversed end-diastolic flow in the umbilical artery is a particularly serious development with a strong correlation with fetal hypoxia and ultimately intrauterine death if the fetus is not delivered (**Figure 4.19**).

An analysis of randomized controlled trials of the use of umbilical Doppler in over 10,000 high-risk pregnancies found that, compared with no Doppler ultrasound, the use of Doppler ultrasound in high-risk pregnancy (especially those complicated by hypertension, SGA or FGR) was associated with a reduction in perinatal deaths from 1.7% to 1.2%. There were also fewer inductions of labour and fewer admissions to hospital without reports of adverse effects. The use of Doppler ultrasound in high-risk pregnancies therefore improves a number of obstetric care outcomes and reduces perinatal deaths.

FETAL VESSELS

Falling oxygen levels in the fetus lead to a redistribution of blood flow to 'essential' organs (such as the brain, heart and adrenal glands) from 'non-essential' organs (such as the kidneys, gastrointestinal tract and long bones) where there is vasoconstriction. Several fetal vessels have been studied and reflect this 'centralization' of flow, often called cerebral redistribution. As hypoxia increases, the pulsatility index in the middle cerebral artery falls, indicating increasing diastolic flow as the cerebral circulation opens up (**Figure 4.20**). At the same time, there is increased resistance in

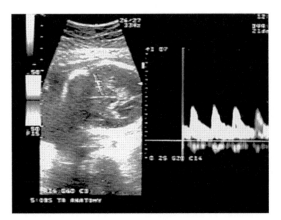

Figure 4.20 Middle cerebral artery Doppler showing increased diastolic flow with possible redistribution to brain in hypoxia.

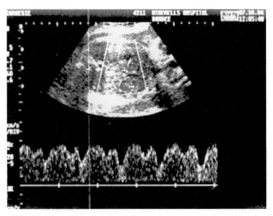

Figure 4.21 Normal ductus venosus Doppler waveform.

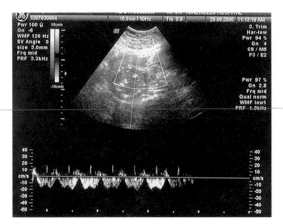

Figure 4.22 Reverse flow in ductus venosus

the fetal aorta reflecting compensatory vasoconstriction in the fetal body. Absent diastolic flow in the fetal aorta implies fetal acidaemia. Perhaps the most sensitive index of fetal acidaemia and incipient heart failure is demonstrated by increasing pulsatility in the central veins supplying the heart, such as the ductus venosus (DV) and inferior vena cava (IVC). The DV shunts a portion of the umbilical vein blood flow directly to the IVC and thence to the right atrium, allowing oxygenated blood from the placenta to bypass the fetal liver. The DV Doppler flow velocity therefore reflects atrial pressure–volume changes during the cardiac cycle. As FGR worsens, there is a direct effect of hypoxia and acidaemia on cardiac function, leading to increased afterload and preload. This leads to a reduced velocity in the DV a-wave owing to increased end-diastolic pressure. A retrograde or 'reversed' DV a-wave signifies the onset of overt cardiac compromise (**Figures 4.21** and **4.22**), and delivery should be considered, as fetal death is imminent.

Measurement of the velocity of blood flow in the middle cerebral artery also gives an indicator of the presence of fetal anaemia. When the fetus is anaemic, the peak systolic blood flow velocity increases. This technique is particularly useful to assess the severity of rhesus isoimmunization disease and in twin-to-twin transfusion syndrome that results in anaemia in the donor twin. Doppler assessment of fetal anaemia has now superseded invasive techniques such as amniocentesis or cordocentesis.

UTERINE ARTERY

Doppler studies of the uterine artery during the first and early second trimester may be used to predict pregnancies at risk of adverse outcome, particularly pre-eclampsia. The proposed pathogenic model of pre-eclampsia is one of incomplete physiological invasion of the spiral arteries by the trophoblast, with a resultant increase in uteroplacental vascular resistance (see **Chapter 9**). This is reflected in the Doppler waveforms obtained from the maternal uterine artery circulation. Doppler ultrasound studies of the uterine arteries may demonstrate markers of increased resistance to flow including the diastolic 'notch' in the waveform (**Figure 4.23**) in early diastole, thought to result from increased vascular resistance in the uteroplacental vascular bed. High-resistance waveform

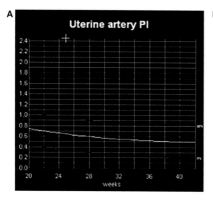
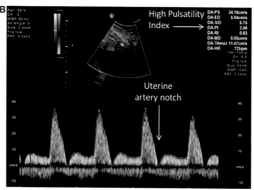

Figure 4.23 (A) Uterine artery waveform with diastolic notch. **(B)** Pulsatility index (PI) above the 97th centile.

patterns are associated with adverse outcomes, including pre-eclampsia, FGR and placental abruption. Among pregnancies at 20–24 weeks' gestation with bilateral notched uterine arteries, 60–70% will subsequently develop one or more of these complications. Consequently, such pregnancies will require close monitoring of fetal growth rate and increased surveillance for the possible development of maternal hypertension and proteinuria.

Uterine artery Doppler evaluation at 20–24 weeks' gestation can be used to stratify pregnant women with risk factors for an SGA baby, for example smoking, chronic hypertension, diabetes and vascular disease, previous SGA baby or stillbirth. Those with a normal uterine artery pulsatility index and normal waveform may be reassured that there is a low probability of an SGA birth. Serial ultrasound to assess fetal growth and umbilical artery Doppler for fetal well-being is recommended if the uterine artery Doppler assessment is abnormal.

CEREBROPLACENTAL RATIO

The cerebroplacental Doppler ratio is a ratio of the pulsatility indices of the middle cerebral artery and the umbilical artery. It is emerging as an important predictor of adverse pregnancy outcome. Fetuses with an abnormal ratio that are appropriately grown for gestational age or have late-onset SGA (>34 weeks' gestation) have a higher incidence of abnormal intrapartum CTG requiring emergency caesarean delivery, a lower cord pH and an increased

admission rate to neonatal intensive care units than fetuses with a normal ratio. In fetuses with early-onset SGA (<34 weeks' gestation), an abnormal ratio is associated with a lower birthweight and an increased rate of adverse neonatal outcome and perinatal death when compared with a normal ratio.

ULTRASOUND AND INVASIVE PROCEDURES

Ultrasound is used to guide invasive diagnostic procedures such as amniocentesis, chorion villus sampling and cordocentesis, as well as therapeutic procedures such as the insertion of fetal bladder shunts or chest drains. If fetoscopy is performed, the endoscope is inserted under ultrasound guidance. This use of ultrasound has greatly reduced the possibility of fetal trauma, as the needle or scope is visualized throughout the procedure and guided with precision to the appropriate place.

THREE- AND FOUR-DIMENSIONAL ULTRASOUND

Both 3D and 4D ultrasound are mainly used as an adjunct to 2D ultrasound, either to interrogate fetal structures that may be difficult to visualize, such as the corpus callosum or fetal spine, or to demonstrate fetal structural abnormalities to the parents, for example cleft lip and palate.

MAGNETIC RESONANCE IMAGING

MRI utilizes the effect of powerful magnetic forces on spinning hydrogen protons, which, when knocked off their axis by pulsed radio waves, produce radio frequency signals as they return to their basal state. The signals reflect the composition of tissue (i.e. the amount and distribution of hydrogen protons) and thus the images provide significant improvement over ultrasound in tissue characterization. Ultrafast MRI techniques enable images to be acquired in less than 1 second to reduce the detrimental effect of fetal motion on image quality. Such technology has led to increased usage of fetal MRI, which provides multiplanar views, better characterization of anatomic details of, for example, the fetal brain and information for planning the mode of delivery and airway management at birth. Fetal MRI is also being used to detect cerebral lesions after fetal interventions. For example, fetal brain MRI may be performed a few weeks after laser fetoscopic coagulation of placental anastomoses in twin-to-twin transfusion syndrome, to examine for acute cerebral ischaemic lesions. MRI is also being used to image placenta accreta spectrum to better define the degree of placental attachment to pelvic organs and for surgical planning.

FURTHER READING

Alfirevic Z, Neilson JP (1996). Doppler ultrasound for fetal assessment in high risk pregnancies. *Cochrane Database of Systematic Reviews*, 4: CD000073.

Lalor JG, Fawole B, Alfirevic Z, Devane D (2008). Biophysical profile for fetal assessment in high risk pregnancies. *Cochrane Database of Systematic Reviews*, 1: CD000038.

SELF-ASSESSMENT

For interactive SBAs and EMQs relating to this chapter, visit www.routledge.com/cw/mccarthy.

CASE HISTORY 1

An 18 year old in her first pregnancy attends for review at the antenatal clinic at 34 weeks' gestation. Her dates were confirmed by ultrasound at booking (12 weeks). She is a smoker. The midwife measures her fundal height at 30 cm. An ultrasound scan is performed because of the midwife's concern that the fetus is SGA, and the measurements are plotted in **Figure 4.24**.

A Do the ultrasound findings support the clinical diagnosis of SGA?

B What additional features/measures on ultrasound assessment could give an indication of fetal well-being?

ANSWERS

A Yes, because the fetal AC is below the 5th centile for gestation. This finding does not give an indication of the well-being of the fetus and is compatible with FGR secondary to placental insufficiency or a healthy, constitutionally small baby.

B The additional features/measures are as follows.

Liquor volume
Amniotic fluid volume is decreased in FGR associated with fetal hypoxia where there may be redistribution of fetal blood flow away from the kidneys to vital structures such as the brain and heart, with a consequent reduction in renal perfusion and urine output.

Doppler ultrasound

Umbilical artery
Waveforms from the umbilical artery provide information on fetoplacental blood flow and placental resistance. Diastolic flow in the umbilical artery increases (i.e. placental resistance falls) throughout gestation. If the resistance index in the umbilical artery rises above the 95th centile of the normal graph, this implies poor perfusion of the placenta, which may eventually result in fetal hypoxia. Absent or reversed end-diastolic flow in the umbilical artery is a particularly serious development, with a strong correlation with fetal hypoxia and intrauterine death.

Fetal vessels
Falling oxygen levels in the fetus may lead to cerebral redistribution, diverting blood from the fetal body to the brain, heart, adrenals and spleen. The middle cerebral artery will show increasing diastolic flow as hypoxia increases, while a rising resistance in the fetal aorta reflects compensatory vasoconstriction in the fetal body. When diastolic flow is absent in the fetal aorta, this implies fetal acidaemia. Increasing pulsatility in the central veins supplying the heart, such as the DV and IVC, is an indicator of fetal acidaemia and impending heart failure; when late diastolic flow is absent in the ductus venosus, fetal death is imminent.

Cardiotocography
Fetal tachycardia, reduced variability in heart rate, absence of accelerations and presence of decelerations identified on a CTG are associated with fetal hypoxia.

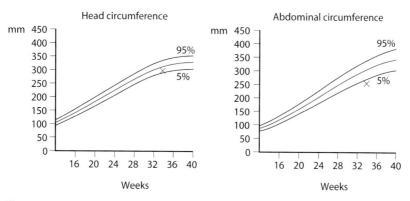

Figure 4.24 Plot of fetal head circumference and fetal abdominal circumference.

CASE HISTORY 2

A 16 year old is admitted to the labour ward at 38 weeks' gestation. She gives a history suggestive of rupture of membranes with meconium staining and is experiencing uterine contractions. She was seen at 10 weeks' gestation for consideration of termination of pregnancy and had a scan at that time that confirmed her gestational age. She opted to continue with the pregnancy but did not attend for antenatal care. She admitted to smoking 20 cigarettes per day. Abdominal examination shows the fetus is in cephalic presentation. The symphysis–fundal height measurement is 30 cm. Vaginal examination confirms that the cervix is 8 cm dilated. A CTG demonstrates a baseline fetal heart rate of 170 bpm with persistent variable decelerations for more than 30 minutes, and fetal scalp pH is 7.14 with a base deficit of 12 mmol/L. A category 1 emergency caesarean section is performed and a male infant weighing 1,900 g is delivered within 20 minutes of the decision. Apgar scores are 3 at 1 minute and 8 at 5 minutes. The placental histology confirms patchy hypoplasia of the distal villous tree and a number of villous infarcts suggesting chronic placental pathology.

From which complications are such severely growth-restricted infants particularly at risk?

ANSWER

Reduced oxygen supply in utero can result in the fetus being stillborn or suffering damage from acute asphyxia. In the latter case, the neonate may demonstrate features of hypoxic ischaemic encephalopathy (HIE), which may lead to death from multi-organ failure. If the infant survives, neurological damage and cerebral palsy may result. Chronic hypoxia in utero can also result in neurological damage without the acute manifestations of HIE. Other consequences of reduced oxygen supply in utero include increased haemopoiesis and cardiac failure. Increased haemopoiesis can in turn result in coagulopathy, polycythaemia and jaundice in the newborn. Neonatal hypothermia and hypoglycaemia are also more common in this type of infant and result from reduced body fat and glycogen stores. Both of these conditions, if untreated, can lead to increased mortality and neurological damage.

Reduced supply of amino acids in utero can impair immune function, increasing the risk of infection in the newborn.

Growth-restricted babies are also at increased risk of chronic diseases such as coronary heart disease, stroke, hypertension and non-insulin-dependent diabetes in adulthood. This is thought to be because the fetal adaptation to undernutrition in utero results in the permanent resetting of homeostatic mechanisms, and this leads to later disease.

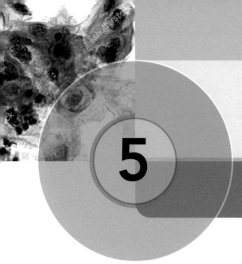

Prenatal diagnosis

ANNA L DAVID

5

Learning Objectives

- Understand why prenatal diagnosis is performed and what conditions can be tested for in the fetus.
- Appreciate the risks and benefits of the invasive prenatal diagnostic tests that can be performed, and realise how to appropriately counsel a pregnant woman and her partner who are considering having such a test.
- Know the various screening tests that are used to predict the risk of having a pregnancy affected by Down syndrome and other aneuploidies.
- Learn about newer, non-invasive methods of prenatal screening and diagnosis based on measurement of cell-free fetal deoxyribonucleic acid (DNA) in the maternal circulation.

INTRODUCTION

Prenatal diagnosis is the identification of a disease in the fetus prior to birth. For some of these conditions, treatment before birth improves neonatal outcome. This chapter will discuss why prenatal diagnostic tests may be performed and the types of non-invasive and invasive tests that are available. It will discuss factors that should be taken into consideration prior to offering testing, and it emphasizes the importance of good communication with pregnant women and their partners/families, as well as multidisciplinary working.

WHY IS PRENATAL DIAGNOSTIC TESTING PERFORMED?

Prenatal diagnosis is usually performed because something leads to the suspicion of disease being present in the fetus. For example:

- *family history* – genetic disease with a known recurrence risk
- *past obstetric history* – rhesus factor D (RhD) alloimmunization
- *serum screening tests* – trisomy 21
- *ultrasound screening* – 12-week dating or 20-week anomaly scan

10.1201/9781003196112-5

Prenatal diagnosis frequently follows a prenatal screening test, whether this is simply the history taking at the booking visit or a more formal screening test such as those offered for Down syndrome, haemoglobinopathies or ultrasound screening.

The attributes of a screening test are as follows:

- *Relevance* – the condition screened for must be relevant and important.
- *Effect on management* – alternative management options must be available, for example planning therapy or offering termination of an affected pregnancy.
- *Sensitivity* – the test must have a high detection rate for the condition.
- *Specificity* – the test must exclude the vast majority who do not have the condition.
- *Predictive value* – the test must predict accurately who does and who does not have the condition.
- *Affordability* – the test should be cheap enough to be cost-effective.
- *Equity* – the test should be available to all.

CLASSIFICATION

Prenatal diagnostic tests can be divided into non-invasive tests and invasive tests. The main non-invasive test is the use of ultrasound scanning to screen for structural fetal abnormalities, such as neural tube defects, gastroschisis, cystic adenomatoid malformation of the lung and renal abnormalities (**Table 5.1**).

Maternal blood can be tested for exposure to viruses (viral serology). If a pregnant woman has no immunoglobulin (Ig)G or IgM for a particular virus early in pregnancy, but then develops IgM and IgG later in pregnancy, it suggests that they have had a clinical or subclinical infection with that virus earlier during pregnancy. Maternal blood is usually only tested if features on ultrasound are suggestive of infection having occurred, for example hydrops or ventriculomegaly, or if there is a history of exposure to a particular virus, for example parvovirus.

Cell-free fetal deoxyribonucleic acid (cffDNA) can be extracted from maternal blood to determine fetal blood group in cases of RhD alloimmunization, to determine the sex of the fetus in X-linked disorders or to diagnose skeletal dysplasias such as achondroplasia. There is much interest in using

Table 5.1 Examples of conditions and their method of diagnosis

Diagnostic test	Condition
Ultrasound diagnosis	Neural tube defect
	Gastroschisis
	Cystic adenomatoid malformation of the lung
	Twin-to-twin transfusion syndrome
Invasive test – CVS or amniocentesis	Down syndrome
	Spina bifida
	Thalassaemia
Invasive test – cordocentesis	Alloimmune thrombocytopaenia
Ultrasound then invasive test	Congenital diaphragmatic hernia
	Exomphalos
	Ventriculomegaly
	Duodenal atresia

CVS, chorion villus sampling.

next-generation sequencing analysis of cffDNA in maternal blood for non-invasive prenatal diagnosis of aneuploidy and of monogenic disorders such as the haemoglobinopathies.

Amniocentesis and chorion (or chorionic) villus sampling (CVS) are the two most common invasive tests and are used to check the karyotype of the fetus or to diagnose single-gene disorders. These tests carry a small risk of miscarriage; therefore, the risk of being affected by the condition and the seriousness of the condition should be severe enough to warrant taking the risk. Rarely, cordocentesis is used as an invasive diagnostic test.

Frequently, non-invasive tests and invasive tests are used together. The ultrasound scan may diagnose a structural problem in the fetus such as a congenital diaphragmatic hernia, but since congenital diaphragmatic hernias are associated with underlying chromosomal abnormalities, an invasive prenatal diagnostic test would then be offered.

INVASIVE TESTING

PRETEST COUNSELLING

Invasive tests are most frequently performed to diagnose aneuploidy, for example Down syndrome, or genetic conditions such as sickle cell disease or thalassaemia. Pregnant women can choose to have, or not to have, invasive testing. This is an important decision that may have lifelong consequences and therefore must be a decision that is fully informed.

For a clinician to discuss the option of invasive testing in a meaningful way, the clinician needs to know important information about the condition to be tested for, the type of test and what the results might indicate.

> **BOX 5.1: Considerations for pretest counselling for prenatal diagnosis**
>
> - The condition suspected and its severity so that the pregnant woman can assess the effect that having a child with this disorder would have on her and her family.
> - That the history is correct – involvement of colleagues from the clinical genetics department is often invaluable.
> - An accurate assessment of the risk of an affected fetus – again involvement of colleagues from the clinical genetics department may be helpful.
> - That a diagnostic test is available – sometimes the mutation has not been identified yet.
> - What sample is needed and how it should be processed.
> - The accuracy and limitations of the particular laboratory test being performed, including culture failure rates and reporting times.
> - Acceptability – some pregnant women feel that they cannot accept the small risk of miscarriage.
> - Whether it is ethical – some genetic mutations may not carry a significant risk of serious disability for an individual, and yet it is possible to offer prenatal diagnosis for them, for example sickle cell disease.

Prior to the test, the clinician should also discuss with the pregnant woman what options would be available to her if the test result showed that the fetus was affected with the condition. This is an important part of the decision-making process and often the partner is included in these discussions. There may be little point doing an invasive test if it will not be of benefit to the pregnant woman or the baby,

especially if it might increase the risk of pregnancy complications.

The three options available are usually to:

1. continue – the information from the test may facilitate plans for care around the time of delivery, or may help the pregnant woman and her family prepare for the birth of a baby with a serious condition
2. influence the decision to terminate the pregnancy
3. terminate, but provide information that may prove useful when counselling about recurrence risks in future pregnancies

Some pregnant women decline invasive testing, as they feel that it would not provide them with useful information and it would put them at an unacceptable risk of miscarriage or preterm birth. To ensure informed consent, the clinician needs to be certain that the pregnant woman understands the procedure, why it is being offered and the risks, limitations and subsequent management options. The clinician also needs to be sure that there is no evidence of duress from others such as family members, the community or religious groups. Informed written consent is advised prior to the procedure as a formal record that the discussion has taken place. This should be in line with existing consent advice from the General Medical Council and the Royal College of Obstetricians and Gynaecologists (RCOG) recommendations.

Invasive prenatal procedures should not be carried out without reviewing available blood-borne virus screening tests such as human immunodeficiency virus (HIV) and hepatitis. If these are declined or unavailable, the pregnant woman should be counselled about the potential risk of vertical transmission of infection to the fetus.

CHORION VILLUS SAMPLING (ALSO KNOWN AS CHORION VILLUS BIOPSY)

Fetal trophoblast cells in the mesenchyme of the villi divide rapidly in the first trimester. A CVS procedure aims to take a sample of these rapidly dividing cells from the developing placenta. This is done either by passing a needle under ultrasound guidance through

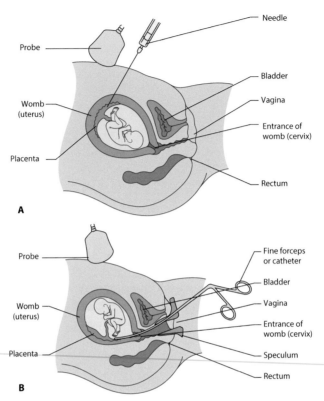

Figure 5.1 Chorionic villus sampling via (**A**) the transabdominal approach and (**B**) the transvaginal approach. (Adapted from the RCOG information leaflet of both approaches.)

the abdominal wall and myometrium into the placenta (**Figure 5.1A**) or by passing a fine catheter (or biopsy forceps) through the cervix into the placenta (**Figure 5.1B**).

An ultrasound scan is performed to:

- confirm that the pregnancy is viable prior to the procedure
- ensure that it is a singleton pregnancy (prenatal diagnosis in multiple pregnancy is more complex)
- confirm gestational age (CVS should not be performed before 10 weeks' gestation)
- localize the placenta and determine whether a transabdominal or transcervical approach is more appropriate

Transabdominal procedures are performed more commonly, but they may not be feasible if the uterus is retroverted or the placenta is low on the posterior wall of the uterus.

The additional overall risk of miscarriage following CVS performed by an appropriately trained operator is likely to be below 0.5%. This is in addition to the background (natural) risk of miscarriage for a first trimester pregnancy. To reduce the risk of technical challenges, CVS should be performed from 11+0 weeks of gestation where possible. CVS can be performed in multiple pregnancies; commonly, a double entry technique is used to reduce the chance of cross-contamination (see **Chapter 7**). The additional risk of miscarriage following CVS in twin pregnancies performed by an appropriately trained operator is likely to be around 1%.

Many laboratories can provide a rapid result for common aneuploidies (T21, 18, 13, X and Y) within 48 hours for a CVS sample. Full culture results to provide a karyotype takes approximately 7–10 days and results for genetic disorders can take varying amounts of time. Many genetics laboratories are moving towards performing microarray analysis on CVS samples to make a diagnosis of aneuploidy, rather than culturing fetal cells for the traditional karyotype. Chromosomal microarray analysis (CMA) is a relatively new technique that identifies submicroscopic abnormalities that are too small to be detected by conventional karyotyping. Like conventional fetal karyotyping, prenatal CMA requires direct testing of fetal tissue and thus can be offered only with CVS, amniocentesis or cordocentesis. There is the potential for complex results and detection of clinically uncertain findings that can result in substantial patient anxiety. Comprehensive pretest counselling is therefore recommended.

Placental mosaicism is sometimes found. This is the occurrence of two different cell types in the same sample; usually, one cell line is normal and one cell line is abnormal. It occurs in <2% of CVS procedures. The mosaic pattern may be present in the placenta and may not occur in the fetus (confined placental mosaicism). Mosaic results should be discussed with the clinical genetics department to get accurate information on the impact this may have on the fetus. If necessary, another fetal tissue (e.g. amniotic fluid) may need to be sampled to make a definitive diagnosis.

AMNIOCENTESIS

Amniotic fluid contains amniocytes and fibroblasts shed from fetal membranes, skin and the fetal genitourinary tract. An amniocentesis procedure takes a sample (15–20 mL) of amniotic fluid that contains these cells. This is done by passing a needle under continuous direct ultrasound control through the abdominal wall and myometrium into the amniotic cavity and aspirating the fluid (**Figure 5.2**).

An initial ultrasound is performed prior to the procedure. The additional overall risk of miscarriage following amniocentesis performed by an appropriately trained operator is likely to be below 0.5% for a procedure performed from 15 weeks of gestation under ultrasound guidance.

Many laboratories can provide a rapid result for common aneuploidies (T21, 18, 13, X and Y) within 48 hours for an amniocentesis sample. Full culture results take approximately 7–10 days and results for genetic disorders take varying amounts of time. CMA is also increasingly being used instead of traditional karyotyping and is becoming available in a similar way to CVS.

Amniotic fluid may be used to check for fetal viral infections, for example cytomegalovirus. In the past, it was also used for biochemical tests, for example alpha-fetoprotein for spina bifida and spectrophotometric tests for RhD haemolytic disease. These have been superseded by ultrasound imaging.

COMPARISON OF CHORION VILLUS SAMPLING AND AMNIOCENTESIS

The advantage of CVS over amniocentesis is that it can be performed earlier in pregnancy, at a stage when surgical termination is possible in the event of a 'bad result', and at a stage in pregnancy before

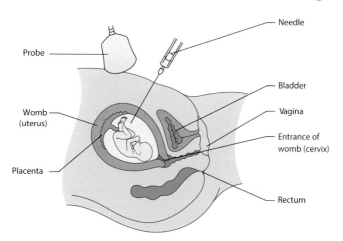

Figure 5.2 Amniocentesis. (Adapted from the RCOG information leaflet.)

67

Table 5.2 Other risks associated with CVS and amniocentesis

Risk	CVS	Amniocentesis
Second sampling/ repeat procedure	Up to 6%	Up to 6%
Blood stained sample	Not applicable	Up to 0.8%
Confined placental mosaicism	<2%	Not applicable
Maternal cell contamination	1–2%	1–2%
Rapid test failure	2%	2%
Failed cell culture	0.5–1%	0.5–1%

Source: Adapted from RCOG Green-top Guideline No 8: Amniocentesis and chorionic villus sampling.
CVS, chorion villus sampling.

there is a need to disclose the pregnancy to family, friends and employers. For some genetic disorders, for example haemoglobinopathies, CVS may be preferred over amniocentesis because it provides a larger sample of DNA for rapid polymerase chain reaction (PCR) analysis. Severe infection, maternal visceral injury and fetal injury are rare risks. Other risks are listed in **Table 5.2**.

CORDOCENTESIS

Cordocentesis is performed when fetal blood is needed, or when a rapid full culture for karyotype is needed. The most common reason for performing a cordocentesis is for suspected severe fetal anaemia or thrombocytopaenia, with availability of immediate transfusion if confirmed.

A needle is passed under ultrasound guidance through the abdominal wall and myometrium and, most commonly, into the umbilical cord at the point where it inserts into the placenta. This point is chosen because the umbilical cord is fixed and does not move. Cordocentesis can be performed from about 20 weeks' gestation. The risk of miscarriage varies with indication and position of the placenta (**Table 5.3**).

Table 5.3 Comparison of invasive tests

Test	CVS	Amniocentesis	Cordocentesis
Gestation from which test can be performed	11 weeks	15 weeks	Around 20 weeks
Miscarriage risk	<0.5%*	<0.5%*	2–5%

* Performed by an appropriately trained operator.
CVS, chorion villus sampling.

BOX 5.2: Care after any invasive test

Following any invasive procedure, the following should take place:

- The sample should be accurately labelled and checked with the patient.
- The sample should be transported promptly and securely to the appropriate laboratory.
- The procedure and any complications should be documented in the medical notes.
- There should be communication with the referring clinician.
- The pregnant woman should avoid strenuous exercise for the next 24 hours.
- The pregnant woman should be advised that, while she may experience some mild abdominal pain, it should be relieved by paracetamol.

- The pregnant woman should be advised that, if she has any fever, bleeding, pain not relieved by paracetamol or leakage of fluid vaginally, she should seek medical advice, and she should be told how to access this.
- The pregnant woman should be given appropriate contact numbers.
- A process for giving results should be agreed, including who will give the results, how they will be given and when the results are likely to be available.
- If the pregnant woman is RhD negative, an appropriate dose of anti-D should be administered (with a Kleihauer test if more than 20 weeks' gestation).
- A plan of ongoing care should be discussed once the results are available.

DOWN SYNDROME AND OTHER ANEUPLOIDIES

In the UK, prenatal diagnosis of Down syndrome is the most common reason for performing invasive prenatal diagnostic testing. Current Down syndrome screening tests can also indicate an increased risk of a fetus having other aneuploidies such as trisomy 13 (Patau syndrome) and trisomy 18 (Edwards syndrome). The NHS Fetal Anomaly Screening Programme in the UK defines the standards that hospitals should adhere to in their screening programmes for aneuploidies (for trisomy 21, 18 and 13). Hospitals are required to regularly report their data on the number of those who are eligible, those who are tested and those who decline screening, as well as the results of the invasive tests and pregnancy outcomes.

Most prenatal diagnostic tests arise following a 'high-risk' screening test. In the UK, the National Institute for Health and Care Excellence (NICE) has recommended that all pregnant women should be offered screening for Down syndrome as part of their routine antenatal care.

Several different screening tests are available, but the UK National Screening Committee recommends combined screening in the first trimester. This test involves the combination of an ultrasound scan to measure the nuchal translucency (NT) and the crown–rump length (CRL) from 11+2–14+1 weeks' gestation, and a blood test between 10+0–14+1 weeks' gestation to measure the levels of human chorionic gonadotrophin (hCG) and pregnancy associated plasma protein-A (PAPP-A) in maternal blood. The eligibility criteria for the combined test is when the CRL is between 45.0 mm and 84.0 mm (**Figure 5.3**).

The NT measurement is the thickness of a collection of fluid under the skin in the nuchal (neck) region of the fetus. Fetuses with Down syndrome tend to have a thicker NT, hence a thick NT measurement increases the risk of the fetus having Down syndrome (**Figure 5.3**).

The risk of Down syndrome increases with maternal age. For each pregnancy, the individual risk can be calculated by taking the age-related risk and then adjusting this risk up or down based on the measurements obtained for the NT, hCG and PAPP-A. Based on their individual screening result, the pregnant woman can then choose whether to have an invasive test or not.

The UK National Screening Committee recommends the quadruple test (hCG, alpha-fetoprotein, unconjugated oestriol and inhibin A) as the screening strategy of choice in the second trimester for those individuals booking later in pregnancy or when it is not possible to measure the NT. The test can be performed between 14+2 and 20+0 weeks' gestation.

Prior to performing the screening test, the pregnant woman should be encouraged to consider what action she would take and how she would feel if she screened positive. It is also important to explain to

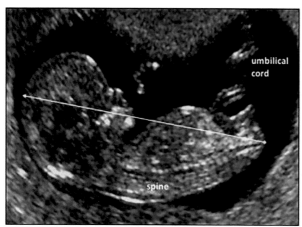
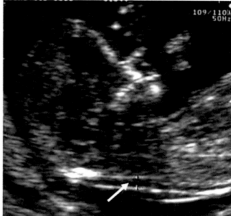

Figure 5.3 Ultrasound images demonstrating the measurement of crown–rump length (left-hand image) and nuchal translucency (arrow, right-hand image).

pregnant women that this initial test is simply a screening test and not a diagnostic test. A low-risk result does not rule out the possibility of Down syndrome completely (even if the result shows a very low risk of 1:10,000, the patient could be the 1 person in 10,000 who has an affected fetus). With a high-risk result of 1:10, 9 out of 10 or 90% of fetuses would be normal. The diagnostic tests available should be explained.

The accuracy of the screening test for Down syndrome can be refined by adding further markers such as measuring the length of the nasal bone, the frontomaxillary nasal angle and looking for the presence of tricuspid regurgitation and at the ductus venosus wave form. These increase the sensitivity of the test and reduce the false-positive rate. However, they are resource intensive and not currently used in the UK Fetal Anomaly Screening Programme. A prenatal diagnostic test such as CVS or amniocentesis must still be performed to reach a definitive diagnosis.

NON-INVASIVE PRENATAL TESTING

Maternal blood contains a mixture of maternal DNA (90%) and placental DNA (10%). In most cases, the placental DNA will be the same as the fetal DNA. The contribution of DNA from the placenta is called cffDNA. This can be detected in the maternal blood as early as 5 weeks of pregnancy. The concentration of cffDNA increases with gestation from around 10% at 10 weeks of gestation. After delivery, the level of cffDNA drops rapidly and is usually undetectable by the first day after birth, making it suitable for pregnancy-specific testing.

The use of cffDNA to screen for Down syndrome and other aneuploidies has now been implemented within the UK NHS Fetal Anomaly Screening Programme and is undergoing evaluation. It is currently being offered on the NHS to all pregnant women who receive a higher chance result (between 1 in 2 and 1 in 150) from either the combined or the quadruple test in both singleton and twin pregnancies. Individuals with a high-risk result can choose to have non-invasive prenatal testing (NIPT) rather than immediately undergo an invasive diagnostic test such as CVS or amniocentesis. Current studies suggest that

NIPT using cffDNA detects around 98% of all babies with Down, Patau and Edwards syndrome. NIPT is not diagnostic, however, and an invasive prenatal diagnostic test is recommended to confirm the result.

NEW DEVELOPMENTS IN PRENATAL DIAGNOSIS

Non-invasive prenatal diagnosis (NIPD) is now becoming available for certain congenital disorders by amplifying the cffDNA using PCR to confirm the fetal genotype. Care must be taken to ensure that there is a sufficient concentration of cffDNA in the maternal blood (the 'fetal fraction') for the test to be accurate. This may mean that the mother's blood needs to be retested later in pregnancy when the fetal fraction of cffDNA is higher. Maternal obesity is associated with a larger blood volume and this may make a conclusive result impossible. Two recent examples of such non-invasive diagnostic tests are for single-gene disorders and to check the fetal blood group.

FETAL SINGLE-GENE DISORDERS

Certain autosomal dominant single-gene disorders can now be diagnosed using cffDNA. The test can be offered when the father is known to be affected by the condition, when there is a risk of recurrence or when the condition is suspected on ultrasound scan. For example, NIPD for the autosomal dominant severe skeletal dysplasias such as achondroplasia and thanatophoric dysplasia that are caused by a mutation in the fibroblast growth factor 3 receptor gene (*FGFR3*) are now offered for routine clinical use in the UK National Genomic Test Directory. Ultrasound findings such as short long bones (<3rd centile), a small narrow chest with normal head and abdominal measurements can indicate an affected fetus. If the mother is unaffected, she will have a normal FGFR3 gene. When a PCR test on the cffDNA in the mother's blood identifies a mutation in the FGFR3 gene, this must have come from the fetus indicating that the fetus is affected. If the PCR test is negative for the FGFR3 mutation, the fetus is unaffected. An invasive prenatal diagnostic test is not necessary to make the diagnosis, and it can be avoided.

FETAL BLOOD GROUP

Similarly, if RhD-positive DNA is amplified from the blood of an RhD-negative pregnant woman, this must have come from the fetus (as the pregnant individual has no RhD-positive DNA of their own), and the test therefore shows that the fetus is RhD positive. In RhD-negative pregnant women with anti-D antibodies, this test is used to determine the blood group of the fetus, as an RhD-positive fetus is at risk of alloimmune haemolytic disease, whereas an RhD-negative fetus is not at risk. Intensive surveillance can be instituted for a pregnancy with an RhD-positive fetus, and the parents of the RhD-negative fetus can be reassured that problems will not occur. This type of NIPD avoids the need for invasive prenatal diagnostic testing, which of itself might increase exposure to sensitizing RhD antigens. Fetal blood group can be determined from samples taken in the first trimester and testing for the common blood group antigens, including rhesus and Kell, can be performed (see the section 'Rhesus isoimmunization' in **Chapter 6**).

NON-INVASIVE PRENATAL DIAGNOSIS FOR ANEUPLOIDY

There is much promising work on NIPD for Down syndrome using cffDNA in the maternal blood. Single-molecule counting methods such as digital PCR are based on the detection of the extra copy of chromosome 21 to distinguish normal cases from trisomy 21 cases. Detecting the different DNA methylation patterns between the maternal and fetal circulating DNA molecules has been proposed as an alternative strategy for the identification of cffDNA sequences. This is based on the ratio of a subset of fetal-specific methylated regions located on chromosome 21 compared with normal cases. These tests have the potential to replace invasive prenatal diagnostic testing for Down syndrome.

WHOLE EXOME SEQUENCING

Gene sequencing is increasingly being applied for prenatal diagnosis. Whole genome sequencing has been studied but is costly and requires large amounts of fetal DNA. The alternative is whole exome sequencing, which focuses on the exons or protein-coding regions of the genome only. Exons account for around 1.5% of the DNA in the genome, comprising approximately 22,000 genes. Importantly, most identified genes implicated in Mendelian disease involve the exons. Studies suggest that prenatal whole exome sequencing may increase the frequency of identification of genetic causes of structural anomalies in fetuses compared with karyotyping or CMA alone. It may be particularly useful in selected fetuses that have multisystem or severe abnormalities such as cardiac or skeletal disorders.

FETAL IMAGING

Fetal magnetic resonance imaging (MRI) is an increasingly used imaging tool in pregnancy and can improve the analysis of central nervous system abnormalities in the fetus, particularly in the differential diagnosis of ventriculomegaly, where ultrasound may not always provide sufficient soft tissue resolution. Fetal MRI is used to confirm eligibility for fetal surgery, such as in fetuses with open spina bifida, when hindbrain herniation ('Chiari II' malformation) is easily detected using MRI. It may also be used to image the fetal brain after laser for twin-to-twin transfusion syndrome in monochorionic multiple pregnancies to detect neurological damage secondary to hypoxia or hypoperfusion (see **Chapter 7**). For abnormalities in the fetal body, MRI is helpful due to the superior soft tissue resolution. Examples include fetal neck masses to aid detection of an intact fetal airway, cloacal abnormalities and congenital diaphragmatic hernia.

Currently, there are some limitations to fetal MRI, as it is sensitive to fetal motion, although fast imaging techniques have overcome this to some extent. In addition, manipulation of images using computerized reconstruction techniques can 'stitch' images together in a three-dimensional (3D) approach to improve resolution. It is hoped that MRI may also provide a better assessment of placental function and oxygenation, which ultrasound is currently unable to provide.

3D and four-dimensional (4D) ultrasound has so far played a limited role as a diagnostic tool. Surface rendering can help in the visualization of cleft lip and palate for parents. Volume rendering allows the volume of an organ, such as the lung for example, to be calculated. 3D ultrasound can also be used in the presence of ventriculomegaly to detect the intact corpus callosum, a structure that is often difficult to visualize with ultrasound.

FURTHER READING

Fetal anomaly screening programme. https:// www.gov.uk/government/publications/ fetal-anomaly-screening-programme-handbook.

NICE (2008). *Antenatal Care for Uncomplicated Pregnancies*. Clinical guideline [CG62]. Last updated: 4 February 2019. https://www.nice.org.uk/guidance/cg62.

SELF-ASSESSMENT

For interactive SBAs and EMQs relating to this chapter, visit www.routledge.com/cw/mccarthy.

CASE HISTORY 1

Ms N is a 22-year-old woman living in the North West of England. She found herself unexpectedly pregnant and had not been taking peri-conceptual folic acid. When she first attended the antenatal clinic, an ultrasound scan showed her to be 19 weeks' pregnant. The fetus was noted to have an abnormal head shape, the cerebellum was described as banana shaped and a myelomeningo-coele was identified in the lumbar region. The fetus had bilateral talipes.

Figure 5.4 shows normal intracranial anatomy imaged in the plane of the thalami to visualize the ventricles (**Figure 5.4A**) and the transcerebellar plane (**Figure 5.4B**). Note

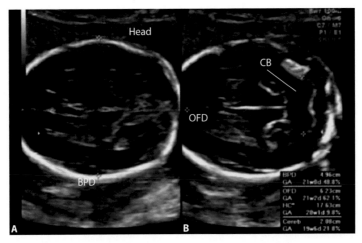

Figure 5.4 Normal cranial anatomy in (**A**) the plane of the thalami to visualize the ventricles and (**B**) the transcerebellar plane. Note the ovoid head shape and the dumb bell-shaped cerebellum. BPD, biparietal diameter; CB, cerebellum; OFD occipitofrontal diameter.

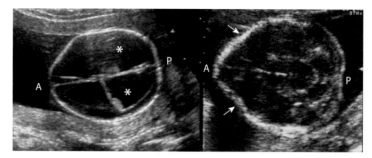

Figure 5.5 Abnormal cranial anatomy in a fetus with a neural tube defect in (**A**) the plane of the thalami to visualize the ventricles marked with asterisks, which are dilated (ventriculomegaly), and (**B**) the transcerebellar plane: note the scalloped head shape anteriorly (lemon shaped) marked by the white arrows and the banana-shaped cerebellum (red arrow). (A, anterior; P, posterior.)

the ovoid head shape and the dumb bell-shaped cerebellum (indicated by white arrow). **Figure 5.5** is a similar plane in Ms N, whose fetus has a neural tube defect.

A How should this patient be managed?
B What is the outlook for the baby/child?
C What options does Ms N have?
D What is the risk of it happening again in a future pregnancy?
E What advice would you give about future pregnancies?

ANSWERS

A A prenatal diagnosis of a neural tube defect has been made on ultrasound scan. Ultrasound scan will detect at least 90% of all neural tube defects. Ms N should be seen by the consultant and the ultrasound findings should be explained to her. She should have the opportunity to discuss the prognosis with a neurosurgeon, and this may be best organized by referring her to a tertiary fetal medicine unit.

B For pregnant women to make decisions about whether to continue with their pregnancy or not, they need an honest and realistic view of the likely outcome for their baby/child. It is always difficult to predict the outlook for the baby/child but lower lesions generally have a better prognosis. The main problems encountered are:
   • problems with mobility – individuals with a neural tube defect tend to become wheelchair bound as they get older
   • continence and voiding – both bladder and bowel
   • low intelligence quotient (IQ)
   • repeated surgery – shunts, bladder and bowel, orthopaedic
   • difficulty forming normal relationships and living independently

C Ms N may choose to continue with the pregnancy with support from healthcare professionals both before and after delivery. Parents who choose to continue with a pregnancy may benefit from contacting a parent support group such as SHINE. Postnatal surgery has until recently been the only option. Fetal surgery is now being offered in the UK and many other countries to repair the myelomeningocoele defect during pregnancy. MRI should be performed to confirm the hindbrain herniation (Chiari II malformation) and to exclude other structural anomalies. Invasive prenatal testing to confirm a normal karyotype is also required. Fetal surgery involves extensive maternal surgery with an associated risk of spontaneous preterm birth. However, there is now outcome data up to 20 years to show benefit for the affected neonate/child of improved mobility and continence. Alternatively, the mother may opt for termination of the pregnancy.

D The risk of recurrence of a neural tube defect is 5% after one affected pregnancy (12% after two affected pregnancies and 20% after three affected pregnancies). Neural tube defects are more common in some geographical areas (e.g. Ireland, Scotland and North West England), if the mother has diabetes or epilepsy, if the mother is taking anti-epileptic medication and in the pregnant population who are obese. Folic acid (400 μg) taken pre-conceptually and for the first trimester reduces the risk of neural tube defects.

E By taking folic acid for at least 3 months pre-conceptually, the risk of recurrence can be reduced. Ms N should take a higher dose of pre-conceptual folic acid (5 mg instead of the usual 400 μg). She should also ensure that she eats healthily and that her weight is normal. Any medication she is taking should be reviewed.

CASE HISTORY 2

Ms G is an 18-year-old woman who had her first scan at 16 weeks' gestation. When the fetal abdomen was scanned, an irregular mass was seen to project from the anterior abdominal wall at the level of the umbilicus, to the right side of the umbilical cord insertion. **Figure 5.6** shows the herniated bowel (indicated by a white arrow) in the amniotic fluid. No other fetal abnormalities were noted.

A How should this patient be managed?
B What should the consultant tell her about the outlook for her baby?
C What plans would you make for delivery?

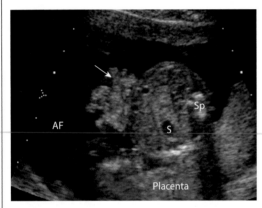

Figure 5.6 Ultrasound image of gastroschisis (arrow). AF, amniotic fluid; S, fetal stomach; Sp, fetal spine.

Table 5.4 Key differences between abdominal wall defects

Exomphalos	Gastroschisis
Membrane covered herniation of abdominal contents – smooth outline	Not membrane covered Free floating bowel loops – irregular outline
Umbilical cord inserts into apex of sac	Herniation lateral (usually to the right) of the cord insertion
Very high incidence of associated abnormalities and genetic syndromes	Relatively low incidence of other abnormalities
High incidence of chromosomal abnormalities – karyotyping should be offered	No increase in incidence of chromosomal abnormalities
May contain stomach, liver, spleen	Usually only small bowel extra-abdominally
Associated with polyhydramnios	Associated with oligohydramnios

ANSWERS

A A prenatal diagnosis of a gastroschisis has been made on ultrasound scan. Ultrasound scan will detect at least 90% of all gastroschisis defects. Ms G should be seen by the consultant and the ultrasound findings should be explained to her. She requires referral to a tertiary unit for ongoing management and planning of delivery. Involvement of a multidisciplinary team would be important.

B The consultant should stress that the majority of babies born with gastroschisis will do well in the long term and lead normal lives. Gastroschisis is not usually associated with any other physical problems or with learning problems (**Table 5.4**). It should be explained that the fetus will need to be monitored regularly during the pregnancy, as fetuses with gastroschisis are often small and may have oligohydramnios. In later pregnancy, the fetal bowel may dilate, which can be associated with bowel

ischaemia and bowel atresia. This can make the postnatal surgery more difficult.

Following delivery, the baby would require an operation to repair the defect. Surgical repair ranges from reduction of bowel and suturing of defect under anaesthetic to the need for a silo. This is a covering placed over the abdominal organs on the outside of the baby. Gradually, the organs are squeezed by hand through the silo into the opening and returned to the body. This method can take up to a week to return the abdominal organs to the body cavity. Severe cases may require bowel resection for atresias or volvulus. Survival rates of up to 97% are found for simple cases and the majority of babies are on full oral feeds by 4 weeks of age. For more complex, severe cases, there is a lower rate of survival with longer hospitalization.

Ms G should be given the opportunity to meet the paediatric surgeons during the pregnancy and visit the paediatric surgical unit. After delivery, she should be encouraged to express breast milk to feed to her baby.

C Induction around 37 weeks' gestation enables delivery to be planned in a unit with appropriate paediatric surgical facilities and may reduce the incidence of stillbirth late in pregnancy. There does

not appear to be any benefit of delivery by caesarean section for babies with gastroschisis. If other organs such as the liver are also herniated, caesarean delivery may be indicated. A normal delivery makes it easier to visit her baby on the paediatric surgical unit in the first few days after birth.

CASE HISTORY 3

Ms E is a 37-year-old woman who attended for her first scan at 18 weeks' gestation. On ultrasound scan, a smooth protrusion could be seen on the anterior abdominal wall of the fetus. It appeared to be covered by a membrane and the umbilical cord inserted into the apex of the protrusion. The sonographer described this as an exomphalos in her report. **Figure 5.7** shows an ultrasound image of an exomphalos with the sac containing the herniated bowel.

A How should this patient be managed?
B What options are available to Ms E?

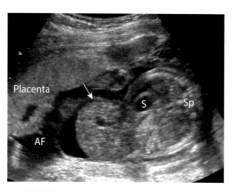

Figure 5.7 Ultrasound image of exomphalos, showing the sac containing the herniated bowel (white arrow). AF, amniotic fluid; S, fetal stomach; Sp, fetal spine.

ANSWERS

A A prenatal diagnosis of an exomphalos has been made on ultrasound scan. Ultrasound scan will detect at least 90% of all exomphalos defects, but this diagnosis cannot be made until after 12 weeks' gestation. Prior to 12 weeks, there is developmental physiological herniation of abdominal contents into the base of the umbilical cord. Ms E should be seen by the consultant and the ultrasound findings should be explained to her. As there is a high incidence of associated abnormalities (in 70–80% of fetuses), she should be referred to a tertiary unit for detailed ultrasound. The consultant should also explain that there is a high chance of chromosomal abnormality (approximately one-third of fetuses) and discuss the option of invasive testing (see **Table 5.3**).

B Ms E's options include:
  * do nothing
  * terminate the pregnancy
  * CVS now and continue if the chromosomes are normal – it is possible that other abnormalities may still be detected on ultrasound later in pregnancy; if the chromosomes are abnormal, she would still have the option of a surgical termination of pregnancy up to 14 weeks' gestation in some hospitals
  * wait until after 15 weeks' gestation, then have an amniocentesis with a lower risk of miscarriage – even if the chromosomes are normal, it is still possible that other abnormalities may be detected on ultrasound later in pregnancy

Ms E chose to have a CVS that showed that the fetus had trisomy 18. She then chose to terminate her pregnancy, as she knew that most fetuses with trisomy 18 either were stillborn or did not live beyond the first few months.

CASE HISTORY 4

Mrs D has a brother with Duchenne muscular dystrophy (DMD). He has been under the care of the clinical geneticists and Mrs D has been tested and found to be a carrier of the gene. She contacts her general practitioner (GP) when she is 7 weeks' pregnant, as she wishes to have testing to see whether the fetus is affected by DMD.

A What are the chances of Mrs D having an affected fetus?

B How should Mrs D be managed?

ANSWERS

A There is a 1:4 chance of an affected fetus. DMD is an X-linked recessive condition. There is a 1:2 chance that any baby will be a girl and a 1:2 chance that it will be a boy. If the fetus is male, there is a 1:2 chance that it has inherited a normal X chromosome from Mrs D (unaffected) and a 1:2 chance that it has inherited the X chromosome carrying the abnormal gene, in which case the boy would be affected. If the fetus is female, there is a 1:2 chance that it will have inherited a normal X chromosome from Mrs D and therefore not be a carrier, and a 1:2 chance that it will have inherited the X chromosome carrying the abnormal gene and therefore be a carrier. A female fetus would not be affected, as this is an X-linked recessive condition and a female fetus would have inherited a normal X chromosome from the father.

B The GP should arrange an urgent referral to the antenatal clinic and also contact the clinical genetics department. Mrs D requires an initial ultrasound scan to confirm that the fetus is viable, to confirm the gestation and to confirm that it is a singleton pregnancy. Testing would be much more complex if this were a twin pregnancy.

Initially, a blood test can be performed on Mrs D to ascertain the sex of the fetus. All fetuses shed small quantities of DNA into the maternal circulation. This can be amplified by a PCR technique. By testing the maternal serum for cffDNA from the Y chromosome, the sex of the fetus can be ascertained. If Y chromosome DNA is found in the maternal serum, it must have come from a male fetus. If no Y chromosome DNA is found, then it is likely that it is a female fetus. However, there is also a small possibility that the test has not worked because there is insufficient cffDNA level in the maternal plasma. It is currently recommended that, before 9 weeks of gestation, two samples should be collected, 1 week apart, to ensure that there is sufficient cffDNA to make a diagnosis.

Mrs D had a blood test at 8 weeks' gestation and a second blood test at 10 weeks that showed that she was carrying a female fetus. As this meant that she would not have an affected baby, she did not need to have any further invasive testing. If the blood test had shown that she was carrying a male fetus, she would then have had a CVS to determine whether this was an affected or unaffected male. By having the blood test, she was able to avoid invasive testing.

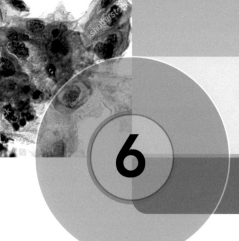

Antenatal obstetric complications

6

SURABHI NANDA

Learning Objectives
- Appreciate the causes and management of minor complications of pregnancy.
- Be able to provide a differential diagnosis and a management plan for abdominal pain in pregnancy.
- Understand the risk factors, presentation and management of venous thromboembolic disease in pregnancy.
- Understand the complications of drug abuse in pregnancy.
- Understand the causes, complications and management of oligohydramnios and polyhydramnios.
- Understand the causes and management of malpresentation in late pregnancy.
- Understand the complications and management of post-term pregnancy.
- Understand the causes, prevention and treatment of haemolytic disease of the fetus and newborn.

INTRODUCTION

There are a variety of complications that can arise during pregnancy. Some of these 'minor' conditions arise because the physiological changes of pregnancy exacerbate many 'irritating' symptoms that in the normal, non-pregnant state would not require specific treatment. While these problems are not dangerous to the pregnant woman, they can be extremely troublesome and incapacitating, and sometimes may mimic symptoms of exacerbation of some pre-existing medical problems, and therefore need to be appropriately differentiated. Some of the more major complications are discussed in detail in other chapters. Here we discuss common complications, including malpresentation, rhesus disease and abnormalities of amniotic fluid production.

10.1201/9781003196112-6

MINOR PROBLEMS OF PREGNANCY

MUSCULOSKELETAL PROBLEMS

BACKACHE

Backache is extremely common in pregnancy and is caused by:

- hormone-induced laxity of spinal ligaments
- a shifting in the centre of gravity as the uterus grows
- additional weight gain

These cause an exaggerated lumbar lordosis. Pregnancy can exacerbate the symptoms of a prolapsed intervertebral disc, occasionally leading to complete immobility. Occasionally, there may be an additional impingement of the sciatic nerve, leading to referred pain along the leg and hip and a further change in posture and gait. Advice should include maintenance of correct posture, avoiding lifting heavy objects (including children), avoiding high heels, regular physiotherapy (including hydrotherapy and Pilates), swimming and simple analgesia (paracetamol or paracetamol–codeine combinations). As these symptoms are usually more pronounced in the third trimester, non-steroidal anti-inflammatory drugs (such as ibuprofen), are not recommended due to the risk of premature closure of ductus arteriosus and oligohydramnios.

SYMPHYSIS PUBIS DYSFUNCTION/ PELVIC GIRDLE PAIN

This is an excruciatingly painful condition most common in the third trimester, although it can occur at any time during pregnancy, especially in multiple/higher order multiple pregnancies. The symphysis pubis joint becomes 'loose', causing the two halves of the pelvis to rub on one another when walking or moving. The condition improves after delivery and the management revolves around simple analgesia. Under a physiotherapist's direction, a low stability belt may be worn.

CARPAL TUNNEL SYNDROME

Compression neuropathies occur in pregnancy due to increased soft-tissue swelling. The most common of these is carpal tunnel syndrome. The median nerve, where it passes through the fibrous canal at the wrist before entering the hand, is most susceptible to compression. The symptoms include numbness, tingling and weakness of the thumb and forefinger, as well as often quite severe pain at night. Simple analgesia and splinting of the affected hand usually help, although there is no realistic prospect of cure until after delivery. Surgical decompression is very rarely performed in pregnancy. Some medical conditions such as multiple sclerosis relapse may present with similar symptoms (usually on one side). Early symptoms of pre-eclampsia may also cause swelling of hands and present with carpal tunnel syndrome.

GASTROINTESTINAL SYMPTOMS

CONSTIPATION

Constipation is common in pregnancy and usually results from a combination of hormonal and mechanical factors that slow gut motility. Concomitantly administered iron tablets may exacerbate the condition. Pregnant women should be given clear explanations, reassurance and advice regarding the adoption of a high-fibre diet. Medications are best avoided but, if necessary, mild (non-stimulant) laxatives such as lactulose may be suggested. Prolonged constipation or symptoms not responding to diet or laxatives should raise suspicion of an underlying pathology, including bowel obstruction.

HYPEREMESIS GRAVIDARUM

Nausea and vomiting in pregnancy are extremely common; 70–80% of pregnant women experience these symptoms early in their pregnancy and approximately 35% of all pregnant women are absent from work on at least one occasion through nausea and vomiting. Although the symptoms are often most pronounced in the first trimester, they are by no means confined to it. Similarly, despite common usage of the term 'morning sickness', in only a minority of cases are the symptoms solely confined to the morning. Nausea and vomiting in pregnancy tends to be mild and self-limited and is not associated with adverse pregnancy outcomes.

Hyperemesis gravidarum (HG), however, is a severe, intractable form of nausea and vomiting that affects 0.3–2.0% of pregnancies. It causes imbalances of fluid and electrolytes, disturbs nutritional intake and metabolism, causes physical and psychological debilitation and is associated with adverse pregnancy outcomes, including an increased risk of preterm birth and low birthweight babies. A recent nationwide survey of over 5,000 participants on HG in the UK showed that nearly 5% of participants terminated a pregnancy and around 50% considered termination owing to HG. Over 25% reported suicidal ideation. The aetiology is unknown and various putative mechanisms have been proposed, including an association with high levels of serum human chorionic gonadotrophin (hCG), oestrogen and thyroxine. The likely cause is multifactorial, although studies are underway to identify biomarkers and gene linkage in HG. Severe cases of HG cause malnutrition and vitamin deficiencies, including Wernicke encephalopathy, and intractable retching predisposes to oesophageal trauma and Mallory–Weiss tears. Treatment includes dietary and lifestyle changes, as well as alternative therapies such as ginger, acupressure, fluid replacement and thiamine supplementation. Antiemetics such as phenothiazines and metoclopramide are safe and are commonly prescribed. Oral corticosteroids are reserved for severe cases that have not responded to standard therapy. The National Institute for Health and Care Excellence (NICE, 2019) has recommended doxylamine/pyridoxine (Xonvea®) for pregnant women with symptoms that have not responded to standard conservative management.

GASTRO-OESOPHAGEAL REFLUX

This is very common. Altered structure and function of the normal physiological barriers to reflux, namely the weight effect of the pregnant uterus and hormonally induced relaxation of the oesophageal sphincter, explain the extremely high incidence in the pregnant population. For the majority of patients, lifestyle modifications such as smoking cessation, frequent light meals, earlier evening meals and lying with the head propped up at night are helpful. When these prove insufficient to control symptoms, medications can be added in a stepwise fashion, starting with simple antacids. Histamine-2 receptor antagonists and proton pump inhibitors have a good safety record in pregnancy and can be used.

HAEMORRHOIDS

Several factors conspire to render haemorrhoids more common during pregnancy, including the effects of circulating progesterone on the vasculature, pressure on the superior rectal veins by the gravid uterus and increased circulating volume. A conservative approach is usually advocated, including local anaesthetic/anti-irritant creams and a high-fibre diet. Never overlook the 'warning' symptoms of tenesmus, mucus, blood mixed with stool and back passage discomfort that may suggest rectal carcinoma; a rectal digital examination should be carried out if these symptoms are suggested.

OBSTETRIC CHOLESTASIS

Obstetric cholestasis (also intrahepatic cholestasis of pregnancy) affects 0.7% of pregnancies with some ethnic variation. It normally presents in the second half of pregnancy with pruritus and abnormal liver function tests, including bile acids (liver function tests), neither of which has an alternative cause and both of which resolve after birth. The clinical importance of obstetric cholestasis lies in the potential fetal risks (with serum bile acids >40 µmol/L), which may include spontaneous preterm birth, iatrogenic preterm birth and fetal death (serum bile acids >100 µmol/L). There can also be morbidity relating to intense pruritus and consequent sleep deprivation. It is normally treated with ursodeoxycholic acid, which improves pruritus and liver function but has not been proven to improve fetal and neonatal outcomes. Pregnant women with obstetric cholestasis are therefore normally offered delivery after 37 weeks' gestation, depending on their symptoms and the rise in their bile acids.

VARICOSE VEINS

Varicose veins may appear for the first time in pregnancy or pre-existing veins may become worse. They are thought to be due to the relaxant effect of progesterone on vascular smooth muscle and the dependent venous stasis caused by the weight of the pregnant uterus on the inferior vena cava.

Varicose veins of the legs may be symptomatically improved with support stockings, avoidance of standing for prolonged periods and simple analgesia. Thrombophlebitis may occur in a large varicose vein, more commonly after delivery. A large superficial varicose vein may bleed profusely if traumatized; the leg must be elevated and direct pressure applied. Vulval and vaginal varicosities are uncommon but symptomatically troublesome; trauma at the time of delivery (episiotomy, tear, instrumental delivery) may also cause considerable bleeding. Above-knee varicose veins are a contributory risk factor for venous thromboembolism.

OEDEMA

This is common, occurring to some degree in approximately 80% of all pregnancies. There is generalized soft-tissue swelling and increased capillary permeability, which allows intravascular fluid to leak into the extravascular compartment. The fingers, toes and ankles are usually worst affected and the symptoms are aggravated by hot weather. Oedema is best dealt with by frequent periods of rest with leg elevation; occasionally, support stockings are indicated. Excessively swollen fingers may necessitate removal of rings and jewellery before they get stuck. It is important to remember that generalized (rather than lower limb) oedema may be a feature of pre-eclampsia, so remember to check the blood pressure and urine for protein. More rarely, severe oedema may suggest underlying cardiac impairment or nephrotic syndrome.

BOX 6.1: Other common 'minor' disorders

- Itching
- Urinary incontinence
- Nosebleeds
- Thrush (vaginal candidiasis)
- Headache
- Fainting
- Visual floaters
- Breast tenderness
- Tiredness
- Altered taste sensation or changes in appetite
- Insomnia
- Leg cramps
- Striae gravidarum and chloasma

PROBLEMS DUE TO ABNORMALITIES OF THE PELVIC ORGANS

FIBROIDS (LEIOMYOMATA)

Fibroids are compact masses of smooth muscle that lie in the cavity of the uterus (submucous), within the uterine muscle (intramural) or on the outside surface of the uterus (subserous). They may enlarge in pregnancy and, in so doing, present problems later on in pregnancy or at delivery (**Figure 6.1**). A large fibroid at the cervix or in the lower uterine segment may prevent descent of the presenting part and obstruct vaginal delivery.

Red degeneration is one of the most common complications of fibroids in pregnancy. As it grows, the fibroid may become ischaemic, which usually presents as acute pain, tenderness over the fibroid and frequent vomiting. If these symptoms are severe, it may precipitate uterine contractions, causing miscarriage or preterm labour. The symptoms usually settle within a few days, but occasionally may require pain relief with simple analgesia including codeine-based compounds and hydration (oral or

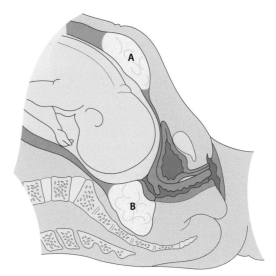

Figure 6.1 Fibroids complicating pregnancy. The tumour in the anterior wall of the uterus (**A**) has been drawn up and out of the pelvis as the lower segment formed, but the fibroid (**B**) arising from the cervix remains in the pelvis and will obstruct labour.

rarely intravenous). The differential diagnosis of red degeneration includes acute appendicitis, pyelonephritis/urinary tract infection, ovarian cyst accident and placental abruption.

A subserous pedunculated fibroid may tort in the same way that a large ovarian cyst can. When this happens, acute abdominal pain and tenderness may make the two difficult to distinguish from one another. In this scenario, a pertinent history followed by ultrasound scan (transvaginal in the first trimester, transabdominal in the second and third) will help aid the diagnosis.

RETROVERSION OF THE UTERUS

In around 15% of the population, the uterus is retroverted. In pregnancy, the uterus grows and a retroverted uterus will normally 'flip' out of the pelvis and begin to fill the abdominal cavity, as an anteverted uterus would. In a small proportion of cases, the uterus remains in retroversion and eventually fills up the entire pelvic cavity; as it does so, the base of the bladder and the urethra are stretched. Retention of urine may occur, classically at 12–14 weeks, and this not only is very painful but may also cause long-term bladder damage if the bladder becomes overdistended. In this situation, catheterization is essential until the position of the uterus has changed.

CONGENITAL UTERINE ANOMALIES

The shape of the uterus is embryologically determined by the fusion of the Müllerian ducts. Abnormalities of fusion may give rise to anything from a sub-septate uterus through to a bicornuate uterus and very rarely to a double uterus with two cervices. These findings are often discovered incidentally at the time of a pelvic operation, such as a laparoscopy, or an ultrasound scan. Confirmatory diagnosis of a uterine anomaly in pregnancy can be tricky.

The usual problems associated with bicornuate uterus are:

- miscarriage
- preterm labour
- preterm premature rupture of membranes (PPROM)

- abnormalities of lie and presentation, and occasionally fetal growth problems
- higher caesarean section rate

Such pregnancies need surveillance in a preterm clinic, with serial cervical length measurements and ultrasound scan in the third trimester to assess growth trajectory, lie and presentation.

OVARIAN CYSTS IN PREGNANCY

Ovarian cysts are common in pregnancy; fortunately, the incidence of malignancy is uncommon in those of childbearing age. The most common types of pathological ovarian cyst are serous cysts and benign teratomas. Physiological cysts of the corpus luteum may grow to several centimetres but rarely require treatment. Asymptomatic cysts may be followed up by clinical and ultrasound examination, but large cysts (for example dermoid cysts) may require surgery in pregnancy.

Surgery is usually postponed until the second or early third trimester, when there is the potential that, if the baby were delivered, it would be able to survive. The major problems are large (>6 cm) ovarian cysts in pregnancy, which may undergo torsion, haemorrhage or rupture, causing acute abdominal pain. The resulting pain and inflammation may lead to a miscarriage or preterm labour. Symptomatic cysts, most commonly due to torsion, will require an emergency laparotomy and ovarian cystectomy or even oophorectomy, if the cyst is torted. A full assessment must include a family history of ovarian or breast malignancy, tumour markers (although these are of limited value in pregnancy) and detailed ultrasound investigation of both ovaries. Surgery in late second and third trimester of pregnancy is normally performed through a midline or paramedian incision, under a regional or sometimes a general anaesthetic; a low transverse suprapubic incision would not allow access to the ovary, as it is drawn upwards in later pregnancy.

CERVICAL AND BREAST CANCERS IN PREGNANCY

Cervical abnormalities are much more difficult to deal with in pregnancy, partly because the cervix itself is more difficult to visualize at colposcopy and also because biopsy may cause considerable bleeding. Cervical carcinoma most commonly arises in poor attenders for cervical screening. The disease is commonly asymptomatic in early stages, but later-stage presentation includes vaginal bleeding (especially post-coital). Examination may reveal a friable or ulcerated lesion with bleeding and purulent discharge. The prospect of cervical carcinoma in pregnancy leads to complex ethical and moral dilemmas concerning whether the pregnancy must be terminated (depending on the stage it has reached) to facilitate either surgical treatment (radical hysterectomy) or chemoradiotherapy. Cervical cancer is discussed in greater detail in **Chapter 16** of *Gynaecology by Ten Teachers*, 21st Edition.

Breast cancer is the most common malignancy complicating pregnancy (accounting for 40% of cases); the current incidence rate is estimated to be 1 in 1,000 pregnancies, with numbers rising due to increasing background incidence of the disease and rising age in the pregnant population. Presentation may be delayed, leading to more advanced clinical staging at diagnosis. Management represents a challenging situation, in which healthcare professionals attempt to maximize the curative approach (surgery, chemotherapy and radiotherapy earlier in gestation) for the patient while minimizing adverse effects on the fetus (growth restriction, fetal anomaly or demise, and preterm delivery).

URINARY TRACT INFECTION

Urinary tract infections (UTIs) are common in pregnancy. Eight per cent of pregnancies have asymptomatic bacteriuria; if this is untreated, it may progress to UTI or even pyelonephritis, with the attendant associations of low birthweight and preterm delivery.

The predisposing factors are:

- history of recurrent cystitis
- renal tract abnormalities: duplex system, scarred kidneys, ureteric damage and stones
- diabetes
- bladder-emptying problems (e.g. multiple sclerosis)

The symptoms of UTI may be different in pregnancy; it occasionally presents as low back pain and general malaise with flu-like symptoms. The classic presentation of frequency, dysuria and haematuria is not often seen. On examination, tachycardia, pyrexia, dehydration and loin tenderness may be present. Investigations should include a full blood count and midstream specimen of urine (MSU) sent for urgent microscopy, culture and sensitivities. If there is a strong clinical suspicion of UTI, treatment with antibiotics should start straightaway. The pregnant woman should be advised to drink plenty of clear fluids and take a simple analgesic such as paracetamol.

The most common organism for UTI is *Escherichia coli*; less commonly implicated are streptococci, *Proteus*, *Pseudomonas* and *Klebsiella* spp. Many laboratories define a UTI as the presence of >10^5 colony-forming units (cfu)/mL. The commonly reported 'heavy mixed growth' is often associated with UTI symptoms and may be treated or the MSU may be repeated after a week, depending on the clinical scenario. The first-line antibiotic for UTI is amoxycillin or oral cephalosporins. If there are two or more proven UTIs in pregnancy, or in individuals with pre-existing medical problems such as multiple sclerosis following one proven UTI, low-dose preventative antibiotic prophylaxis is usually recommended.

Pyelonephritis is characterized by dehydration, a very high temperature (>38.5°C), systemic disturbance and occasionally shock. This requires urgent and aggressive treatment including intravenous fluids, opiate analgesia and intravenous antibiotics (such as cephalosporins or gentamicin). In addition, renal function should be determined, with at least baseline urea and electrolytes, and the baby must be monitored with cardiotocography (CTG). Recurrent UTIs in pregnancy require MSUs to be sent to the microbiology laboratory at each antenatal visit, and low-dose prophylactic oral antibiotics may be prescribed. Investigation should take place after delivery, unless frank haematuria or other symptoms suggest that an urgent diagnosis is essential. Investigations might include a renal ultrasound scan, renal dimercapto succinic acid (DMSA) function scan, creatinine clearance, intravenous urogram and cystoscopy.

ABDOMINAL PAIN IN PREGNANCY

Abdominal pain is one of the most common minor disorders of pregnancy; the problem is in distinguishing pathological from 'physiological' pain. There are many possibilities to exclude and, in addition, the anatomical and physiological changes of pregnancy may alter 'classical' presenting symptoms and signs, making clinical diagnosis challenging. The causes listed in **Box 6.2**, 'Causes of abdominal pain in pregnancy', are not exhaustive, but cover most possible diagnoses. The crucial point to make is that certain conditions are potentially so dangerous or debilitating (e.g. acute appendicitis), and may be masked by the altered anatomy and physiology of pregnancy, that clinicians may need to perform investigations (X-rays, computed tomography (CT) or magnetic resonance imaging (MRI) scans) and arrange invasive assessments to make a diagnosis. Avoiding these investigations (mostly for the fear of an adverse impact on pregnancy), and therefore risking not making an early diagnosis, means that treatment for a serious and life-threatening condition may be delayed.

VENOUS THROMBOEMBOLISM

Venous thromboembolism (VTE) is the most common cause of direct maternal death in the UK. In the most recent Confidential Enquiries into Maternal Deaths and Morbidity report (2017–2019), there were 32 fatalities, giving a maternal mortality rate of 0.89 per 100,000, more than twice that of the next most common cause (genital tract sepsis).

Pregnancy is a hypercoagulable state because of an alteration in the thrombotic and fibrinolytic systems. There is an increase in clotting factors VIII, IX and X and fibrinogen levels, and a reduction in protein S and antithrombin III concentrations. The net result of these changes is thought to be an evolutionary response to reduce the likelihood of haemorrhage following delivery.

The physiological changes predispose pregnant women to thromboembolism and this is further exacerbated by venous stasis in the lower limbs due to the weight of the gravid uterus placing pressure on

---

BOX 6.2: Causes of abdominal pain in pregnancy

Obstetric conditions

Early pregnancy (<24 weeks)
- Ligament stretching
- Miscarriage
- Ectopic pregnancy
- Acute urinary retention due to retroverted gravid uterus
- Ovarian hyperstimulation

Later pregnancy (>24 weeks)
- Labour
- Placental abruption
- Severe pre-eclampsia and/or haemolysis, elevated liver enzymes and low platelets (HELLP) syndrome
- Uterine rupture
- Chorioamnioitis

Pregnancy-unrelated conditions

Uterine/ovarian causes
- Torsion or degeneration of fibroid
- Ovarian cyst accident

Urinary tract disorders
- Urinary tract infection (acute cystitis and acute pyelonephritis)
- Renal colic

Gastrointestinal disorders
- Medical gastric/duodenal ulcer
- Acute appendicitis, pancreatitis, gastroenteritis, cholecystitis
- Intestinal obstruction or perforation

Medical causes
- Sickle cell disease (abdominal crisis)
- Diabetic ketoacidosis
- Acute intermittent porphyria
- Pneumonia (especially lower lobe)
- Pulmonary embolus
- Malaria

---

the inferior vena cava in late pregnancy and immobility, particularly in the puerperium.

Pregnancy is associated with a 6–10-fold increase in the risk of VTE compared with the non-pregnant situation. Without thromboprophylaxis, the incidence of non-fatal pulmonary embolism (PE) and deep vein thrombosis (DVT) in pregnancy is about 0.1% in developed countries; this increases following delivery to around 1–2% and is further increased following emergency caesarean section.

THROMBOPHILIA

Some individuals are predisposed to thrombosis through changes in the coagulation/fibrinolytic system that may be inherited or acquired (see **Box 6.3**, 'Risk factors for thromboembolic disease'). There is growing evidence that both heritable and acquired thrombophilias are associated with a range of adverse pregnancy outcomes, particularly recurrent fetal loss. The major hereditary forms of thrombophilia currently recognized include deficiencies of the endogenous anticoagulants protein C, protein S and antithrombin III, and abnormalities of procoagulant factors, factor V Leiden (caused by a mutation in the factor V gene) and the prothrombin mutation

G20210A. It seems probable that there are still some thrombophilias not yet discovered or described. Heritable thrombophilias are present in at least 15% of Western populations.

Acquired thrombophilia is most commonly associated with antiphospholipid syndrome. Antiphospholipid syndrome is the combination of lupus anticoagulant with or without anticardiolipin antibodies, with a history of recurrent miscarriage and/or thrombosis. It may (or, more commonly, may not) be associated with other autoantibody disorders such as systemic lupus erythematosus.

If thrombophilic disorders are taken together, more than 50% of cases of pregnancy-related VTE are associated with a thrombophilia. It is therefore vital that individuals with a history of thrombotic events are screened for thrombophilia. The presence of thrombophilia, with a history of thrombotic episode(s), means that prophylaxis should be considered for pregnancy.

BOX 6.3: Risk factors for thromboembolic disease

Pre-existing

- Age (>35 years)
- Thrombophilia
- Obesity (body mass index ≥30 kg/m²) either pre-pregnancy or early pregnancy
- Previous thromboembolism
- Severe varicose veins
- Smoking
- Paraplegia
- Medical comorbidities (e.g. cancer, heart failure, active systemic lupus erythematosus, inflammatory bowel disease or polyarthropathy, nephrotic syndrome, type I diabetes mellitus with nephropathy, sickle cell disease, intravenous drug use)

Specific to pregnancy

- Multiple gestation
- Current pre-eclampsia
- Parity ≥3 (an individual becomes para 3 after their third delivery)
- Caesarean section, especially if emergency
- Prolonged labour (>24 hours)
- Midcavity forceps or rotational operative delivery

- Damage to the pelvic veins
- Sepsis
- Prolonged bed rest
- Stillbirth
- Preterm birth
- Post-partum haemorrhage (>1 L/requiring transfusion)

New onset/transient

- Any surgical procedure in pregnancy or puerperium except immediate repair of the perineum (e.g. appendicectomy, post-partum sterilization)
- Bone fracture
- Hyperemesis
- Ovarian hyperstimulation syndrome (first trimester only)
- In vitro fertilisation (IVF)
- Admission or immobility (≥3 days' bed rest)
- Current systemic infection (requiring intravenous antibiotics or admission to hospital, e.g. pneumonia, pyelonephritis, post-partum wound infection)
- Long-distance travel (>4 hours)

DIAGNOSIS OF ACUTE VENOUS THROMBOEMBOLISM

Clinical diagnosis of VTE is unreliable. Therefore, anyone suspected of having a DVT or PE should be investigated promptly.

DEEP VEIN THROMBOSIS

The most common symptoms are pain in the calf with varying degrees of redness or swelling. While legs are often swollen during pregnancy, unilateral symptoms should ring alarm bells. The signs are few, except that often the calf is tender to gentle touch. It is mandatory to ask about symptoms of PE (see the next section, 'Pulmonary embolus'), as an individual with PE might present initially with a DVT.

Compression ultrasound has a high sensitivity and specificity in diagnosing proximal thrombosis in the non-pregnant population and should be the first investigation used in a suspected DVT. Calf veins are often poorly visualized; however, it is known that a thrombus confined purely to the calf veins with no extension is very unlikely to give rise to a PE.

Venography is invasive, requiring the injection of contrast medium and the use of X-rays. It does, however, allow excellent visualization of veins both below and above the knee.

PULMONARY EMBOLUS

It is crucial to recognize PE, as missing the diagnosis could have fatal implications. The most common presentation is of mild breathlessness or inspiratory chest pain in a pregnant woman who is not cyanosed but may be slightly tachycardic (>90 beats per minute [bpm]) with a mild pyrexia (37.5°C). Rarely, massive PE may present with sudden cardiorespiratory collapse (see **Chapter 14**).

If PE is suspected, initial electrocardiogram, chest X-ray and arterial blood gases should be performed to exclude other respiratory diagnoses. However, these investigations are insufficient on their own to exclude or diagnose PE and it may be sensible to investigate the lower limbs for evidence of DVT by ultrasound, and if positive treat with a presumptive diagnosis of PE. If all the tests are normal but a high clinical suspicion of PE remains, a ventilation–perfusion (VQ) scan or CT pulmonary angiogram should be performed. In both cases, the radiation to the fetus is below the threshold considered potentially dangerous to the fetus.

A low-level D-dimer, commonly used as a screening test for thromboembolic disease in the non-pregnant population, suggests the absence of a DVT or PE, and no further objective tests are necessary. An increased level of D-dimer suggests that thrombosis may be present and an objective diagnostic test for DVT and/or PE should be performed. In pregnancy, however, D-dimer can be elevated due to the physiological changes in the coagulation system, limiting its clinical usefulness as a screening test in this situation. To some extent, D-dimer retains its negative predictive value in the pregnant and non-pregnant population but is not a reliable diagnostic test of acute PE in pregnancy.

TREATMENT OF VENOUS THROMBOEMBOLISM

Management of acute VTE should involve a multidisciplinary team including senior physicians, obstetricians and radiologists. Low-molecular-weight heparins (LMWHs) are the treatment of choice. They do not cross the placenta and have been shown to be at least as safe and effective as unfractionated heparin in the treatment of VTE, but with lower and fewer haemorrhagic complications in the initial treatment of non-pregnant subjects on unfractionated heparin. In addition, LMWH is safe and easy to administer. Affected individuals are taught to inject themselves and can continue on this treatment for the duration of their pregnancy. Warfarin is given orally and prolongs the prothrombin time, and is rarely recommended for use in pregnancy (exceptions include individuals with mechanical heart valves), as it crosses the placenta and can cause limb and facial defects in the first trimester and fetal intracerebral haemorrhage in the second and third trimesters. However, following delivery, people can choose to convert to warfarin (with the need for stabilization of the doses initially and frequent checks of the international normalized ratio) or remain on LMWH. Both warfarin and LMWH are safe in breastfeeding. Newer anticoagulants such as fondaparinux (a direct factor Xa inhibitor) and lepirudin (a direct thrombin inhibitor) are not licensed for use in pregnancy or breastfeeding. Graduated elastic stockings should be used for the initial treatment of DVT and should be worn for 2 years following a DVT to prevent post-thrombotic syndrome. Pregnant women with severe acute PE should be managed on an individual basis regarding the use of intravenous unfractionated heparin, thrombolytic therapy or thoracotomy and surgical embolectomy.

PREVENTION OF VENOUS THROMBOEMBOLISM IN PREGNANCY AND POST-PARTUM

The Royal College of Obstetricians and Gynaecologists (RCOG) has recently released updated guidelines on the prevention of thrombosis and embolism in pregnancy and the puerperium (Green-top Guideline No 37a, 2015) and these are summarized in **Figure 6.2**.

⊙⊶ KEY LEARNING POINTS

- Screening for thrombophilias should be carried out in those with a strong family or personal history of VTE.
- Rapid treatment of suspected VTE in pregnancy should be commenced while awaiting diagnosis.
- LMWHs are the treatment of choice.
- Graduated compression stockings should be fitted and worn for 2 years to reduce the incidence of post-thrombotic syndrome.
- Individuals with previous VTE should be offered pre-pregnancy counselling.

SUBSTANCE ABUSE IN PREGNANCY

Approximately one-third of adults who access drug services are of reproductive age. There are approximately 6,000 births to problem drug users in the UK each year (about 1% of all deliveries). Multidisciplinary care is often necessary to optimize outcomes because the financial, psychological, social and domestic problems associated with drug

---

BOX 6.4: Problems frequently encountered among drug addicts

- Social problems: housing, crime, children in care or abused.
- Coexistent addictions: alcohol and smoking.
- Malnutrition: especially iron and vitamins B and C.
- Risk of viral infections (e.g. human immunodeficiency virus (HIV), hepatitis B/C or other common sexually transmitted infections).
- Specific fetal and neonatal risks.

---

misuse are often greater than the physical and medical concerns.

Opioids, especially heroin, remain the most commonly used drugs in the UK, although many drug users take combinations of drugs that often include cocaine or crack cocaine. Amphetamines, benzodiazepines and cannabis are also common.

Most problem drug users smoke tobacco and are heavy users of alcohol and cannabis. Taking drugs in combination greatly increases the unpredictability of their effect on the user. Intravenous injection of drugs also puts drug users at greater risk of infection with blood-borne viruses (hepatitis B and C and HIV). Many drug users live in disadvantaged communities in conditions of poverty and social exclusion. Many have had poor parenting experiences, poor education and significant mental health problems. The aims of management are to stabilize the mother's drug-taking habits and ensure contact with social/care workers and psychiatric/drug liaison services as appropriate.

It is important not to try to reduce the opiate dose too rapidly in pregnancy. Sudden detoxification ('cold turkey') can be dangerous for the baby, especially in the third trimester when even mild withdrawal is associated with fetal stress, fetal distress and still-birth; the principle is to administer the lowest effective dose of methadone liquid in three divided doses every day.

Screening for infections such as hepatitis B and HIV is routinely offered in the UK. In many cases, multidisciplinary case conferences should be held to make arrangements and decisions for when the baby is delivered.

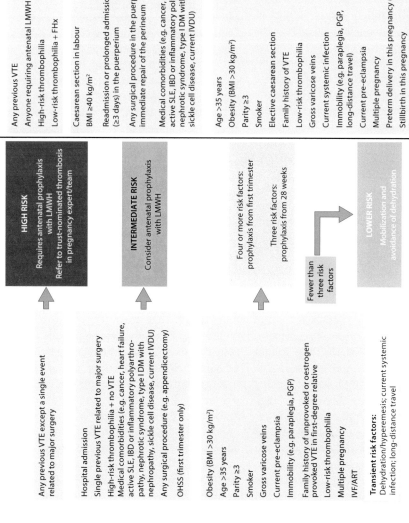

Antenatal assessment and management (to be assessed at booking and repeated if admitted)

Postnatal assessment and management (to be assessed on delivery suite)

HIGH RISK
Requires antenatal prophylaxis with LMWH
Refer to trust-nominated thrombosis in pregnancy expert/team

Any previous VTE except a single event related to major surgery

INTERMEDIATE RISK
Consider antenatal prophylaxis with LMWH

Hospital admission
Single previous VTE related to major surgery
High-risk thrombophilia + no VTE
Medical comorbidities (e.g. cancer, heart failure, active SLE, IBD or inflammatory polyarthro-pathy, nephrotic syndrome, type I DM with nephropathy, sickle cell disease, current IVDU)
Any surgical procedure (e.g. appendicectomy)
OHSS (first trimester only)

Four or more risk factors: prophylaxis from first trimester

Three risk factors: prophylaxis from 28 weeks

Obesity (BMI >30 kg/m²)
Age >35 years
Parity ≥3
Smoker
Gross varicose veins
Current pre-eclampsia
Immobility (e.g. paraplegia, PGP)
Family history of unprovoked or oestrogen provoked VTE in first-degree relative
Low-risk thrombophilia
Multiple pregnancy
IVF/ART

Transient risk factors:
Dehydration/hyperemesis; current systemic infection; long-distance travel

Fewer than three risk factors

LOWER RISK
Mobilization and avoidance of dehydration

HIGH RISK
At least 6 weeks' postnatal prophylactic LMWH

Any previous VTE
Anyone requiring antenatal LMWH
High-risk thrombophilia
Low-risk thrombophilia + FHx

INTERMEDIATE RISK
At least 10 days' postnatal prophylactic LMWH
NB If persisting or >3 risk factors consider extending thromboprophylaxis with LMWH

Caesarean section in labour
BMI ≥40 kg/m²
Readmission or prolonged admission (≥3 days) in the puerperium
Any surgical procedure in the puerperium except immediate repair of the perineum
Medical comorbidities (e.g. cancer, heart failure, active SLE, IBD or inflammatory polyarthropathy; nephrotic syndrome, type I DM with nephropathy, sickle cell disease, current IVDU)

Two or more risk factors

Age >35 years
Obesity (BMI >30 kg/m²)
Parity ≥3
Smoker
Elective caesarean section
Family history of VTE
Low-risk thrombophilia
Gross varicose veins
Current systemic infection
Immobility (e.g. paraplegia, PGP, long-distance travel)
Current pre-eclampsia
Multiple pregnancy
Preterm delivery in this pregnancy (<37 weeks)
Stillbirth in this pregnancy
Midcavity rotational or operative delivery
Prolonged labour (>24 hours)
PPH >1 litre or blood transfusion

Fewer than two risk factors

LOWER RISK
Early mobilization and avoidance of dehydration

Antenatal and postnatal prophylactic dose of LMWH
Weight <50 kg = 20 mg enoxaparin/2,500 units dalteparin/3,500 units tinzaparin daily
Weight 50–90 kg = 40 mg enoxaparin/5,000 units dalteparin/4,500 units tinzaparin daily
Weight 91–130 kg = 60 mg enoxaparin/7,500 units dalteparin/7,000 units tinzaparin daily
Weight 131–170 kg = 80 mg enoxaparin/10,000 units dalteparin/9,000 units tinzaparin daily
Weight >170 kg = 0.6 mg/kg/day enoxaparin/75 u/kg/day dalteparin/75 u/kg/day tinzaparin

APL, antiphospholipid antibodies (lupus anticoagulant, anticardiolipin antibodies, β₂-glycoprotein 1 antibodies); ART, assisted reproductive technology; BMI based on booking weight; DM, diabetes mellitus; FHx, family history; gross varicose veins, symptomatic; above knee or associated with phlebitis/oedema/skin changes; high-risk thrombophilia, antithrombin deficiency, protein C or S deficiency, compound or homozygous for low-risk thrombophilias; IBD, inflammatory bowel disease; immobility, ≥ 3 days; IVDU, intravenous drug user; IVF, *in vitro* fertilisation; LMWH, low-molecular-weight heparin; long-distance travel, >4 hours; low-risk thrombophilia, heterozygous for factor V Leiden or prothrombin G20210A mutations; OHSS, ovarian hyperstimulation syndrome; PGP, pelvic girdle pain with reduced mobility; PPH, postpartum haemorrhage; thrombophilia, inherited or acquired; VTE, venous thromboembolism.

Figure 6.2 Obstetric thromboprophylaxis risk assessment and management. (Adapted from RCOG (2015), Green-top Guideline No 37a.)

ALCOHOL

There is much debate about what a 'safe' dose of alcohol is during pregnancy. What is likely is that an intake of less than 100 g per week (approximately two drinks per day; for example, two medium glasses of wine or one pint of beer) is not associated with any adverse effects. Doses greater than this have been related to fetal growth restriction (FGR). Massive doses, in excess of 2 g/kg of body weight (17 drinks per day), have been associated with fetal alcohol syndrome. However, the syndrome is not seen consistently in infants born to heavy consumers of alcohol and occurs only in approximately 30–33% of children born to those who drink about 2 g/kg of body weight per day (equivalent to approximately 18 units of alcoholic drink per day). The differing susceptibility of fetuses to the syndrome is thought to be multifactorial and reflects the interplay of genetic factors, social deprivation, nutritional deficiencies and tobacco and other drug abuse, along with alcohol consumption.

If alcohol abuse is suspected, it may be necessary to involve social workers and arrange for formal psychiatric/addiction assessment. It is extremely difficult to 'test' for alcohol abuse, as even markers such as mean corpuscular volume and gamma-glutamyl transpeptidase (GGT) are not reliable in pregnancy. Malnutrition is very likely in heavy alcohol abuse and requires B vitamin supplements and iron. A common problem is that many of those who abuse alcohol and other drugs not only do not take their medicines but also default antenatal appointments.

SMOKING AND PREGNANCY

Smoking acutely reduces placental perfusion. Overall perinatal mortality is increased, babies are smaller at delivery and there is a higher risk of placental abruption in smokers than in non-smokers. It is estimated that a baby will weigh less than its target weight by a multiple of 15 g times the average number of cigarettes smoked per day; smoking fewer than five cigarettes per day has a barely discernible obstetric effect and quitting by 15 weeks' gestation reduces the risk as much as quitting before pregnancy. In the UK, it is now a recommended practice to offer and test carbon monoxide levels in addition to offering smoking cessation at booking and each subsequent visit, as a part of the Saving Babies Lives Care Bundle for maternity care.

OLIGOHYDRAMNIOS AND POLYHYDRAMNIOS

Amniotic fluid is produced almost exclusively from fetal urine from the second trimester onwards. It serves a vital function in protecting the developing baby from pressure or trauma, allowing limb movement (and hence normal postural development) and permitting the fetal lungs to expand and develop through breathing.

OLIGOHYDRAMNIOS

Too little amniotic fluid (oligohydramnios) is commonly defined as an amniotic fluid index (AFI) less than the 5th centile for gestation. The AFI is an ultrasound estimation of amniotic fluid derived by adding together the deepest vertical pool in four quadrants of the abdomen. The AFI (in cm) is therefore associated with some degree of error. In general, however, it is possible to differentiate subjectively on ultrasound between 'too much', 'too little' and 'normal looking'. Another objective assessment is to measure the deepest vertical pool and, if below the 5th centile, to then measure the AFI. Causes of oligohydramnios and anhydramnios are summarised in **Table 6.1**.

Oligohydramnios may be suspected antenatally following a history of clear fluid leaking from the vagina; this may represent PPROM (see **Chapter 8**). Clinically, on abdominal palpation, the fetal poles may be very obviously felt and 'hard', with a small-for-gestational age uterus.

The fetal prognosis depends on the cause of oligohydramnios, but both pulmonary hypoplasia and limb deformities (contractures, talipes) are common to severe early-onset (<24 weeks' gestation) oligohydramnios. Renal agenesis and bilateral multicystic kidneys carry a lethal prognosis, as life after birth is impossible without functioning kidneys. In this situation, the fetal lungs would probably be hypoplastic; this may also be true of severe urinary tract obstruction. Oligohydramnios due to FGR/uteroplacental insufficiency is usually of a less severe degree and less commonly causes limb and lung problems.

Table 6.1 Possible causes of oligohydramnios and anhydramnios

Too little production	Diagnosed by
Renal agenesis	Ultrasound: no renal tissue, no bladder
Multicystic kidneys	Ultrasound: enlarged kidneys with multiple cysts, no visible bladder
Urinary tract abnormality/obstruction	Ultrasound: kidneys may be present, but urinary tract dilatation
FGR and placental insufficiency	Clinical: reduced SFH, reduced fetal movements, possibly abnormal CTG Ultrasound: FGR, abnormal fetal Doppler wave forms
Drugs (e.g. NSAIDs)	Withholding NSAIDs may allow amniotic fluid to reaccumulate
Congenital infections	Ultrasound: other structural defects
Post-term pregnancy	Clinical: reduced SFH, reduced fetal movements, possibly abnormal CTG Ultrasound: possibly FGR, abnormal fetal Doppler wave forms, reduced liquor
PPROM	Speculum examination: pool of amniotic fluid on posterior blade

CTG, cardiotocography; FGR, fetal growth restriction; NSAID, non-steroidal anti-inflammatory drug; PPROM, preterm premature rupture of membranes; SFH, symphysis–fundal height.

POLYHYDRAMNIOS

Polyhydramnios is the term given to an excess of amniotic fluid (i.e. AFI >95th centile for gestation on ultrasound estimation). It may present as severe abdominal swelling and discomfort. On examination, the abdomen will appear distended out of proportion to the gestation (increased symphysis–fundal height [SFH]). Furthermore, the abdomen may be tense and tender and the fetal poles will be hard to palpate. The condition may be caused by maternal, placental or fetal conditions, and if severe or increasing polyhydramnios, may precipitate preterm labour.

BOX 6.5: Causes of polyhydramnios

Maternal
- Diabetes
- Placental (e.g. chorioangioma)
- Arteriovenous fistula

Fetal
- Multiple gestation (in monochorionic twins, it may be twin-to-twin transfusion syndrome)
- Idiopathic
- Oesophageal atresia/tracheo-oesophageal fistula
- Duodenal atresia
- Neuromuscular fetal condition (preventing swallowing)
- Anencephaly
- Fetal congenital infections or chromosomal abnormalities/genetic syndromes

The management of polyhydramnios is directed towards establishing the cause (and hence determining fetal prognosis), relieving the discomfort of the mother (if necessary by amniodrainage) and assessing the risk of preterm labour due to uterine overdistension.

Polyhydramnios due to diabetes needs urgent investigation, as it often suggests high blood glucose levels. In this context, polyhydramnios should correct itself when glycaemic control is optimized.

Twin-to-twin transfusion syndrome is a rare cause of acute polyhydramnios in the recipient sac of monochorionic twins. It is associated with oligohydramnios and a small baby in the other sac. The condition may be rapidly fatal for both twins; amniodrainage and removal by fetoscopic laser ablation of the placental vascular connections are two therapeutic modalities employed in dealing with this condition. This is discussed further in **Chapter 7**.

FETAL MALPRESENTATION AT TERM

Malpresentation is a presentation that is not cephalic. Breech presentation is the most commonly encountered malpresentation and occurs in 3–4% of term pregnancies, but is more common at earlier gestations.

Similarly, oblique and transverse positions are not uncommon antenatally. They become a problem only if the baby (or first presenting baby in a multiple gestation) is not cephalic by 37 weeks' gestation.

BREECH PRESENTATION

There are three types of breech: the most common is extended (frank) breech (**Figure 6.3A**), less common is a flexed (complete) breech (**Figure 6.3B**) and least common is footling breech, in which a foot presents at the cervix (**Figure 6.3C**). Cord and foot prolapse are risks in this situation.

ANTENATAL MANAGEMENT OF BREECH PRESENTATION

If a breech presentation is clinically suspected at or after 36 weeks, this should be confirmed by ultrasound scan. The scan should document fetal biometry, amniotic fluid volume, the placental site and the position of the fetal legs, and look for any anomalies previously undetected.

> **BOX 6.6: Predisposing factors for breech presentation**
>
> **Maternal**
> - Fibroids
> - Congenital uterine abnormalities (e.g. bicornuate uterus)
> - Uterine surgery
>
> **Fetal/placental**
> - Multiple gestation
> - Prematurity
> - Placenta praevia
> - Abnormality (e.g. anencephaly or hydrocephalus)
> - Fetal neuromuscular condition
> - Oligohydramnios
> - Polyhydramnios

The three management options available at this point should be discussed with the pregnant woman. These are external cephalic version (ECV), vaginal breech delivery and elective caesarean section. A previous large multicentre randomized controlled trial suggested that planned vaginal delivery of a breech

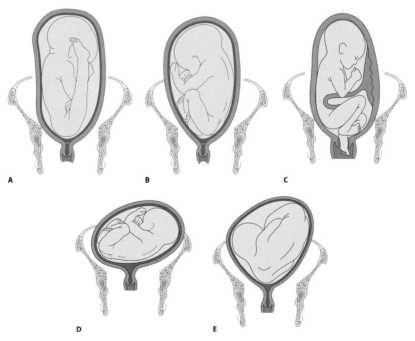

Figure 6.3 (**A**) Frank breech (also known as extended breech) presentation with extension of the legs. (**B**) Breech presentation with flexion of the legs. (**C**) Footling breech presentation. (**D**) Transverse lie. (**E**) Oblique lie.

presentation is associated with a 3% increased risk of death or serious morbidity to the baby. Although this trial did not evaluate long-term outcomes, it has led to the recommendation that the best method of delivering a term breech singleton is by planned caesarean section. Despite this, either by choice or as a result of precipitous labour, a small proportion of pregnant women with breech presentations will opt to deliver vaginally. It therefore remains important that clinicians and hospitals are prepared for vaginal breech delivery.

EXTERNAL CEPHALIC VERSION

ECV is a relatively straightforward and safe technique for singleton breech pregnancies and has been shown to reduce the number of caesarean sections due to breech presentations. Success rates vary according to the experience of the operator but, in most units, are around 50% (and are higher in the multiparous population who tend to have lax abdominal musculature).

The procedure is performed at or after 37 completed weeks' gestation by an experienced obstetrician at or near delivery facilities. ECV should be performed with a tocolytic (e.g. nifedipine) to improve the success rate. The pregnant woman is laid flat with a left lateral tilt, having ensured that she has emptied her bladder and is comfortable. With ultrasound guidance, the breech is elevated from the pelvis and one hand is used to manipulate this upwards in the direction of a forwards roll while the other hand applies gentle pressure to flex the fetal head and bring it down to the pelvis (**Figure 6.4**).

The procedure can be mildly uncomfortable for the patient and should last no more than 10 minutes. If the procedure fails, or becomes difficult, it is abandoned. A fetal heart rate trace must be performed before and after the procedure and it is important to administer anti-D if the patient is rhesus negative.

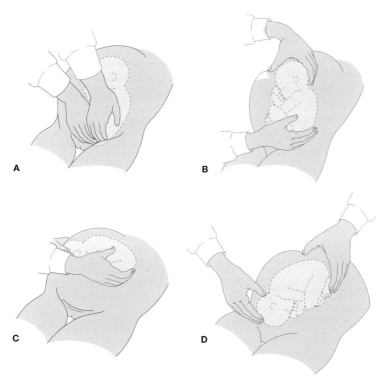

Figure 6.4 External cephalic version. (**A**) The breech is disengaged from the pelvic inlet. (**B**) Version is usually performed in the direction that increases flexion of the fetus and makes it do a forwards somersault. (**C**) On completion of version, the head is often not engaged for a time. (**D**) The fetal heart rate should be checked after the external version has been completed.

to be adequate and an estimated fetal weight of <3,500 g (ultrasound or clinical measurement).

- There should be no evidence of hyperextension of the fetal head, and fetal abnormalities that would preclude safe vaginal delivery (e.g. severe hydrocephalus) should be excluded.

Management of labour

- Fetal well-being and progress of labour should be carefully monitored.
- An epidural analgesia is not essential but may be advantageous; it can prevent pushing before full dilatation.
- Fetal blood sampling from the buttocks may be considered but used with caution. FBS may provide an accurate assessment of the acid–base status (when the fetal heart rate trace is suspect).
- There should be an operator experienced in delivering breech babies available in the hospital.

Although much emphasis is placed on adequate case selection prior to labour, a survey of outcomes of undiagnosed breech presentations in labour managed by experienced medical staff showed that safe vaginal delivery can be achieved.

Technique

A vaginal breech delivery should be characterized by 'masterly inactivity' (hands-off). Problems are more likely to arise when the obstetrician tries to speed up the process by pulling on the baby, and this should be avoided.

Delivery of the buttocks

In most circumstances, full dilatation and descent of the breech will have occurred naturally. When the buttocks become visible and begin to distend the perineum, preparations for the delivery are made. The buttocks will lie in the anterior–posterior diameter. Once the anterior buttock is delivered and the anus is seen over the fourchette (and no sooner than this), an episiotomy can be cut.

Delivery of the legs and lower body

If the legs are flexed, they will deliver spontaneously. If extended, they may need to be delivered using the Pinard manoeuvre. This entails using a finger to flex

MODE OF DELIVERY

If ECV fails, or is contraindicated, and caesarean section is not indicated for other reasons, then pregnant women should be counselled regarding elective caesarean section and planned vaginal delivery. Although evidence suggests that it is probably safer for breech babies to be delivered by caesarean section, there is still a place for a vaginal breech delivery in certain circumstances. Individual choice and the failure to detect breech presentation until very late in labour mean that obstetricians need to be expert in the skills of breech vaginal delivery and aware of the potential complications.

PRE-REQUISITES FOR VAGINAL BREECH DELIVERY

Feto-maternal

- The presentation should be either extended (hips flexed, knees extended) or flexed (hips flexed, knees flexed but feet not below the fetal buttocks).
- There should be no evidence of feto-pelvic disproportion with a pelvis clinically thought

the leg at the knee and then extend at the hip, first anteriorly then posteriorly. With contractions and maternal effort, the lower body will be delivered. Usually a loop of cord is drawn down to ensure that it is not too short.

Delivery of the shoulders

The baby will be lying with the shoulders in the transverse diameter of the pelvic midcavity. As the anterior shoulder rotates into the anterior–posterior diameter, the spine or the scapula will become visible. At this point, a finger gently placed above the shoulder will help to deliver the arm. As the posterior arm/shoulder reaches the pelvic floor, it too will rotate anteriorly (in the opposite direction). Once the spine becomes visible, delivery of the second arm will follow. This can be imagined as a 'rocking boat' with one side moving upwards and then the other. The Lovset manoeuvre essentially copies these natural movements (**Figure 6.5**). However, it is unnecessary

and meddlesome to do routinely (one risks pulling the shoulders down but leaving the arms higher up, alongside the head).

Delivery of the head

The head is delivered using the Mauriceau–Smellie–Veit manoeuvre: the baby lies on the obstetrician's arm with downward traction being levelled on the head via a finger in the mouth and one on each maxilla (**Figure 6.6**). Delivery occurs with first downwards and then upwards movement (as with instrumental deliveries). If this manoeuvre proves difficult, forceps need to be applied. An assistant holds the baby's body upwards while the forceps are applied in the usual manner (**Figure 6.7**).

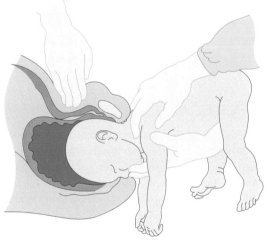

Figure 6.6 Mauriceau–Smellie–Veit manoeuvre for delivery of the head.

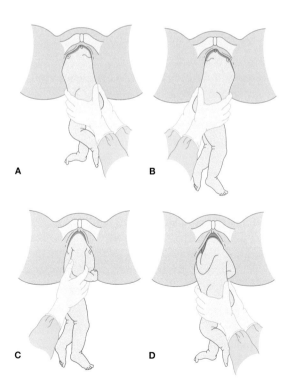

Figure 6.5 Lovset manoeuvre. (**A**) Turning the infant to bring down the anterior shoulder. (**B**) Downward traction and descent of shoulders along the midline (sacral-pubic) axis. (**C**) Delivering the anterior arm and shoulder. (**D**) Delivering the posterior arm and shoulder.

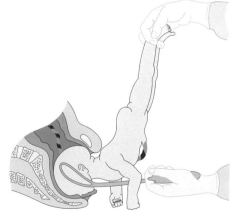

Figure 6.7 Delivery of the aftercoming head with forceps.

93

Complications

The greatest fear with a vaginal breech is that the baby will get 'stuck'. Interference in the natural process by the inappropriate use of oxytocic agents or by trying to pull the baby out (breech extraction) will paradoxically increase the risk of obstruction occurring. When delay occurs, particularly with delivery of the shoulders or head, the presence of an experienced obstetrician will reduce the risk of death or serious injury.

> ### ⊙━ KEY LEARNING POINTS
>
> - Breech presentation: ECV should be offered at 36–37 weeks in selected individuals.
> - Elective caesarean section is safer than vaginal delivery for a baby presenting by the breech at or close to term.
> - Planned or unexpected vaginal breech deliveries should be attended by experienced clinicians.

OTHER FETAL MALPRESENTATIONS

A transverse lie occurs when the fetal long axis lies perpendicular to that of the maternal long axis and classically results in a shoulder presentation (see **Figure 6.3D**). An oblique lie occurs when the long axis of the fetal body crosses the long axis of the maternal body at an angle close to 45° (see **Figure 6.3E**).

Anyone presenting at term with a transverse or oblique lie is at potential risk of cord prolapse following spontaneous rupture of the membranes, and prolapse of the hand, shoulder or foot once in labour. In most cases, the pregnant woman is multiparous with a lax uterus and abdominal wall musculature, and gentle version of the baby's head in the clinic or on the ward will restore the presentation to cephalic. If this does not occur or the lie is unstable (alternating between transverse, oblique and longitudinal), it is important to think of possible uterine or fetal causes of this.

The diagnosis of transverse or oblique lie might be suspected by abdominal inspection: the abdomen often appears asymmetrical. The SFH may be less than expected and, on palpation, the fetal head or buttocks may be in the iliac fossa. Palpation over the pelvic brim will reveal an 'empty' pelvis.

It goes without saying that labour with the baby's lie anything other than longitudinal will not result in a vaginal birth; this is one situation in which, if caesarean section is not performed, both the pregnant woman and the baby are at considerable risk of morbidity and mortality. The only exception to this is for exceptionally preterm or small babies, where vaginal delivery may occur irrespective of lie or presentation.

A pregnant woman with an unstable lie at term should be admitted to the antenatal ward. The normal plan would be to deliver by caesarean section if the presentation is not cephalic in early labour or if spontaneous rupture of the membranes occurs. In the multiparous, an unstable lie will often correct itself in early labour (as long as the membranes are intact).

POST-TERM PREGNANCY

A pregnancy that has extended to or beyond 42+0 weeks' gestation is defined as a prolonged or post-term pregnancy. Accurate dating remains essential for the correct diagnosis and should ideally involve a first-trimester ultrasound estimation of crown–rump length.

Post-term pregnancy affects approximately 10% of all pregnancies and the aetiology is unknown. Post-term pregnancy is associated with increased risks to both the fetus and the mother, including an increased risk of stillbirth and perinatal death, and prolonged labour and caesarean section.

Fetal surveillance and induction of labour are two strategies employed that may reduce the risk of adverse outcome. Unfortunately, there are no known tests that can accurately predict fetal outcome post-term; an ultrasound scan may give temporary reassurance if the amniotic fluid and fetal growth are normal. Similarly, a CTG should be performed at and after 42 weeks.

Immediate induction of labour or delivery post-term should take place if there is:

- reduced amniotic fluid on scan
- reduction in fetal growth
- reduced fetal movements
- abnormal CTG
- maternal hypertension or any other medical or obstetric complication

Induction of labour is discussed further in **Chapter 12**.

When counselling the parents regarding waiting for labour to start naturally after 42 weeks, it is important that the pregnant woman is aware that no test can guarantee the safety of the baby and that perinatal mortality is increased (at least twofold) beyond 42 weeks. A labour induced post-term is more likely to require caesarean section; this may partly be due to the reluctance of the uterus to contract properly and the possible compromise of the baby leading to abnormal CTG. NICE recommends regular surveillance with ultrasound and CTG when patients chose to continue the pregnancy beyond 42+0 weeks, after informed discussion.

VAGINAL BLEEDING IN PREGNANCY

Bleeding in pregnancy is common but invariably causes anxiety. It should always be investigated to rule out significant and dangerous causes; in many cases of minor bleeding, a cause is never found.

Vaginal bleeding at less than 24 weeks' gestation is defined as a threatened miscarriage and the causes and management are described in more detail in **Chapter 5** of *Gynaecology by Ten Teachers*, 21st Edition. Vaginal bleeding from 24 weeks to delivery of the baby is defined as an antepartum haemorrhage (APH). The causes of APH are placental or local. The incidence of APH is 3%. It is estimated that 1% is attributable to placenta praevia, 1% is attributable to placental abruption and the remaining 1% is from other causes.

BOX 6.9: Causes of APH

Placental causes
- Placental abruption
- Placenta praevia
- Vasa praevia

Local causes
- Cervicitis
- Cervical ectropion
- Cervical carcinoma
- Cervical polyp
- Vaginal trauma
- Vaginal infection

APH must always be taken seriously, and anyone presenting with a history of fresh vaginal bleeding must be investigated promptly and properly. The key questions are whether the bleeding is placental and whether the bleeding is compromising the pregnant woman and/or fetus. A pale, tachycardic pregnant woman looking anxious with a painful, firm abdomen, underwear soaked in fresh blood or blood/staining along the legs, and reduced fetal movements needs emergency assessment and management for a possible placental abruption. A pregnant woman having had a small post-coital bleed with no systemic signs or symptoms represents a different end of the spectrum.

HISTORY

- How much bleeding is there?
- Triggering factors (e.g. post-coital bleed)
- Is the bleeding associated with pain or contractions?
- Is the baby moving?
- Last cervical smear (date and normal or abnormal)
- Is there known vasa praevia (bleeding in such scenarios risks severe fetal compromise)?

EXAMINATION

- Pulse, blood pressure
- Is the uterus soft or tender and firm?
- Fetal heart auscultation/CTG
- Speculum vaginal examination, with particular importance placed on visualizing the cervix (having established that placenta is not a praevia, preferably using a portable ultrasound machine)

INVESTIGATIONS

- Depending on the degree of bleeding, full blood count, clotting and, if suspected praevia/abruption, cross-match 6 units of blood
- Ultrasound (fetal size, presentation, amniotic fluid, placental position and morphology)

MANAGEMENT

If there is minimal bleeding and the cause is clearly local vaginal bleeding, symptomatic management may be given (e.g. antifungal preparations for candidiasis), as long as there is reasonable certainty that cervical carcinoma is excluded by smear history and direct visualization of the cervix. The management of significant APH is described in detail in **Chapter 14**.

RHESUS ISOIMMUNIZATION

Blood groups are defined in two ways. First, there is the ABO group, allowing four different permutations of blood group (O, A, B and AB). Second, there is the rhesus system, which consists of C, D and E antigens. The importance of these blood group systems is that a mismatch between the fetus and mother can mean that, when fetal red cells pass across to the maternal circulation, as they do to a greater or lesser extent during pregnancy, sensitization of the maternal immune system to these fetal 'foreign' red blood cells may occur and subsequently give rise to haemolytic disease of the fetus and newborn (HDFN). The rhesus system is the one most commonly associated with severe haemolytic disease.

AETIOLOGY OF RHESUS DISEASE

The rhesus system comprises at least 40 antigens, the most clinically important of which are C, D and E. They are coded on two adjacent genes that sit within chromosome 1. One gene codes for antigen polypeptides C/c and E/e while the other codes for the D polypeptide (rhesus antigen). The d (little d) antigen has not been identified, so it is probable that individuals who are D negative lack the antigen altogether, as opposed to those with c (little c) or e (little e), where c is the allelic antigen of C and e is the allelic antigen of E. Antigen expression is usually dominant, whereas those who have a negative phenotype are either homozygous for the recessive allele or have a deletion of that gene (**Figure 6.8**). In practice, only anti-D and anti-c regularly cause HDFN and anti-D is much more common than anti-c.

The occurrence of HDFN as a result of rhesus isoimmunization involves three key stages (**Figure 6.9**). First, a rhesus-negative mother must conceive a baby who has inherited the rhesus-positive

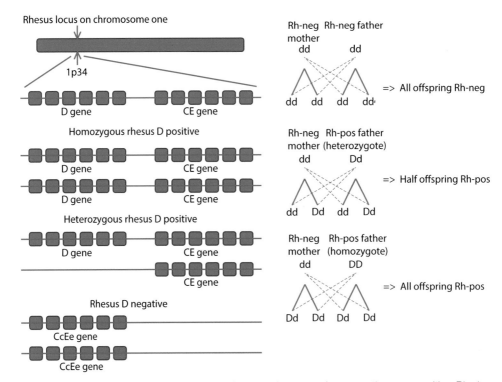

Figure 6.8 The parental genotype determinants of rhesus phenotype. (neg, negative; pos, positive; Rh, rhesus.)

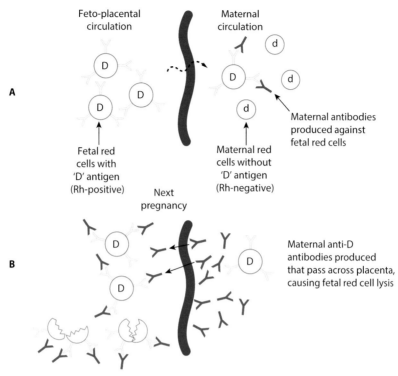

Figure 6.9 The mechanism of rhesus sensitization (**A**) and fetal red cell destruction (**B**). (Rh, rhesus.)

phenotype from the father. Second, fetal cells must gain access to the maternal circulation in a sufficient volume to provoke a maternal antibody response. Finally, maternal antibodies must cross the placenta and cause immune destruction of red cells in the fetus.

Rhesus disease does not affect a first pregnancy, as the primary response is usually weak and consists primarily of immunoglobulin (Ig)M antibodies that do not cross the placenta. However, in a subsequent pregnancy with a rhesus-positive baby, rhesus-positive red cells pass from the baby to the maternal circulation and cause maternal resensitization (see **Figure 6.9**). On this occasion, the B-cells produce a much larger response, this time of IgG antibodies that can cross the placenta to the fetal circulation. If these antibodies are present in sufficient quantities, fetal haemolysis may occur, leading to such severe anaemia that the fetus may die unless a transfusion is performed.

PREVALENCE OF RHESUS DISEASE

The prevalence of D-rhesus negativity is 15% in the UK Caucasian population, but lower in all other ethnic groups. Approximately 55% of UK Caucasian males are heterozygous for the D antigen; therefore, around two-thirds of rhesus-negative mothers would be expected to carry a rhesus-positive fetus. Rhesus disease is most common in countries where anti-D prophylaxis is not widespread, such as the Middle East and Russia.

BOX 6.10: Potential sensitizing events for rhesus disease

- Miscarriage
- Termination of pregnancy
- APH
- Invasive prenatal testing (chorion villus sampling, amniocentesis and cordocentesis)
- Delivery

PREVENTING RHESUS ISOIMMUNIZATION

The process of isoimmunization can be prevented by the intramuscular administration of anti-D immunoglobulins to a mother. Anti-D immunoglobulins 'mop up' any circulating rhesus-positive cells before an immune response is excited in the mother. It is normal practice to administer anti-D as soon as possible after any potential sensitizing events that may cause feto-maternal haemorrhage and preferably within 72 hours of exposure to fetal red cells. However, if, exceptionally, this deadline cannot be met, some protection may still be offered if anti-D Ig is given up to 10 days after the sensitizing event. The exact dose is determined by the gestation at which sensitization has occurred and the size of the feto-maternal haemorrhage. A Kleihauer test of maternal blood determines the proportion of fetal cells present in the maternal sample. It relies on the ability of fetal red blood cells to resist denaturation by alcohol or acid and it allows calculation of the size of the feto-maternal transfusion and the amount of extra anti-D Ig required.

BOX 6.11: Management of sensitizing events in the rhesus-negative pregnant woman

- In the first trimester of pregnancy, because the volume of fetal blood is so small, it is unlikely that sensitization would occur, and anti-D is only indicated following ectopic pregnancy, molar pregnancy, therapeutic termination of pregnancy and in cases of uterine bleeding where this is repeated, heavy or associated with abdominal pain. The dose that should be given is 250 IU.
- For potentially sensitizing events between 12 and 20 weeks' gestation, a minimum dose of 250 IU should be administered within 72 hours of the event and a Kleihauer test should be performed. Further anti-D can be given if indicated by the Kleihauer test.
- For potentially sensitizing events after 20 weeks' gestation, a Kleihauer test is required and, pending the result, a minimum anti-D Ig dose of 500 IU should be administered within 72 hours of the event. Further anti-D can be given if indicated by the Kleihauer test.

A small number of rhesus-negative individuals become sensitized during pregnancy despite the administration of anti-D at delivery and without a clinically obvious sensitizing event. The likelihood is that a small feto-maternal haemorrhage occurs without any obvious clinical signs; therefore, prophylactic anti-D would reduce the risk of isoimmunization from this event. Current UK guidelines suggest that all rhesus-negative pregnant women who have not been previously sensitized should be offered routine antenatal prophylaxis with anti-D, either with a single-dose regimen at around 28 weeks or a two-dose regimen given at 28 and 34 weeks' gestation.

BOX 6.12: Signs of fetal anaemia

Note: Clinical and ultrasound features of fetal anaemia do not usually become evident unless fetal haemoglobin is more than 5 g/dL less than the mean for gestation or the fetal haemoglobin is less than 6 g/dL.

- Polyhydramnios
- Enlarged fetal heart
- Ascites and pericardial effusions
- Hyperdynamic fetal circulation (can be detected by Doppler ultrasound by measuring increased velocities in the middle cerebral artery or aorta)
- Reduced fetal movements
- Abnormal CTG with reduced variability, eventually a 'sinusoidal' trace

MANAGEMENT OF RHESUS DISEASE IN A SENSITIZED PREGNANT WOMAN

Once a pregnant woman who is D-rhesus negative has been sensitized to the D-rhesus antigen, no amount of anti-D will ever turn the clock back. In a subsequent pregnancy, close surveillance is required. Rhesus disease gets worse with successive pregnancies, so it is important to note the severity of the disease in previous pregnancies. The management depends on the clinical scenario.

The father of the next baby is D-rhesus negative. In this situation, there is no risk that the baby will be D-rhesus positive and therefore there is no chance of rhesus disease.

The father of the next baby is D-rhesus positive. He may be heterozygous and, in this situation, determining the paternal phenotype is useful in anticipating the likely fetal phenotype and, thus, the potential for development of HDFN. However, it is important to bear in mind that there are issues regarding paternal testing, and assuming paternity runs the risk of false prediction. Notwithstanding this issue, paternal blood grouping is frequently used and often useful. In addition, non-invasive fetal blood group genotyping using cell-free fetal deoxyribonucleic acid (cffDNA) from maternal blood samples taken between 16 and 25 weeks' gestation have made it possible to determine the fetal rhesus genotype type and this is now recommended for the risk assessment and subsequent surveillance plan of the fetus at risk of HDFN.

In a sensitized pregnant woman, if the father is D-rhesus positive or unknown, standard management involves monitoring antibody levels every 2–4 weeks from booking. Antibody levels or quantity can be described using the titre or by using international units (IU) as a standard quantification method. The titre simply refers to the number of times a sample has been diluted before the amount of antibody becomes undetectable; titre of 2, 4, 8, 16, 32, 64, 128, etc. Each time a sample is tested, it should be checked in parallel with the previous sample to ensure the detection of significant changes in the antibody level. However, titrations of anti-D do not correlate well with the development of HDFN, and the standard quantification method (IU/mL) gives more clinically relevant levels (**Table 6.2**).

If antibody levels rise, the baby should be examined for signs of anaemia. In the past, the bilirubin concentration of amniotic fluid was determined optically to give an indirect measure of fetal haemolysis. This involved an invasive procedure with the attendant risks of miscarriage/preterm labour and further boosting of the alloimmune response. Now, middle cerebral artery (MCA) Doppler peak systolic velocity (PSV) measurements are used to correlate reliably with fetal anaemia. The sensitivity

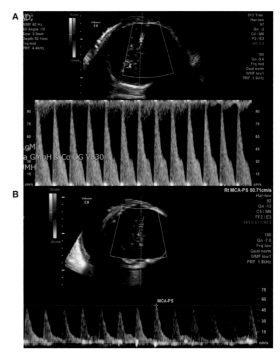

Figure 6.10 Middle cerebral artery Doppler waveform analysis of (**A**) a fetus with anaemia secondary to rhesus disease demonstrating an increased peak systolic velocity and (**B**) the same fetus 48 hours following an intrauterine transfusion.

of MCA PSV is reported at 100% with a false-positive rate of 12% (**Figure 6.10**).

A fetus with a raised MCA PSV has a high probability of anaemia. These cases are not common and the treatment should be in, or guided by, tertiary fetal medicine centres. Treatment options include delivery (if later gestation) or intrauterine transfusion (IUT). Delivery of an anaemic, rapidly haemolysing premature baby is a significant risk and should not be undertaken lightly, and must take place in a unit where adequate neonatal expertise is available, and generally not be before 36–37 weeks' gestation, unless there are specific reasons, such as no available expertise for IUT.

IUT is life-saving in a severely anaemic fetus that is too premature for delivery to be contemplated. The aim is to restore haemoglobin levels, reversing or preventing hydrops or death. A side effect is that transfusion will also suppress fetal erythropoiesis, which reduces the concentration of antigen-positive cells available for haemolysis. Blood can be

Table 6.2 Anti-D-rhesus titration

Anti-D level	Outcome
<4 IU/mL	HDFN unlikely
4–15 IU/mL	Moderate risk of HDFN
>15 IU/mL	High risk of hydrops fetalis

HDFN, haemolytic disease of the fetus and newborn.

transfused into a fetus in various ways depending on the gestation, the site of the cord insertion and the clinical situation. Routes of administration include:

- umbilical vein at the point of the cord insertion (ideally through the placenta and not through the amniotic sac)
- intrahepatic vein
- peritoneal cavity (not as effective but some blood is absorbed and this may be the only option, for example in early gestations)
- fetal heart

Once a decision has been made that the fetus is severely anaemic and requires a blood transfusion, the invasive procedure aims to first take a sample to confirm the anaemia and then infuse the blood during a single puncture.

Transfused blood is:

- rhesus-D negative
- cross-matched with a maternal sample
- densely packed (haemoglobin usually around 30 g/L) so that small volumes are used
- white cell depleted and irradiated
- screened for infection including cytomegalovirus

AT DELIVERY

If the baby is known to be anaemic or has had multiple transfusions, a neonatologist must be present at delivery should exchange transfusion be required. Blood must therefore always be ready for the delivery. All babies born to rhesus-negative individuals should have cord blood taken at delivery for a blood count, blood group and indirect Coombs test.

ABO INCOMPATIBILITY

ABO blood group isoimmunization may occur when the mother is blood group O and the baby is blood group A or B. Anti-A and anti-B antibodies are present in the maternal circulation naturally, usually secondary to sensitization against A or B substances in food or bacteria. This means that ABO incompatibility may occur in a first pregnancy. In this situation, anti-A or anti-B antibodies may pass to the fetal circulation, causing fetal haemolysis and anaemia. However, most anti-A and anti-B antibodies are mainly IgMs that do

> ### 🔑 KEY LEARNING POINTS
>
> - Rhesus disease gets worse with successive pregnancies.
> - If the father of the fetus is rhesus negative, the fetus cannot be rhesus positive.
> - If the father of the fetus is rhesus positive, he may be a heterozygote (50% likelihood that the baby is D-rhesus positive) or a homozygote (100% likelihood).
> - Non-invasive prenatal testing for fetal D genotype in pregnancy is now recommended for risk assessment of the fetus for HDFN.
> - Anti-D is given only as prophylaxis and is useless once sensitization has occurred.
> - Prenatal diagnosis for karyotype or attempts at determining fetal blood group by invasive testing (e.g. chorion villus sampling) may make the antibody levels higher in those who are already sensitized.

not cross the placenta. In addition, A and B antigens are not fully developed in the fetus. Therefore, ABO incompatibility generally causes mild haemolytic disease of the baby, but may sometimes explain unexpected jaundice in an otherwise healthy term infant.

NEW DEVELOPMENTS

When a fetus is at risk of HDFN in a sensitized rhesus-negative mother, the genotype of the fetus is very important. When the father is heterozygous for rhesus-D, there is a 50% chance that the fetus will be rhesus positive. In this situation, it is important to establish the fetal blood group to determine whether or not the baby is at risk. This can now be done non-invasively by examining cffDNA present in a maternal blood sample. Accuracies close to 100% are reported for rhesus genotyping.

A similar approach can be used to prevent unnecessary prophylaxis. Currently in the UK, all rhesus-negative pregnant women are offered anti-D. However, the disadvantage of this approach is that approximately 40% of D-negative people who are carrying a rhesus-negative child will be given routine prophylactic anti-D unnecessarily. This equates to approximately 40,000 pregnant women in the UK who are receiving prophylaxis unnecessarily each year. Fetal blood group genotyping using cffDNA from maternal blood samples taken between 16 and 25 weeks' gestation have made it possible to determine the fetal rhesus genotype type. Routine fetal rhesus typing for all rhesus-negative pregnant women has been introduced in Denmark and the Netherlands to allow selective use of anti-D, and is being widely adopted in the UK.

FURTHER READING

Qureshi H, Massey E, Kirwan D, et al. (2014). BCSH guideline for the use of anti-D immunoglobulin for the prevention of haemolytic disease of the fetus and newborn. *Transfusion Medicine*, 24:8–20. https://doi.org/10.1111/tme.12091.

RCOG (1999). Green-top guideline No 20b: The management of breech presentation. https://www.rcog.org.uk/globalassets/documents/guidelines/gtg-no-20b-breech-presentation.pdf.

RCOG (2006). Green-top guideline No 20a: External cephalic version and reducing the incidence of breech presentation. https://www.rcog.org.uk/globalassets/documents/guidelines/gt20aexternalcephalicversion.pdf.

RCOG (2015). Green-top guideline No 37a: Reducing the risk of venous thromboembolism during pregnancy and the puerperium. https://www.rcog.org.uk/globalassets/documents/guidelines/gtg-37a.pdf.

SELF-ASSESSMENT

For interactive SBAs and EMQs relating to this chapter, visit www.routledge.com/cw/mccarthy.

CASE HISTORY

The community midwife refers a 25-year-old woman in her second pregnancy to the antenatal clinic at 37 weeks' gestation. Clinical examination has shown the fetus to be in a breech position. An ultrasound scan confirms an extended breech presentation. You are asked to counsel this woman as to the possible options that are available for her management.

A What are the available options?
B What are the advantages and risks of each option?

ANSWERS

A There are three available management options that need to be discussed with this woman. These are:
1. elective caesarean section
2. ECV
3. vaginal breech delivery
B First, a brief history should be taken to determine whether there are any factors in the history that would be a contraindication to vaginal breech delivery or ECV.

The Term Breech Trial demonstrated that there was reduction in the perinatal mortality and morbidity with elective caesarean section over vaginal breech delivery. However, there are some factors that would increase and decrease the strength of the recommendation for a caesarean section, such as previous obstetric history and the presence of a large or small baby (an ultrasound will help with this).

ECV is carried out at 36–37 weeks' gestation, but can be done as far as in early labour (with intact membranes). The procedure has been shown to reduce the number of caesarean sections due to breech presentation. Contraindications to ECV are placenta praevia, oligohydramnios, previous caesarean section, multiple gestation and pre-eclampsia. The risks of the procedure, which need to be outlined, are placental abruption, premature rupture of the membranes, cord accident, transplacental haemorrhage and fetal bradycardia.

Vaginal breech delivery is still an acceptable option if the mother understands the increased risks to the fetus. There are a number of factors that increase the likelihood of a successful vaginal beech delivery: normal sized baby, flexed neck, multiparous, deeply engaged breech and positive mental attitude of the woman.

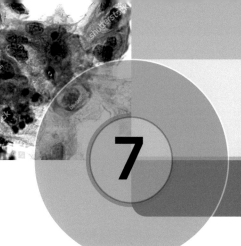

Multiple pregnancy

7

ASMA KHALIL

Learning Objectives
- Understand the classification of multiple pregnancies.
- Understand the risk factors for multiple pregnancies and why the prevalence has increased.
- Understand the increased complications that occur in multiple pregnancies.
- Understand the antenatal care in the presence of a multiple pregnancy.

INTRODUCTION

Up until 2014, the rates of multiple pregnancies were reported to be rising globally, such that 1 in every 29 births in the USA was a twin birth. This high prevalence of multiple pregnancy was attributed predominantly to advancing age in the pregnant population and increasing use of assisted fertility techniques, with rates of multiple pregnancy being directly proportional to the number of embryos transferred. Recently, the rates of multiple births have shown a declining trend owing to advancement in in vitro fertilization (IVF) techniques and guidelines from regulatory bodies advising single embryo transfer. Regardless of chorionicity and amnionicity, complications in multiple pregnancies are higher than for singleton pregnancies and include preterm birth, fetal growth restriction (FGR), cerebral palsy and

stillbirth. The maternal risks are also increased and include hypertensive and thromboembolic disease and antepartum and post-partum haemorrhage.

EPIDEMIOLOGY

The incidence of multiple pregnancy varies worldwide, with rates varying from approximately 6 per 1,000 births in Japan to rates of approximately 40 per 1,000 births in Nigeria. In the UK, the rates of multiple pregnancy are approximately 16 per 1,000 births. The majority (97–99%) of these are twin pregnancies, with the remainder being predominantly triplet pregnancies. Increasing maternal age is one of the key risk factors for multiple pregnancy, with multiple pregnancy occurring in approximately 1 in 10 individuals aged over 45 giving birth in the UK. Assisted conception is also responsible for the

10.1201/9781003196112-7

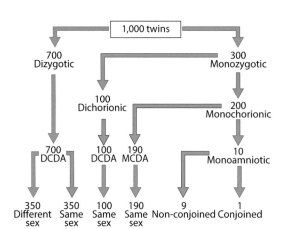

Figure 7.1 Incidence of monozygotic and dizygotic twin pregnancies. (DCDA, dichorionic diamniotic; MCDA, monochorionic diamniotic.)

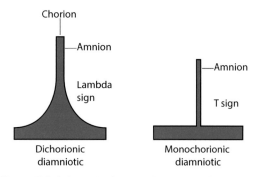

Figure 7.2 Schematic diagram showing chorionicity in dichorionic and monochorionic twin pregnancies. In the dichorionic type, there is an extension of placental tissue into the base of the inter-twin membrane, forming the lambda sign, whereas in monochorionic, the inter-twin membrane is thin and has no extension of the chorionic tissue, forming the 'T' sign.

increasing incidence of multiple pregnancies, with approximately one in five successful IVF procedures resulting in multiple pregnancy. In the USA, over one-third of twin pregnancies and approximately 80% of triplet (and higher order) pregnancies occur following treatment for infertility. **Figure 7.1** shows the relative contributions of the different types of twins to a hypothetical random selection of 1,000 twin pairs.

AETIOLOGY

Multiple pregnancy may be classified according to:

- number of fetuses – twins, triplets, quadruplets, etc.
- number of fertilized eggs – zygosity
- number of placentae – chorionicity
- number of amniotic cavities – amnionicity

Twin pregnancy may be dizygotic (70%) or monozygotic (30%). Dizygotic twins (non-identical) occur from ovulation and subsequent fertilization of two oocytes. This results in dichorionic diamniotic twins, where each fetus has its own placenta and amniotic cavity. Although they always have two functionally separate placentae (dichorionic), the placentae can become anatomically fused together and appear to the naked eye as a single placental mass. They always have separate amniotic cavities (diamniotic) and the two cavities are separated by a thick three-layer membrane (fused chorion in the middle with amnion on either side; **Figure 7.2**). The fetuses can be either same-sex or different-sex pairings.

Monozygotic (identical) pregnancies result from fertilization of a single ovum with subsequent division of the zygote. If the zygote splits shortly after fertilization, the twins will each have a separate placenta and thus will be dichorionic diamniotic. Monochorionic diamniotic (20%) pregnancies occur when division of the zygote occurs between days 4 and 8 postfertilization. The vast majority of monochorionic twins have two amniotic cavities (diamniotic) but the dividing membrane is thin, as it consists of a single layer of amnion alone (see **Figure 7.2**).

Monochorionic monoamniotic (1%) pregnancy occurs when division occurs between days 8 and 12 postfertilization and, finally, conjoined twins occur when division of the zygote happens after day 13.

ANTENATAL CARE IN THE PRESENCE OF A MULTIPLE PREGNANCY

According to the National Institute for Health and Care Excellence (NICE) guidelines, treatment and care should take into account a pregnant woman's needs and preferences.

Owing to an increased risk of pregnancy complications, pregnant women with multiple pregnancies that involve a shared amnion should be offered individualized care in a tertiary-level fetal medicine unit. This care should involve the following:

- Pregnant women with multiple pregnancies should be cared for by a multidisciplinary team consisting of a core team of named specialist obstetricians, specialist midwives and ultrasonographers.
- Ultrasound assessment is recommended to date the pregnancy, to perform first trimester screening and to monitor growth. Abdominal palpation or symphysis–fundal height measurements should not be used to detect or predict FGR.

Those managing twin pregnancies should remember the following:

- Gestation and mode of delivery depends on the type of multiple pregnancy.
- Pregnant women with multiple pregnancies should receive the same advice about diet, lifestyle and nutritional supplements as in routine antenatal care.
- Pregnant women with multiple pregnancies are at higher risk of anaemia than those with singleton pregnancies and a full blood count should be checked at 20 and 28 weeks' gestation and supplementation with iron, folic acid or vitamin B12 initiated.
- There is no benefit in using untargeted administration of corticosteroids. Instead, corticosteroids should be administered when preterm delivery (<34 weeks' gestation) is indicated or suspected.

COMPLICATIONS OF MULTIPLE PREGNANCY

All of the physiological changes of pregnancy, including increased cardiac output, volume expansion, relative haemodilution, diaphragmatic splinting, weight gain and lordosis, are exaggerated in multiple gestations. This results in much greater stresses being placed on maternal reserves. The 'minor' symptoms of pregnancy may be exaggerated, such as nausea, vomiting and heartburn. However,

for individuals with pre-existing health problems, such as cardiac disease, a multiple pregnancy may substantially increase their risk of morbidity.

One of the most common complications of dichorionic diamniotic pregnancies (with significant perinatal morbidity as well as mortality) is preterm delivery, either spontaneous or iatrogenic due to the occurrence of other adverse pregnancy complications such as pre-eclampsia or FGR (**Figure 7.3**). Overall, approximately 60% of twin pregnancies result in spontaneous birth before 37 weeks' gestation. In 15% of cases, delivery will be very preterm (before 32 weeks of gestation). For monochorionic twins, the chance of preterm delivery is increased even further, with 12% born before viability and 25% delivering between 24 and 32 weeks. With two or more babies resulting from each delivery, multiple gestations account for 20–25% of neonatal intensive care unit admissions. Unfortunately, screening tools for preterm labour (such as home uterine activity monitoring, serial cervical length assessment, fetal fibronectin, etc.) have poor predictive performance. Therefore, pregnant women should be educated about the symptoms and signs of preterm labour so that they can seek timely care and so appropriate intervention, such as antenatal corticosteroids and magnesium sulphate for neuroprotection, can be instituted. In addition to the other complications of twin pregnancy described earlier, monochorionic diamniotic pregnancies are also at risk of complications specific to monochorionicity – commonly twin-to-twin

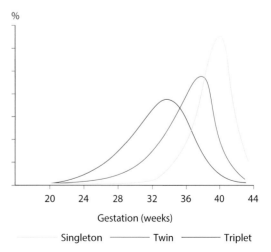

Figure 7.3 Gestational age distribution at delivery of singleton, twin and triplet pregnancies.

transfusion syndrome (TTTS) and, more rarely, twin anaemia–polycythaemia sequence (TAPS).

PERINATAL MORTALITY

Overall perinatal mortality for monochorionic twins is estimated to be 30 per 1,000 (compared with 3.8 per 1,000 among dichorionic twins). The overall infant mortality rate for twins is approximately 5.5 times higher than for singletons, mainly as a result of extreme prematurity. The survival at any given gestation is similar for singletons and multiple pregnancies. The stillbirth rate is 12 per 1,000 twin births and 31 per 1,000 triplet births. This compares with about 5 in 1,000 singleton pregnancies. With the increasing use of early pregnancy scanning, it has been recognized that up to 25% of twins may suffer an early demise and subsequently 'vanish' well before they would have previously been detected. After the first trimester, the intrauterine death of one fetus in a twin pregnancy may be associated with a poor outcome for the remaining co-twin. Maternal complications such as disseminated intravascular coagulation have been reported, but the incidence of this appears to be very low. In dichorionic twins, the second or third trimester intrauterine death of one fetus may be associated with the onset of labour, although, in most cases, the pregnancy would continue uneventfully and result in delivery at term. By contrast, the fetal death of one twin in monochorionic twins may result in immediate complications in the survivor. These include death (15% risk) or brain damage (30% risk) with subsequent neurodevelopmental handicap. Acute hypotensive episodes, secondary to placental vascular anastomoses with resultant haemodynamic volume shifts and acute release of vasoactive substances into the survivor's circulation, have been implicated.

FETAL GROWTH RESTRICTION

FGR in multiple pregnancies can be attributed to placental insufficiency (dichorionic twins) or to unequal placental sharing with unequal blood flow across placental vascular anastomoses (monochorionic twins). Compared with singletons, the risk of FGR is higher in each individual twin alone and is substantially raised in the pregnancy as a whole. For growth-restricted fetuses, the antenatal care focuses on prediction of the severity of impaired fetal oxygenation and determining the appropriate time for delivery. This can be reasonably achieved by careful and systematic ultrasonographic assessment of fetal growth velocity and fetal Doppler assessments such as umbilical artery, middle cerebral artery and ductus venosus (DV) studies. In singletons, this is a balance between the relative risks of intrauterine death and the risk of neonatal death or handicap from elective iatrogenic preterm delivery. The situation is much more complicated in twin pregnancies. The potential benefit of expectant management or elective delivery for the small fetus must also be weighed against the risk of the same policy for the normally grown co-twin. In a dichorionic pregnancy, each fetus runs twice the risk of low birthweight and there is a 25% chance that at least one of the fetuses will be small for gestational age. The chance of suboptimal fetal growth for monochorionic twins is almost double that for dichorionic twins. In dichorionic twin pregnancies where one fetus has growth restriction, elective preterm delivery may lead to iatrogenic complications of prematurity in the previously healthy co-twin. In general, delivery should be avoided before 28–30 weeks' gestation, even if there is evidence of imminent intrauterine death of the smaller twin; however, this may not be applicable in the management of monochorionic twins.

The death of one of a monochorionic twin pair may result in either death or handicap of the co-twin because of acute hypotension secondary to placental vascular anastomoses between the two circulations. As the damage potentially happens at the moment of death of the first twin, the timing of delivery may be a very difficult decision. Below 30 weeks' gestation, the aim is to prolong the pregnancy as far as possible without risking the death of the growth-restricted twin.

COMPLICATIONS UNIQUE TO MONOCHORIONIC TWIN PREGNANCIES

TWIN-TO-TWIN TRANSFUSION SYNDROME

Unique to monochorionic pregnancy is a complication involving the development of abnormal unbalanced vascular anastomoses leading to the development of

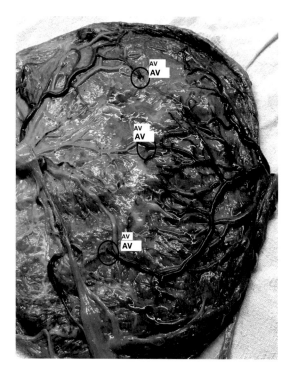

Figure 7.4 Placental injection of a typical uncomplicated monochorionic diamniotic placenta showing arteriovenous (AV) anastomosis. There appears to be equal sharing of the placental territory and the twins delivered at 36 weeks.

TTTS. Although vascular connections are found in nearly all monochorionic twins (**Figure 7.4**), approximately 10–15% of monochorionic diamniotic pregnancies and 5% of monoamniotic pregnancies will subsequently develop TTTS. Four types of vascular connections have been identified in monochorionic pregnancies: arteriovenous (AV), venoarterial, arterioarterial (AA) and venovenous.

If the connections are unbalanced, with more AV connections occurring in one direction than the other, alterations in the hydrostatic and osmotic forces occur, resulting in the manifestations seen in TTTS. An equal number of bidirectional anastomoses results in balanced connections, and TTTS does not occur under these circumstances. AA anastomoses are protective against the development of TTTS.

TTTS may be diagnosed and graded in severity according to the widely accepted Quintero staging system, which is based on ultrasonographic assessment:

- *Stage I*: Oligohydramnios and polyhydramnios sequence, and the bladder of the donor twin is visible. Doppler assessments in both twins are normal. **Figure 7.5** shows a schematic diagram of stage I TTTS.
- *Stage II*: Oligohydramnios and polyhydramnios sequence, but the bladder of the donor is not visualized. Doppler assessments in both twins are normal.
- *Stage III*: Oligohydramnios and polyhydramnios sequence, non-visualized bladder and abnormal Doppler assessments. There is absent/reversed end-diastolic velocity in the umbilical artery, reversed flow in a-wave of the DV or pulsatile flow in the umbilical vein in either fetus.

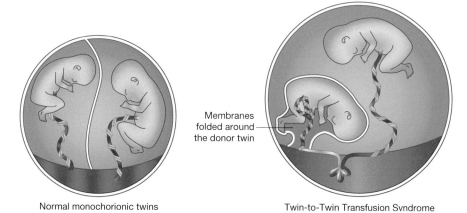

Normal monochorionic twins

Membranes folded around the donor twin

Twin-to-Twin Transfusion Syndrome

Figure 7.5 Schematic diagram showing stage I Twin-to-Twin transfusion syndrome.

- *Stage IV*: One fetus or both fetuses show signs of hydrops.
- *Stage V*: One fetus or both fetuses have died.

Infrequently, the evolution of features of TTTS might not occur sequentially as described by Quintero staging.

TAPS is a rarer chronic form of TTTS in which a large inter-twin haemoglobin difference occurs but the oligohydramnios polyhydramnios sequence that is observed with TTTS is not seen. It is thought to occur from residual small (<1 mm) unidirectional AV anastomoses without accompanying AA anastomoses. TAPS may occur spontaneously (3%) or more frequently after laser surgery for TTTS (13%). The small

residual anastomoses lead to gradual development of anaemia in one twin and polycythaemia in the other twin. As the vessels are small, this allows haemodynamic compensation, which is thought to be why the characteristic oligohydramnios polyhydramnios pattern does not occur. Severe polycythaemia can occur, leading to fetal and placental thrombosis and hydrops fetalis in the anaemic twin. Rarely, mirror syndrome – the combination of fetal hydrops and maternal pre-eclampsia – has been reported.

Serial ultrasound is recommended to assess growth in multiple pregnancies. According to the International Society of Ultrasound in Obstetrics and Gynecology (ISUOG) guidelines on multiple pregnancy, all monochorionic pregnancies must have 2-weekly ultrasound monitoring, starting from 16 weeks for early detection of complications such as TTTS, TAPS and selective FGR (**Figure 7.6**), thereby enabling early intervention to optimize outcomes. The risk of developing TTTS in monochorionic twins reduces after 26 weeks. Likewise, dichorionic twin pregnancies must have monthly growth scans to detect discordant growth (**Figure 7.7**).

Treatment of twin-to-twin transfusion syndrome

When TTTS is suspected or diagnosed, a referral should be made to a tertiary maternal fetal unit.

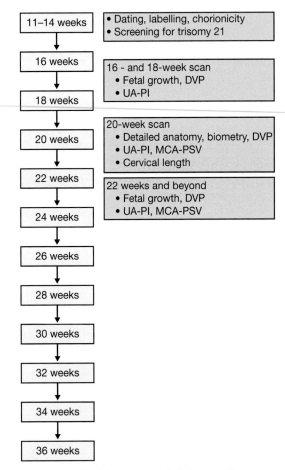

Figure 7.6 ISUOG recommended ultrasound monitoring pathway for monochorionic twin pregnancies. (DVP, deepest vertical pocket; MCA-PSV, middle cerebral artery peak systolic velocity; UA-PI, umbilical artery pulsatility index.)

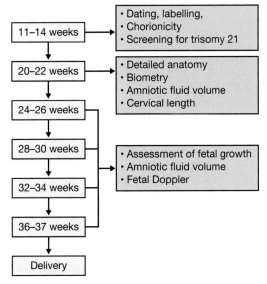

Figure 7.7 ISUOG recommended ultrasound monitoring pathway for uncomplicated dichorionic twin pregnancies.

When TTTS is confirmed, management options include expectant management, fetoscopic laser ablation of vascular anastomoses, amnioreduction, septostomy and selective feticide. Fetoscopic laser ablation is now generally considered the definitive treatment of severe (defined as Quintero stage II or above) TTTS between 16 and 26 weeks' gestation. Above 26 weeks, delivery may be considered. These recommendations are based on the results of a meta-analysis that demonstrated that fetuses undergoing laser ablation rather than amnioreduction were twice as likely to survive and had an 80% reduction in neurological morbidity (overall survival odds ratio (OR) 2.04, 95% confidence interval (CI) 1.52–2.76; neonatal death OR 0.24, 95% CI 0.15–0.40; and neurological morbidity OR 0.20, 95% CI 0.12–0.33).

The procedure is performed under local anaesthetic with intravenous sedation, with regional anaesthesia or occasionally under general anaesthesia. Under ultrasound guidance, a 2–3-mm diameter fetoscope is introduced into the amniotic cavity of the recipient twin. The location of the dividing twin membrane between the two amniotic cavities at the placental interface and the placental insertions of the umbilical cords are visualized. AV anastomoses are ablated using laser energy. Following the laser therapy, the fetoscope is removed and an amnioreduction is performed until the amniotic fluid volume appears normal by ultrasound assessment.

TWIN ANAEMIA–POLYCYTHAEMIA SEQUENCE

TAPS is another unique but rare complication of monochorionic pregnancies. TAPS is a form of slow chronic transfusion that is believed to occur via small (<1 mm) AV anastomoses and results in highly discordant haemoglobin concentrations in the twin pair (**Figure 7.8**). The donor twin becomes anaemic while the recipient twin suffers from polycythaemia. TAPS can occur spontaneously (up to 3% of cases) or could be iatrogenic after laser therapy (up to 13% of cases). Doppler assessment of fetal MCA PSV (Middle cerebral artery Peak systolic velocity) is valuable for antenatal diagnosis of TAPS. The management options for TAPS include expectant management, early delivery, laser therapy, intrauterine transfusion of the anaemic twin with/without partial exchange

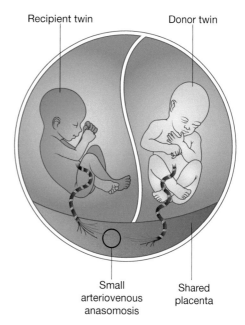

Figure 7.8 Twin anaemia–polycythaemia sequence. Schematic diagram showing a plethoric polycythaemic twin and the pale anaemic twin. Note the small arteriovenous anastomosis supplying the polycythaemic twin.

transfusion of the polycythaemic twin. The choice would depend on gestational age at diagnosis, stage of TAPS, the pregnant woman's preference and technical feasibility of intrauterine therapy.

TWIN REVERSED ARTERIAL PERFUSION

Twin reversed arterial perfusion (TRAP) sequence or acardiac twin (**Figure 7.9**) is another rare complication of monochorionic placentation, which comprises a twin with an absent or a non-functional heart, perfused in a retrograde manner by the normal (pump) twin through an AA anastomosis. Historically, the prevalence of TRAP sequence has been reported to be about 1% of monozygotic twins. The pump twin is subjected to a hyperdynamic circulation, which eventually may result in progressive high output cardiac failure and in utero demise. Studies report that, in nearly a third to a half of pregnancies with TRAP sequence, the pump twins die in utero if left untreated. Therefore, various intrauterine procedures to arrest the circulation of the acardiac twin have been tried, ranging from cord occlusion using

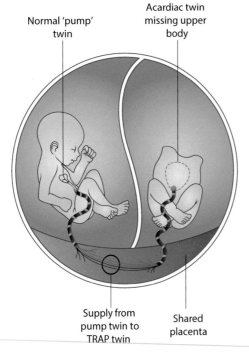

Normal 'pump' twin

Acardiac twin missing upper body

Supply from pump twin to TRAP twin

Shared placenta

Figure 7.9 Schematic diagram showing a normally formed pump twin with a twin reversed arterial perfusion (TRAP) twin.

coils or ligation to fetoscopic procedures that coagulate the cord supplying the acardiac twin using monopolar or bipolar diathermy and coagulation of placental anastomosis using laser. The optimum timing of such interventions remains undefined. Traditionally, fetal interventions were preferred after 16 weeks of gestation due to the reported increased risk of fetal loss and talipes equinovarus with early amniocentesis performed before obliteration of the coelomic cavity. A few studies have suggested conservative management with delayed intervention after 16 weeks if there is development of poor prognostic markers, such as rapid growth of the acardiac twin (estimated weight >50% of the pump twin), or development of features of cardiac failure or hyperdynamic circulation in the pump twin.

MONOCHORIONIC MONOAMNIOTIC TWIN PREGNANCY

Monoamniotic twin pregnancies result from division of a single fertilized oocyte. The incidence of monoamniotic twins is approximately 1 in 10,000

pregnancies. It is the least common pattern of placentation but is associated with high morbidity and mortality due to the high rate of perinatal mortality that occurs secondary to cord accidents resulting in fetal loss or neurological morbidity. Monochorionic monoamniotic (MCMA) twins have an increased risk of congenital anomalies including neural tube defects and abdominal wall and urinary tract malformations. Even though the excess fetal loss reported in MCMA twin pregnancies was believed to be secondary to cord entanglement, the majority is related to fetal abnormalities. Cord entanglement is present in nearly all MCMA twin pregnancies (**Figure 7.10**). Discordant birthweight affects approximately 20% of surviving monoamniotic twin pairs without congenital anomalies. As a result, close surveillance with ultrasound is essential. MCMA pregnancies are monitored closely with antenatal fetal surveillance and delivery by caesarean section generally at 32–34 weeks' gestation. The ideal method for surveillance (whether in- or outpatient) is unclear. In some countries, patients are hospitalized from 28 weeks' gestation and fetal heart auscultation is performed several times daily using cardiotocography in an effort to detect signs of cord compression. However, there is an absence of evidence regarding the superiority of any method of surveillance over another. Perinatal mortality occurs in approximately 20% of fetuses and infants.

ANTENATAL CARE

The NICE guidelines recommend that pregnant women with uncomplicated dichorionic twin pregnancies be offered at least eight antenatal appointments with a healthcare professional from the core team. **Table 7.1** provides an overview of care for different types of multiple pregnancies, as recommended by NICE 2019 guidelines. Routine antenatal care for all pregnant women involves screening for hypertension and gestational diabetes. These conditions occur more frequently in twin pregnancies than in singleton pregnancies and there is also a higher risk of other problems (such as antepartum haemorrhage and thromboembolic disease); however, the management is the same as for a singleton. Owing to the increased fetoplacental demand

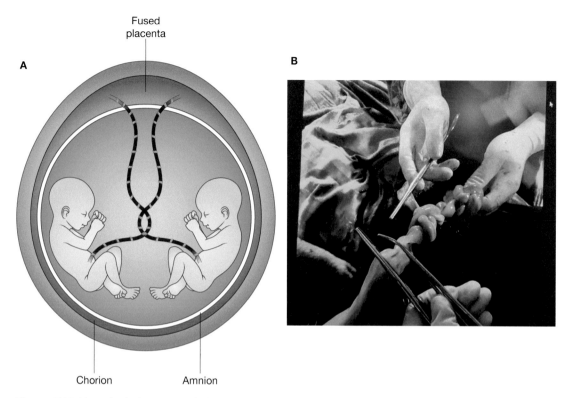

Fused placenta

A

B

Chorion   Amnion

Figure 7.10 Monochorionic monoamniotic twin pregnancy. (**A**) Schematic diagram of a monochorionic monoamniotic twin pregnancy with cord entanglement. (**B**) Cord entanglement was confirmed at the time of caesarean delivery at 33 weeks.

for iron and folic acid, many would recommend routine (as opposed to selective) supplementation in multiple pregnancies. Minor symptoms of pregnancy are more common, but management is again unchanged compared to singletons.

SCREENING IN MULTIPLE PREGNANCY

Pregnant women with multiple pregnancy should be offered a first trimester scan when the crown–rump length (CRL) measures 45–84 mm, which equates to approximately 11 weeks 0 days to 13 weeks 6 days. The purpose of this is fourfold, namely to:

1. accurately estimate gestational age
2. determine chorionicity
3. screen for Down syndrome
4. label the fetuses

Gestational age is assessed by measuring the CRL. In the case of discrepant CRL, generally the larger CRL is used to avoid underestimating FGR. Pregnancies conceived by assisted reproductive technology should be dated using the conception date. Chorionicity is determined by assessing the number of placental masses and assessing the lambda or T-sign and membrane thickness (see **Figure 7.2**). At this stage, the fetuses are mapped and it is documented clearly which fetus is where to ensure consistency with future scans throughout pregnancy; for example, triplet two maternal upper right side. With dichorionic pregnancies, the risk of Down syndrome is calculated for each baby. With monochorionic pregnancies, the risk of Down syndrome is calculated for the pregnancy as a whole. Assessment of the a-wave in the DV at 11–13 weeks' gestation may help identify monochorionic pregnancies at risk of severe TTTS, as reversed a-wave is associated with an increased risk of developing severe TTTS,

Table 7.1 An overview of care for different types of multiple pregnancies, as recommended by NICE 2019 guidelines

Care	Dichorionic diamniotic twins	Monochorionic diamniotic twins	Monochorionic monoamniotic twins	Trichorionic trimniotic triplets	Dichorionic or monochorionic triamniotic triplets
Recommended number of antenatal appointments	At least eight antenatal appointments	At least 11 antenatal appointments	Individualized care, consultant led	At least nine antenatal appointments	At least 11 antenatal appointments
Antenatal care	Specialist team	Specialist team	Specialist team	Specialist team	Specialist team
Timing of delivery	Offer planned birth at 37 weeks	Offer planned birth at 36 weeks	Offer planned birth at 32–33 weeks	Offer planned birth at 35 weeks	Individualized plan for delivery
Mode of delivery	Planned vaginal birth and planned caesarean section are both safe choices for them and their babies if the pregnancy remains uncomplicated and has progressed beyond 32 weeks, the first baby is in a cephalic (head-first) presentation and there is no significant size discordance between the twins	Planned vaginal birth and planned caesarean section are both safe choices for them and their babies if the pregnancy remains uncomplicated and has progressed beyond 32 weeks, the first baby is in a cephalic (head-first) presentation and there is no significant size discordance between the twins	Offer a caesarean section to women with a monochorionic monoamniotic twin pregnancy	Offer a caesarean section to women with a triplet pregnancy	Offer a caesarean section to women with a triplet pregnancy

as well as other complications including aneuploidy. However, due to high false-positive rates, this is not widely advocated or must be interpreted with caution. First-trimester ultrasound markers have been found to be poor predictors of TTTS, selective FGR and intrauterine demise in monochorionic twin pregnancy. Both amniocentesis and chorion villous sampling (CVS) can be performed in twin pregnancies, but, in dichorionic pregnancies, CVS is the preferred method for prenatal diagnosis, as it provides first-trimester diagnosis and the possibility of safer, earlier, selective termination if needed.

ANOMALY SCAN

Fetuses of multiple pregnancies have higher rates of congenital anomalies than singleton fetuses. Monozygotic twins are two or three times more likely to have structural defects than dizygotic twins or singleton fetuses. These include midline anomalies such as anencephaly and holoprosencephaly. In general, only one fetus is affected by the congenital malformations, should they occur. In 5–20% of cases, the defect is present in both twins. Multiple gestations with an abnormality in one fetus can be managed expectantly or by selective fetocide of the affected twin. In cases when the abnormality is non-lethal but may well result in disability, the parents may need to decide whether the potential burden of a disabled child outweighs the risk of loss of the normal twin from fetocide-related complications, which occur after 5–10% of procedures. In cases when the abnormality is lethal, it may be best to avoid such risk to the normal fetus, unless the condition itself threatens the survival of the normal twin. Anencephaly is a good example of a lethal abnormality that can threaten the survival of the normal twin. At least 50% of pregnancies affected by anencephaly are complicated by polyhydramnios, which can lead to the spontaneous preterm delivery of both babies.

Fetocide in monochorionic pregnancies carries increased risk and requires a more invasive technique, such as cord occlusion/intrafetal laser, with such techniques associated with a higher complication rate. As there are potential vascular anastomoses between the two fetal circulations, intracardiac injections cannot be employed. In twins, like in singletons, the risk for chromosomal abnormalities increases with maternal age. The rate of spontaneous dizygotic twinning also increases with maternal age. Many pregnant women undergoing assisted conception techniques (that increase the chance of dizygotic twinning) are also older than the mean age of the pregnant population. Chromosomal defects may be more likely in a multiple pregnancy for various reasons, and couples should be counselled accordingly.

GROWTH ASSESSMENTS

Multiple pregnancies are at high risk of FGR. As a result, fetal weight should be calculated from 20 weeks' gestation at a maximum of 4-week intervals. A growth discrepancy of 25% or greater should be considered clinically significant, a tertiary referral opinion should be sought and additional monitoring or delivery should be planned, depending on gestation.

Other indications for a tertiary-level fetal medicine opinion include discordant fetal growth, fetal anomaly, TRAP, TTTS or single intrauterine demise.

DELIVERY

A care plan should be discussed and made with the patient, ideally throughout pregnancy, with a clear delivery plan discussed and documented early in the third trimester. This is essential, as multiple pregnancies have a high prevalence of preterm delivery. The discussion with the patient should include the desired mode for delivery, the gestation for induction of labour if there is no spontaneous onset of labour, the process for delivery of twin 1 and twin 2 including internal podalic version, the risk of caesarean section, complications following delivery including post-partum haemorrhage, the desire to breastfeed or not and neonatal care for the babies if born preterm.

INTRAPARTUM MANAGEMENT

General management of a patient with twin pregnancy in labour involves:

- antenatal education and a pre-agreed birth plan
- continuous fetal heart monitoring

- two neonatal resuscitation trolleys, two obstetricians and two paediatricians available, with the special care baby unit and anaesthetist informed well in advance of the delivery
- analgesia, ideally in the form of an early epidural, to allow for internal podalic version (if needed) for twin 2
- a standard oxytocin solution for augmentation prepared, run through an intravenous giving-set and clearly labelled 'for augmentation', for use for delivery of the second twin
- oxytocin infusion in anticipation of post-partum haemorrhage
- portable ultrasound

With uncomplicated dichorionic diamniotic pregnancies, vaginal delivery is advocated, provided the presenting twin is cephalic. The risk of requiring emergency caesarean section for delivery of the second twin following vaginal delivery of the first twin is approximately 4%.

If the second twin is non-vertex, which occurs in about 40% of twins, a vaginal delivery can be safely considered. If the second twin is a breech, the membranes can be ruptured once the breech is fixed in the birth canal. A breech extraction may be performed if fetal distress occurs or if a footling breech is encountered, but this requires considerable expertise. Complications are less likely if the membranes are not ruptured until the feet are held by the operator. When the fetus is transverse, external cephalic version can be successful in more than 70% of cases. The fetal heart rate should be closely monitored, and ultrasound can be helpful to demonstrate the final position of the baby. If external cephalic version is unsuccessful, and assuming that the operator is experienced, an internal podalic version can be undertaken (**Figure 7.11**).

Internal podalic version is performed by identifying a fetal foot through intact membranes. The foot is grasped and pulled gently and continuously into the birth canal. The membranes are ruptured as late as possible. This procedure is easiest when the transverse lie is with the back superior or posterior. If the back is inferior or if the limbs are not immediately palpable, ultrasound may help to show the operator where they would be found. This will minimize the unwanted experience of bringing down a fetal hand in the mistaken belief that it is a foot.

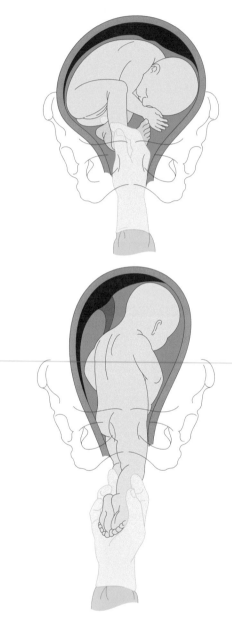

Figure 7.11 Internal podalic version.

Generally, with dichorionic twin pregnancies, delivery from 37 weeks' gestation is advocated.

Pregnant women with uncomplicated monochorionic twin pregnancies should be offered elective delivery from 36 weeks' gestation, and this should be performed after a course of antenatal corticosteroids has been given. However, this approach carries a 1.5% risk of late in utero death for monochorionic twins.

Continuing uncomplicated twin pregnancies beyond 38 weeks' gestation increases the risk of intrauterine fetal death. The indications for instrumental delivery of the second twin are the same as for singletons.

HIGHER-ORDER MULTIPLES

The incidence of spontaneous triplet pregnancy is 1 in 6,000–8,000 births. Triplets are associated with high morbidity and mortality. According to UK data, they have an average gestation of 34 weeks at delivery, an average birthweight of 1.8 kg and a cerebral palsy rate of 26.7 per 1,000 live births. When performing first trimester screening in monochorionic triplet pregnancies, the risk of Down syndrome should be calculated for each baby in dichorionic and trichorionic triplet pregnancies. NICE recommends that pregnant women with uncomplicated monochorionic triamniotic and dichorionic triamniotic triplet pregnancies be offered at least 11 antenatal appointments with a healthcare professional from the core team. It is not recommended to prolong pregnancy beyond 36 weeks' gestation.

MULTIPLE PREGNANCY SUPPORT GROUPS

Twin pregnancies are associated with a number of financial, personal and social costs for families that continue long beyond the neonatal period. A significant contribution to these costs comes from the increased incidence of disability, largely secondary to preterm delivery. Several specialized support groups for multiple pregnancy exist. In the UK, these include the Twins Trust (previously known as Twins and Multiple Birth Association [TAMBA]) and the Multiple Birth Foundation. All parents expecting twins should be given contact details for such resources locally.

☞ KEY LEARNING POINTS

- Multiple pregnancies are associated with increased incidence of pregnancy complications, such as pre-eclampsia, gestational diabetes, anaemia and post-partum haemorrhage.
- Preterm birth, growth restriction and stillbirth are key causes of the raised fetal morbidity and mortality associated with multiple pregnancies.
- Maternal morbidity and mortality is also increased in multiple pregnancies.
- Early ultrasound assessment is key in the management of multiple pregnancy, as it can correctly classify the type of pregnancy according to chorionicity and amnionicity, allowing risk to be stratified.

FURTHER READING

FIGO Working Group on Good Clinical Practice in Maternal-Fetal Medicine (2019). Good clinical practice advice: Management of twin pregnancy. *International Journal of Gynecology & Obstetrics*, 144(3): 330–337.

Khalil A, Rodgers M, Baschat A, Bhide A, Gratacos E, Hecher K, et al. (2016). ISUOG Practice Guidelines: Role of ultrasound in twin pregnancy. *Ultrasound in Obstetrics & Gynecology*, 47(2): 247–263.

NICE (2019). *Twin and Triplet Pregnancy*. NICE guideline [NG137]. https://www.nice.org.uk/guidance/ng137/chapter/Recommendations.

Royal College of Obstetricians and Gynaecologists (2017). Green-top Guideline No 51: Management of monochorionic twin pregnancy. *BJOG: An International Journal of Obstetrics & Gynaecology*, 124(1): e1–45.

SELF-ASSESSMENT

For interactive SBAs and EMQs relating to this chapter, visit www.routledge.com/cw/mccarthy.

CASE HISTORY 1

Ms B is 38 weeks' gestation in her second pregnancy. This is a dichorionic diamniotic pregnancy that has been uncomplicated to date. Ms B presents contracting every 5 minutes. Twin 1 (the presenting twin) is cephalic and twin 2 is cephalic. Her first pregnancy was a term delivery, delivered 11 months previously as a spontaneous vaginal delivery. On examination, Ms B is 6 cm dilated and both fetal heart recordings are reassuring. An epidural has just been inserted and is providing good analgesia.

A What would you do next?

Ms B's waters rupture and she proceeds to have a spontaneous vaginal delivery. On delivering twin 1, the abdomen is palpated and ultrasound confirms that twin 2 is cephalic. The fetal heart rate remains reassuring.

B How would you proceed?

After 25 minutes of reassuring heart monitoring, Ms B is contracting once every 10 minutes. Fetal heart monitoring remains reassuring.

C How would you proceed?

The membranes surrounding twin 2 rupture. Vaginal examination reveals that Ms B remains fully dilated. However, twin 2 is now transverse with its back upwards. The fetal heart tracing shows prolonged fetal decelerations.

D How would you proceed?

ANSWERS

A There is no indication to intervene in this situation. Ms B has laboured spontaneously and is progressing quickly. Fetal heart rate is reassuring. Allow labour to progress naturally. Continue fetal monitoring.

B Again, there is no indication to intervene. Ms B has successfully delivered twin 1. Waiting allows the head of twin 2 to descend, which will increase the likelihood of a spontaneous vaginal delivery.

C There are now two options. The first option would be to perform an amniotomy to rupture the membranes of twin 2, which will likely increase the frequency of contractions, allowing twin 2 to be delivered. The second option would be to start oxytocin infusion to try to increase the frequency of contractions and allow delivery of twin 2 to proceed. As the membranes are intact, one must be cautious with the use of oxytocin; therefore, the ideal option is to perform a vaginal examination and, when a contraction occurs (which will push the fetal head into the pelvis), perform artificial rupture of the membranes. Oxytocin may be used at this stage to augment contractions.

D This is now an obstetric emergency. Ensure senior obstetric help is present. There are two options on how to manage this situation. The first option is to perform internal podalic version as described in this chapter by performing vaginal examination; follow the fetal spine towards the legs and, on palpating a foot, apply gentle traction to the foot to encourage delivery of the fetus by breech extraction. The second option is to transfer the mother to the operating theatre and perform a category 1 caesarean section. As Ms B is multiparous, internal podalic version and breech extraction would be the quickest way to deliver twin 2 and ensure a quick recovery for Ms B. External cephalic version would be a third option, but, in the presence of a non-reassuring fetal heart rate, this would be contraindicated.

CASE HISTORY 2

Ms S is 16 weeks' gestation in her second pregnancy. This is a monochorionic diamniotic pregnancy that was conceived through IVF. Ms S has an ultrasound scan that shows twin 1 with normal growth and polyhydramnios. Twin 2 has oligohydramnios with no bladder visualized. There is reversed end-diastolic velocity in the umbilical artery and reversed flow in a-wave of the DV. What is the diagnosis and what would your management be?

ANSWER

This monochorionic diamniotic pregnancy is now complicated by TTTS. This is now Quintero stage III and should be referred to a fetal medicine unit with the capacity to perform laser ablation treatment as a means to prevent any further deterioration.

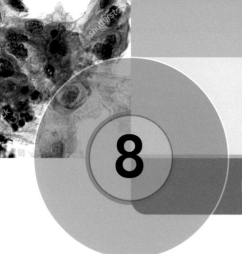

Preterm labour

8

DAVID LISSAUER

Learning Objectives
- Be aware of the extent of the problem of prematurity in the UK and globally.
- Know about the causes of prematurity.
- Understand the prevention and clinical management of preterm labour.

INTRODUCTION

Preterm labour (PTL) is the onset of labour before 37 weeks of pregnancy. This chapter will provide an overview of PTL in the UK and globally. It includes a description of the causes, prevention and clinical management of PTL.

WHY DOES PRETERM LABOUR OCCUR?

In contrast with other species, in which preterm delivery is uncommon, PTL and preterm delivery are relatively common in human pregnancy. A possible explanation lies in human evolution, specifically involving bipedalism and encephalization. Bipedalism (upright posture) is associated with a narrower pelvis. Encephalization (increased brain volume) is associated with a larger head size (**Figure 8.1**). Each has the potential to increase the chance of obstructed labour and the death of both the mother and the baby. Consequently, evolution would favour the emergence of earlier delivery, potentially explaining why PTL is more common in humans than other species.

OVERVIEW OF PRETERM LABOUR

The proportion of infants born preterm varies widely between different countries. In the UK, 7.4% of births were preterm in 2020 (i.e. more than 55,000 infants). However, this figure is only 5.9% in Sweden and Japan, but is 10.2% in the USA (**Figure 8.2**).

The countries with the highest numbers of preterm births are India (3,519,947; prematurity rate 13.6%), followed by China (1,168,126; prematurity

10.1201/9781003196112-8

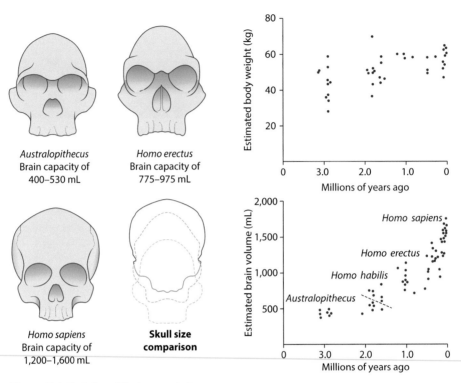

Figure 8.1 Evolution of the human skull.

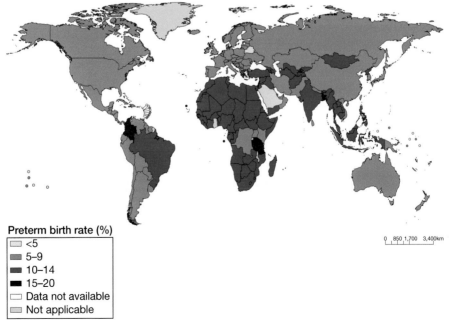

Figure 8.2 Estimated preterm birth rates in 2014. (From Chawanpaiboon S, et al. (2019). *Lancet Global Health*, 7(1): E37–E46. https://doi.org/10.1016/S2214-109X(18)30451-0. With permission from Elsevier.)

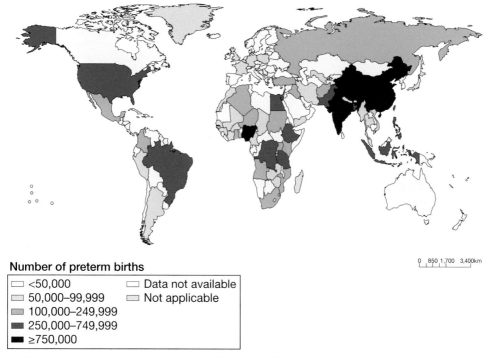

Number of preterm births

- ☐ <50,000
- ☐ 50,000–99,999
- ☐ 100,000–249,999
- ☐ 250,000–749,999
- ☐ ≥750,000
- ☐ Data not available
- ☐ Not applicable

0 850 1,700   3,400km

Figure 8.3 Estimated numbers of preterm births in 2014. (From Chawanpaiboon S, et al. (2019). *Lancet Global Health*, 7(1): E37–E46. https://doi.org/10.1016/S2214-109X(18)30451-0. With permission from Elsevier.)

rate 6.9%), Nigeria (803,178; prematurity rate 11.4%) and Bangladesh (603,698; prematurity rate 19.1%) (**Figure 8.3**).

Worldwide, 5 million children under 5 years of age died in 2020. Almost half (47%) died in the neonatal period, and this proportion is increasing over time. Prematurity is now the single leading cause of deaths in under-5s, with 1.1 million of the 15 million preterm infants dying each year. Most neonatal deaths are in low- and middle-income countries; 43% are in sub-Saharan Africa and 36% are in central and southern Asia.

Of the births that were preterm in England and Wales in 2021:

- 6% were extremely preterm (before 28 weeks)
- 10% were very preterm (between 28 and 32 weeks)
- 83% were moderately preterm (between 32 and <37 weeks)

With decreasing gestation, mortality increases. In high-income countries, a baby born at 24 weeks now has a 50% chance of surviving, and resuscitation

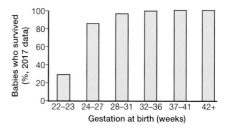

Figure 8.4 Survival by gestational age in the UK, showing the high survival of infants from 24 weeks' gestation or age. (Data from MBRRACE-UK (2019). *Perinatal Mortality Surveillance Report*.)

may be considered and performed for babies as early as 22 or 23 weeks' gestation (**Figure 8.4**). To achieve these impressive survival rates, these extremely preterm infants require neonatal intensive care for survival. They are often in hospital for many weeks or months, and many have complex medical needs. This may cause a great deal of stress and anxiety for the parents and family. Neonatal intensive care is also very expensive.

Although the survival of extremely preterm infants has increased, the proportion with long-term

119

problems has remained substantial. A follow-up of a national cohort of children at 6.5 years who had been born extremely preterm (<27 weeks' gestational age) in Sweden found that 69% survived and 66% of the survivors had no or mild disability, 20% had moderate disability and 14% had severe disability. Cerebral palsy was identified in 9.5%, blindness was identified in 2% and hearing impairment was identified in 2%.

The most common impairments of extremely preterm infants are learning difficulties; their risk rises as gestation at birth decreases, and learning difficulties become increasingly evident during school years. Many children have difficulties with motor function and the processing that underpins learning and thinking (executive processing). This manifests as difficulty with fine motor skills, concentration, abstract reasoning and processing several tasks simultaneously. Deficits in working memory and speed of processing information underpin many of the difficulties. The increase in special educational needs at school age with decreasing gestation is shown in **Figure 8.5**. The degree of cognitive impairment remains stable through childhood (**Figure 8.6**). Children born extremely preterm have more behavioural disorders then their term peers. By adult life,

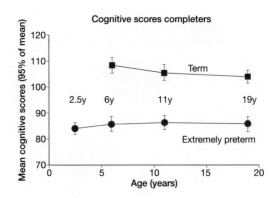

Figure 8.6 Cognitive scores remain stable throughout childhood up to 19 years for extremely preterm children evaluated at each of four time points. (EPICure study. Adapted from Linsell L, Johnson S, Wolke D, et al. (2018). *Archives of Disease in Childhood*, 103(4): 363–370. Published under CC BY 4.0.)

educational attainment and employment are modest compared with term-born young adults and they are less likely to have formed relationships or become parents, but self-rating over a range of areas shows that the majority are contented.

Globally, morbidity from prematurity in low- and middle-income countries is mainly in infants born at 28–37 weeks' gestation and is considerable. Estimates of the global burden of neurodevelopmental impairment among preterm infants are shown in **Figure 8.7**.

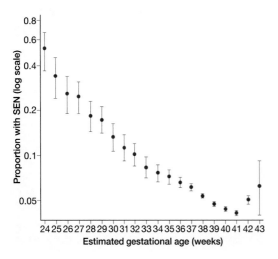

Figure 8.5 Prevalence of special educational needs (SEN) by gestational age at birth, showing an increased proportion not only at extreme prematurity but also at 34 to 39 weeks compared with full-term births. Data based on 407,503 school-aged children in Scotland in 2005. (From MacKay DF, et al. (2010). *PLOS Medicine*, 7(6): e10000289. Published under CC BY 4.0.)

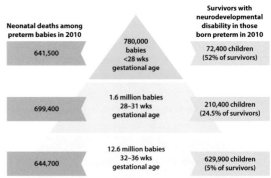

Figure 8.7 Global mortality and mobility of preterm births. Estimates of global burden of mortality and morbidity for the 15 million preterm infants born in 2010 (11% of all 135 million births). (From Blencowe H, Lee ACC, Cousens S, et al. (2013). *Pediatric Research*, 73(Suppl. 1): 17–34. With permission from Springer Nature.)

CAUSES

Preterm delivery can be categorized into:

- spontaneous labour with intact membranes (35%)
- preterm premature rupture of the membranes (PPROM) (25%)
- labour induction or elective caesarean delivery for maternal or fetal indications (25%)
- multiple pregnancy (15%)

In view of the wide variation in prematurity rates between populations, it is not surprising that a wide variety of social and medical risk factors have been identified. They include:

- previous preterm delivery
- short interpregnancy interval (<6 months)
- maternal age, with risk increased if <20 or >35 years old
- maternal nutrition – low body mass index increases the risk of spontaneous preterm delivery, whereas obesity increases the risk of preterm delivery for medical reasons, especially diabetes mellitus and pre-eclampsia
- smoking, including passive and environmental air pollution
- substance misuse

- ethnicity – in the UK, the prematurity rate among Black mothers is higher than that among White mothers
- multiple births
- maternal medical conditions, pregnancy complications and fetal conditions (**Figure 8.8**)
- maternal stress
- socio-economic deprivation

Some of these risk factors increase the risk of infection, inflammation or uterine stretch in pregnancy but the mechanisms of action of many are poorly understood.

There is growing evidence of the association between stress and PTL (e.g. with major life events) and the increased prevalence of PTL among the poor and socially marginalized, as well as among those living in stressful socio-demographic conditions (such as loss of employment, housing or a partner). Prematurity is more common among pregnant women self-reporting increased stress or anxiety. The biochemical pathway through which maternal stress acts is uncertain, but it may involve a premature increase in circulating corticotrophin-releasing hormone.

The prematurity rate is also affected by differences in obstetric management between countries. Examples include differences in the proportion of multiple births, which varies with different assisted reproductive therapy practices and has a marked effect

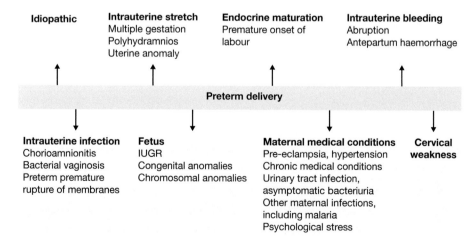

Figure 8.8 Medical conditions associated with prematurity. (From Lissauer T, Fanaroff A, Miall L, et al. (2020). *Neonatology at a Glance*, 4th edn. Wiley Blackwell. With permission. IUGR, Intrauterine growth restriction.)

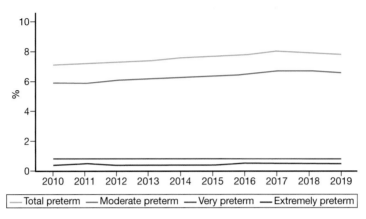

Figure 8.9 Rate of preterm births in England and Wales from 2010 to 2019. (From Office for National Statistics.)

on prematurity rate, and differences in the approach to early elective delivery for medical complications.

The rate of preterm birth overall has risen gradually in England and Wales over the last number of years, from 7% in 2010 to 8% in 2017, although there was a slight fall to 7.8% in 2019 (**Figure 8.9**).

BIOPHYSICAL OR MEDICAL CAUSES OF PRETERM LABOUR

CERVICAL WEAKNESS

Cervical weakness is classically associated with painless premature cervical dilatation and is suggested by a history of painless second-trimester pregnancy loss. There is almost certainly an overlap between cervical weakness and other factors such as ascending infection, as, during pregnancy, the cervix not only acts as a physical obstacle, keeping the pregnancy in the uterus, but also acts as a barrier to ascending infection through the synthesis of a thick mucus plug in the cervical canal that has bactericidal properties. Several studies have demonstrated a strong relationship between cervical length and the risk of preterm birth, and a previous history of cervical surgery is a risk factor for cervical weakness.

INFECTION

Infection of the fetal membranes (chorioamnionitis) is a major cause of preterm birth, particularly in deliveries before 32 weeks' gestation. It is associated with a threefold increase in the risk of preterm birth and a fourfold increase in the risk if the membranes are ruptured. In most cases, infection ascends from the vagina, although the route of infection may be transplacental or introduced during invasive procedures. Cervical weakness, resulting in early shortening, as described earlier, can predispose to ascending bacterial infection. However, it is possible for vaginal pathogens to ascend through a normal cervix. Overall, 33% of all pregnancies delivered after PPROM are complicated by infection. This rate rises the earlier the PPROM occurs, with positive amniotic fluid cultures found in 83% of babies delivered weighing <1 kg, which approximates to a gestation of <28 weeks. Abnormal vaginal flora, for example bacterial vaginosis, affects 16% of pregnant women and is associated with PPROM and PTL, with a greater risk the earlier in gestation it is identified (relative risk: 5–7.5 if identified <16 weeks' gestation). The relationship with preterm birth is not direct, as antibiotic treatment of bacterial vaginosis does not consistently reduce the risk of preterm birth. The current recommendations are to screen those at high risk of preterm delivery for bacterial vaginosis and treat those found to be positive.

UTERINE DISTENSION FROM MULTIPLE PREGNANCY AND POLYHYDRAMNIOS

Overall, 56% of multiple births deliver before 37 weeks and 10–15% deliver before 32 weeks. Consequently, although multiple pregnancies make up only 2% of the pregnant population, they contribute disproportionately to preterm births and, consequently, to neonatal intensive care unit admissions. The risk of preterm birth rises with fetal number, with triplets delivering, on average, at 32 weeks and quadruplets delivering at 28 weeks. Multiple pregnancies have an increased risk of pre-eclampsia, fetal growth restriction and other medical complications of pregnancy, explaining the observation in one study that, of the twins delivered preterm, 24% were for medical reasons and 76% were after PTL or PPROM.

Polyhydramnios, the presence of too much amniotic fluid, also increases the risk of PTL and PPROM, although the effect is not as great as with twins, with preterm birth occurring in between 7% and 25% of fetuses, depending on the severity. Severe polyhydramnios can be managed with amniodrainage, but this may itself precipitate PTL and/or PPROM. Alternatively, non-steroidal anti-inflammatory drugs (NSAIDs) may be used, as they reduce fetal urine production, but flow through the ductus arteriosus has to be closely monitored, as the inhibition of prostagladin E production may result in premature ductal closure.

UTERINE MÜLLERIAN ANOMALIES

Congenital Müllerian anomalies are often unrecognized but are estimated to occur in up to 4% of women of reproductive age. They occur as a consequence of abnormal embryologic fusion and canalization of the Müllerian ducts and result in an abnormally formed uterine cavity, which can range from an arcuate uterus, which results in minimal fundal cavity indentation, to complete failure of fusion resulting in uterine didelphys (**Figure 8.10**). These anomalies are associated with adverse pregnancy outcome in

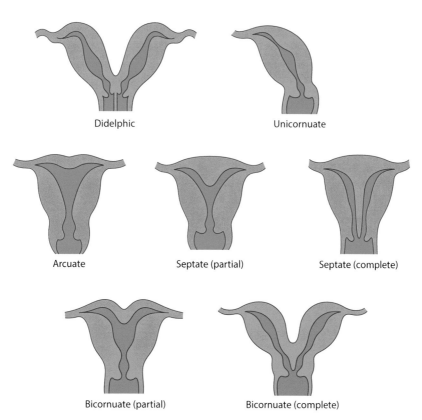

Didelphic

Unicornuate

Arcuate

Septate (partial)

Septate (complete)

Bicornuate (partial)

Bicornuate (complete)

Figure 8.10 Schematic diagram of different types of congenital uterine anomalies. Uterine Müllerian anomalies are associated with an increased risk of preterm delivery.

up to 25% of pregnant women, including first- and second-trimester miscarriage, PPROM, preterm birth, fetal growth restriction, breech presentation and caesarean section.

HAEMORRHAGE

Antepartum haemorrhage and placental abruption may lead to spontaneous PTL. The presence of a subchorionic haematoma in early pregnancy increases the risk of later PPROM, either through an effect of thrombin on membrane strength or through the occurrence of infection in the haematoma. Acute bleeding leads to the release of thrombin that directly stimulates myometrial contractions. Placental abruption complicates 1% of all pregnancies and the effects depend primarily on its severity and the gestational age when it occurs. Risk factors include pre-eclampsia and hypertension, previous abruption, trauma, smoking, cocaine use, multiple pregnancy, polyhydramnios, thrombophilias, advanced maternal age and PPROM. When an abruption involves 50% or more of the placenta, it is frequently associated with fetal death.

PREDICTION OF PRETERM BIRTH

PAST OBSTETRIC HISTORY

Having a previous preterm birth increases the risk fourfold of a further preterm birth in a subsequent pregnancy when compared with someone who has had a previous birth at term. If a pregnant woman has two preterm births, she is at a 6.5 times greater risk of a subsequent preterm birth (**Table 8.1**). Other

Table 8.1 Risk of preterm delivery in subsequent pregnancies

First delivery	Second delivery	Relative risk of preterm labour
Term		1
Preterm		4
Term	Term	0.5
Preterm	Term	1.3
Term	Preterm	2.5
Preterm	Preterm	6.5

factors that increase the risk of preterm birth are previous PPROM, previous use of cerclage, a known uterine variant and intrauterine adhesions. Many risk scoring systems for predicting preterm birth rely heavily on previous obstetric history as a key factor and are therefore not useful in a first pregnancy.

ULTRASOUND MEASUREMENT OF CERVICAL LENGTH

Cervical length measured by transvaginal ultrasound has been shown to be more accurate than transabdominal ultrasound or digital examination. There is a direct relationship between cervical length and the risk of preterm birth (**Figure 8.11**). Cervical length surveillance with serial measurement of cervical length throughout the second trimester and early third trimester is now used to monitor individuals at high risk of preterm birth (**Figure 8.12**). The combination of cervical length and obstetric history can predict 80% of extremely early spontaneous preterm birth (10% screen-positive rate). However, universal cervical length screening of all pregnant women has not been approved in the UK, as it has not been shown to be cost-effective.

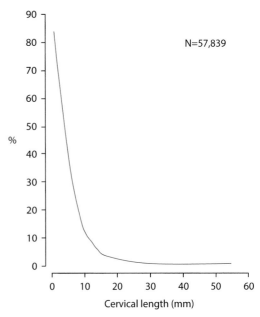

Figure 8.11 Cervical length and the risk of preterm (<34 weeks) delivery.

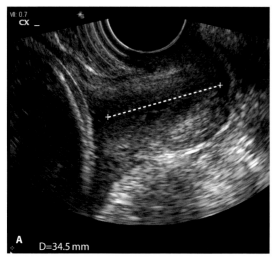

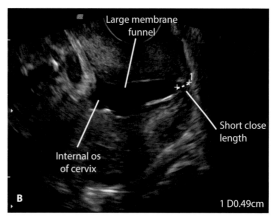

Figure 8.12 (**A**) Normal cervix. (**B**) Cervical length and funnelling on ultrasound.

PREVENTION OF PRETERM DELIVERY

In those found to be at high risk of preterm birth, two interventions are currently available: progesterone and cervical cerclage.

PROGESTERONE

Progesterone has been known to be important in maintaining pregnancy for more than 80 years and is thought to promote uterine quiescence and inhibit the production of proinflammatory cytokines and prostaglandins within the uterus. Many studies have been carried out to investigate the use of progesterone in preventing preterm birth. In pregnancies at high risk of preterm birth, there is some evidence that progesterone is effective in reducing the risk. However, the evidence is conflicting, with the largest randomized trial to date (OPPTIMUM) not showing any benefit of vaginal progesterone. However, systematic reviews that look at the totality of the previous trials suggest that progesterone may be effective, and the evidence is strongest for vaginal progesterone. On this basis, current National Institute for Health and Care Excellence (NICE) guidance recommends offering vaginal progesterone to pregnant women at high risk of preterm birth, such as those with both a history of preterm birth and a short cervix. It can also be considered in pregnant women who have either a history of preterm birth or a short cervix.

CERVICAL CERCLAGE

Transvaginal cervical cerclage may be placed in three different circumstances: following three or more mid-trimester losses or preterm deliveries (history-indicated cerclage), when the cervix shortens (usually <25 mm) in those with a history of cervical surgery or previous preterm birth (ultrasound-indicated cerclage) or when the cervix is dilating in the absence of contractions (emergency cerclage). The exact mechanism by which cerclage helps to prevent or delay PTL is not entirely understood. It is likely, however, that cerclage provides structural support to a weakened cervix and enhances the cervical immunological barrier by improving retention of the mucus plug and preventing ascending infection by maintaining cervical length. Similar to progesterone, cervical cerclage does not appear to reduce the risk of preterm birth in multiple pregnancies. The different types of cerclage are described in **Table 8.2** and an ultrasound image of a cervical cerclage in situ is shown in **Figure 8.13**.

A transabdominal cerclage is usually inserted following a failed vaginal cerclage or extensive cervical surgery. The effectiveness of transabdominal cerclage compared with expectant management or transvaginal cerclage is not clear. Any potential

Table 8.2 Types of cerclage

Type	Description
McDonald transvaginal cerclage	Transvaginal purse-string suture inserted at the cervicovaginal junction without bladder mobilization
Shirodkar (high transvaginal) cerclage	Transvaginal purse-string suture inserted following bladder mobilization, to allow insertion above the level of cardinal ligaments
Transabdominal cerclage	Suture inserted at the cervicoisthmic junction via laparotomy or laparoscopy. Transabdominal cerclages can be inserted either pre-conceptionally or in the first trimester of pregnancy

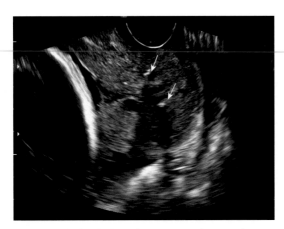

Figure 8.13 Cervical cerclage seen on ultrasound (arrows).

benefits of transabdominal cerclage must be weighed against its increased operative risks. Patients must undergo two operations: one for suture insertion and the other for caesarean section.

MANAGEMENT OF PRETERM LABOUR

Up to 70% of pregnant women who present to the labour ward with threatened PTL will not deliver during that admission, and up to 50% will deliver at term. Deciding who is and who is not in PTL has been helped by testing the cervicovaginal fluid levels of fetal fibronectin (fFN), a glycoprotein found in cervicovaginal fluid, amniotic fluid, placental tissue and the interface between the chorion and decidua. It acts like glue at the maternal–fetal interface and its presence in cervicovaginal fluid between 22 and 36 weeks' gestation has been shown to be a predictor of preterm birth. Negative fFN testing has a very high negative predictive value, enabling most individuals with threatened PTL and a negative fFN test to be sent home. Those with a positive fFN test can be admitted for tocolysis and corticosteroid therapy to promote fetal lung maturation.

TOCOLYTICS

Tocolytics are used to delay delivery long enough for corticosteroid administration to improve neonatal lung function and, if necessary, for in utero transfer to a maternity department with a neonatal intensive care unit. The guidelines for PTL from NICE (2019) state that if tocolytics are administered for the medical treatment of PTL, the first choice should be a calcium channel blocker (nifedipine) or, otherwise, an oxytocin receptor antagonist (OTR-A; atosiban). However, a recent review and network meta-analysis comparing all of the trials of different agents for tocolysis found that prostaglandin (PG) inhibitors and calcium channel blockers are most likely the best therapy for PTL on the basis of delaying delivery by 48 hours, and reducing neonatal mortality, neonatal respiratory distress syndrome (RDS) and maternal side effects. The different types of tocolytics are discussed briefly in the following sections.

CALCIUM CHANNEL BLOCKERS

The effects of calcium channel blockers (e.g. nifedipine) in relaxing the contractions of the human myometrium have been known for several years. Comparing nifedipine with other tocolytics (including beta-sympathomimetics, NSAIDs, magnesium sulphate and OTR-A), no significant reductions were shown in birth within 48 hours of treatment or in perinatal mortality. However, side-effects (including headache, hypotension and dyspnoea), discontinuation due to side effects, and reduction in the incidence of neonatal RDS, necrotizing enterocolitis, intraventricular haemorrhage and neonatal jaundice were least for OTR-A, intermediate for nifedipine and greatest for beta-sympathomimetics.

BETAMIMETICS

Beta-agonists (ritodrine, salbutamol and terbutaline) are predominantly β2 adreno-receptor agonists, which mediate myometrial relaxation by stimulating cyclic adenyl monophosphate production. They are effective in delaying delivery, but do not improve neonatal outcome or ultimate preterm birth rates. Furthermore, they have significant maternal side effects, which means that they are rarely used in the context of threatened PTL in the UK, although globally they are still widely used. The most serious side effect is pulmonary oedema, with an estimated incidence among treated patients of 1:350–1:400. Maternal deaths from acute cardiopulmonary compromise are described, with greater risks if beta-agonists are given in large fluid volumes, in multiple pregnancies and in individuals with cardiac disease.

MAGNESIUM SULPHATE

Magnesium sulphate is widely used in obstetrics in the prevention and treatment of eclampsia. It is also used as fetal neuroprotection in pregnant women in established PTL or planned preterm birth, as it has been shown to reduce the risk of cerebral palsy. It can also be used as a tocolytic, as it decreases the frequency of depolarization of smooth muscle by modulating calcium uptake and results in the inhibition of uterine contractions. It is widely used for this purpose in some countries, but the evidence for it prolonging pregnancy is lacking.

NON-STEROIDAL ANTI-INFLAMMATORY DRUGS

The first NSAID to be widely used in the management of PTL was indomethacin. It is a reversible, non-specific competitive cyclooxygenase inhibitor. Although effective in delaying preterm birth, NSAIDs do have adverse fetal effects, as PG synthesis is responsible for the maintenance of a patent ductus arteriosus and inhibition can lead to its premature closure. This can

occur as early as the late second trimester, with the incidence increasing markedly from 32 weeks. This may lead to persistent pulmonary hypertension in the fetal circulation of the neonate. Indomethacin has also been associated with an increased risk of necrotizing enterocolitis and neonatal renal dysfunction. The latter probably occurs because inhibition of fetal PG synthesis reduces renal perfusion and fetal urine output, resulting in reversible oligohydramnios. Therefore, it is normally used only prior to 32 weeks' gestation.

OXYTOCIN RECEPTOR ANTAGONISTS

OTRs play an important role in the onset and progression of labour. The OTR-A atosiban is a competitive antagonist of oxytocin and vasopressin, binding to both the OTR and the vasopressin receptors within the myometrium. Administration of atosiban results in a dose-dependent inhibition of uterine contractility and oxytocin-mediated PG release. Atosiban is 46–48% plasma protein bound, and only a small amount appears to cross the placenta into the fetal circulation. Treatment with atosiban has been shown to prevent labour after 24 hours, 48 hours and 7 days in comparison with placebo.

CORTICOSTEROID THERAPY

The administration of corticosteroids has the greatest influence on preterm neonatal outcome. Although the use of surfactant therapy in neonates has also had a major impact on the incidence and consequences of RDS, antenatal corticosteroids are still associated with significant reduction in neonatal mortality, principally through reduced rates of RDS and intraventricular haemorrhage. A 2006 *Cochrane Database Review* confirmed significant reductions in the risks of mortality, RDS and intraventricular haemorrhage in preterm infants of 31%, 44% and 46%, respectively, after a single course of corticosteroids. Their mechanism of action is complex; they affect not only fetal lung maturation, but also fetal growth, organ system maturation, fetal brain development, immune function and the fetal hypothalamic–pituitary–adrenocortical axis. Currently, betamethasone or dexamethasone is recommended; both are able to cross the placenta in their active form and have comparable properties. Some dexamethasone preparations contain a sulphite preservative that has been linked with neurotoxicity and should be avoided.

However, enthusiasm for their use has been tempered by recent concerns, namely based on animal and some human data showing that repeated antenatal doses could lead to a decrease in birthweight, brain size and abnormal neuronal development. However, the long-term outcomes related to their use have been largely positive and, overall, antenatal corticosteroid treatment has been associated with less developmental delay in childhood than no corticosteroid treatment and a trend towards fewer children having cerebral palsy. While 30 years' follow-up showed no clinical differences in adults who were exposed in utero to betamethasone, there are no comparable data for dexamethasone.

ANTIBIOTICS

Despite a clear link between bacterial infection and preterm birth, the results of antibiotic treatment as an attempt to prevent PTL have been disappointing. The ORACLE trials focused on the use of antibiotics in PPROM (over 4,000 participants) and spontaneous PTL with intact membranes (over 6,000 participants). These trials demonstrated that, in singleton pregnancies with PPROM, erythromycin improved neonatal outcomes, but that antibiotic treatment in the presence of intact membranes had no benefit. As a result of these trials, 10 days of erythromycin has been adopted as the treatment of choice for PPROM in many obstetric units in the UK.

MANAGEMENT OF PRETERM PREMATURE RUPTURE OF MEMBRANES

PPROM occurs in approximately 2% of all pregnancies and accounts for up to one-third of preterm deliveries. Fifty per cent of pregnant women give birth within 1 week and 75% give birth within 2 weeks of PPROM. The earlier in pregnancy that PPROM occurs, the shorter the interval to birth. Although postnatal survival following PPROM is directly related to birthweight and gestational age at delivery,

in pregnancies complicated by PPROM prior to 23 weeks, pulmonary hypoplasia may develop, leading to an increased risk of neonatal death, even if delivery occurs at later gestational ages. Pulmonary hypoplasia following PPROM occurs in approximately 50% of cases with PPROM at 19 weeks, falling to about 10% at 25 weeks. The presence of amniotic fluid greater than 2 cm on ultrasound is associated with a lower incidence of pulmonary hypoplasia.

PPROM is diagnosed through clinical history and the demonstration of a pool of liquor in the vagina on speculum examination. If pooling of amniotic fluid is not observed, then further information can be obtained by performing an insulin-like growth factor binding protein-1 test or placental alpha-microglobulin-1 test of vaginal fluid. Management balances the risk of prematurity (if delivery is encouraged) with the risk of maternal and fetal infection (if delivery is delayed). In general, conservative management is followed in PPROM before 34 weeks' gestation unless there is evidence of chorioamnionitis and immediate induction of labour is advised in pregnant women after 37 weeks' gestation.

Conservative management includes intensive clinical surveillance for signs of chorioamnionitis including regular recording of the pregnant woman's temperature, heart rate, cardiotocography and biochemistry, with a rising white cell count or a rising C-reactive protein indicating development of chorioamnionitis. Lower genital tract swabs are routinely taken, but cultures do not correlate well with the risk of chorioamnionitis. In the majority of cases of PPROM, there is time for administration of corticosteroids and in utero transfer to a maternity department with a neonatal intensive care unit before the onset of PTL. Tocolysis is contraindicated due to the increased risk of maternal and fetal infection in patients with PPROM.

DELIVERY

When a pregnant woman is in PTL, decision-making is helped by detailed assessment of gestation, fetal and maternal well-being and is informed by knowledge of gestation-specific local neonatal outcomes. Depending on pregnancy gestation, tocolysis may be indicated to enable completion of antenatal corticosteroids, magnesium sulphate to be given and antibiotic therapy, if indicated. Delivery at a perinatal centre to avoid subsequent transfer and separation of the infant and mother should be considered. Decision-making by the obstetrician should involve the neonatologist and parents, as difficult decisions may be required, balancing the risk to the mother or fetus of continuing the pregnancy with the risk of prematurity.

With regard to mode of delivery, vaginal delivery is preferred unless the fetus is compromised, when caesarean delivery may be indicated. For assisted vaginal delivery at less than 34 weeks, forceps rather than vacuum devices are preferred, as there is less risk of trauma to the infant. For breech presentation, there is controversy about optimal mode of delivery; if before 26 weeks, most are delivered vaginally, but after this gestation they are often delivered by caesarean section. The neonatal team should be present at delivery. Unless the infant requires immediate resuscitation, clamping of the cord should be delayed, as this brings significant neonatal benefits. These include a reduced need for subsequent blood transfusions and potentially also a reduction in the incidence of necrotizing enterocolitis and intraventricular haemorrhage in the neonate. Infants <32 weeks' gestation are usually delivered into a plastic bag (wrap) to avoid hypothermia, which compromises outcome.

FURTHER READING

Lissauer T, Fanaroff AA, Miall L, Fanaroff J (2020). *Neonatology at a Glance*, 4th edn. Wiley Blackwell.

NICE (2015). *Preterm Labour and Birth*. NICE guideline [NG25]. Last updated: 10 June 2022. https://www.nice.org.uk/guidance/ng25.

Ohuma E, Moller A-B, Bradley E, et al. (2023) National, regional, and global estimates of preterm birth in 2020, with trends from 2010: a systematic analysis. *Lancet*, 402: 1261–1271.

Opondo C, Jayaweera H, Hollowell J, Li Y, Kurinczuk JJ, Quigley MA (2020). Variations in neonatal mortality, infant mortality, preterm birth and birth weight in England and Wales according to ethnicity and maternal country or region of birth: an analysis of linked national data from 2006 to 2012. *Journal of Epidemiology and Community Health*, 74(4): 336–345. http://dx.doi.org/10.1136/jech-2019-213093.

Royal College of Obstetricians and Gynaecologists (RCOG) (2022). Green-top guideline No 75: Cervical cerclage. *BJOG: An International Journal of Obstetrics & Gynaecology*, 129(7): 1178–1210. https://obgyn.onlinelibrary.wiley.com/doi/full/10.1111/1471-0528.17003.

Serenius F, Ewald U, Farooqi A, et al. (2016). Neurodevelopmental outcomes among extremely preterm infants 6.5 years after active perinatal care in Sweden. *JAMA Pediatrics*, 170(10): 954–963. https://doi.org/10.1001/jamapediatrics.2016.1210.

Smith R (2007). Parturition. *New England Journal of Medicine*, 356(3): 271–283.

Williams TC, Drake AJ (2019). Preterm birth in evolutionary context: A predictive adaptive response? *Philosophical Transactions of the Royal Society B: Biological Sciences*, 374: 20180121. http://dx.doi.org/10.1098/rstb.2018.0121.

World Health Organization (2023). Preterm birth – WHO Fact Sheet. https://www.who.int/news-room/fact-sheets/detail/preterm-birth.

⊙⟲ KEY LEARNING POINTS

- PTL has multiple causes.
- Worldwide, preterm delivery is the most common cause of mortality of children under 5 years of age.
- Screening with transvaginal ultrasound can detect individuals at high risk of preterm delivery.
- Progesterone reduces the risk of preterm birth in pregnant women with a short cervix.
- Cervical cerclage reduces the risk of preterm birth in high-risk pregnant women.
- Antenatal corticosteroids reduce the risk of neonatal RDS.
- Tocolysis may be used to allow time for antenatal steroids to be given.
- Magnesium sulphate given to the mother prior to delivery provides neuroprotection for the fetus.

SELF-ASSESSMENT

For interactive SBAs and EMQs relating to this chapter, visit www.routledge.com/cw/mccarthy.

CASE HISTORY 1

Mrs L, a 41-year-old Black woman, attends your clinic for a booking visit. This is her second pregnancy. Her first child was born at 26 weeks' gestation following premature rupture of the membranes. This was an unplanned pregnancy and her last delivery was 4 months ago. She is a smoker and has a history of gestational diabetes.

Identify the key risk factors for preterm delivery and prepare a plan for management during the pregnancy.

ANSWER

Mrs L is a very high-risk pregnancy with a significant risk of very preterm delivery again. Her main risk factors are her age, ethnicity, previous extreme preterm delivery, smoking and associated medical condition of diabetes. Her management should involve all of the following: consideration for cervical cerclage, smoking cessation services, referral to social work and perinatal medicine clinic for management of her pregnancy, and commencement of aspirin. Her past medical obstetric notes should also be obtained and reviewed to ascertain the previous events leading to preterm delivery.

CASE HISTORY 2

Ms K presents at 31 weeks' gestation with a story of leaking of fluid for 12 hours. She is not having any pains.

A What investigations would you do?

B Discus your management plan.

ANSWERS

A The critical investigation here is a speculum examination to examine for pooling of liquor in the posterior fornix. This confirms PPROM.

B Ongoing management of this pregnancy involves the following: informing the neonatal unit as the risk of preterm delivery is very high; administration of corticosteroids; consideration of the administration of magnesium sulphate; confirmation via ultrasound of the presenting part; admission to hospital; review by a consultant neonatologist; and commencement of oral erythromycin. She should be managed within a perinatal medicine team with multidisciplinary input.

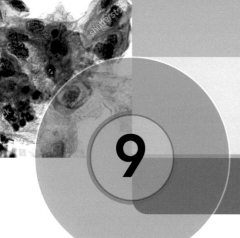

9

Hypertensive disorders of pregnancy

LOUISE C KENNY

Learning Objectives

- Understand the classification of hypertension in pregnancy.
- Appreciate and be able to differentiate between the different risks associated with various types of hypertensive disorders in pregnancy.
- Understand the pathophysiology of pre-eclampsia.
- Be aware of the clinical presentation of pre-eclampsia and understand the principles of management.
- Understand the long-term risks to both the pregnant woman and the baby from pre-eclampsia.

INTRODUCTION

Hypertension is common in pregnancy. Approximately 1 in 10 pregnancies will be complicated by one or more episodes of raised blood pressure prior to delivery. In the majority of cases, the cause is a benign condition called gestational hypertension, which is not associated with adverse outcomes. However, in a third of cases (approximately 3% of pregnancies overall), the cause is pre-eclampsia. Pre-eclampsia is a leading cause of mortality in pregnancy. The World Health Organization estimates that, globally, between 50,000 and 75,000 pregnant women die of this condition each year. Pre-eclampsia is frequently accompanied by fetal growth restriction (FGR), and both pre-eclampsia and FGR result in increased rates of preterm delivery, causing considerable perinatal morbidity and mortality. It is also now clear that

pre-eclampsia has long-term consequences for the pregnant woman, as it predisposes to long-term cardiovascular disease.

As the population entering pregnancy is doing so at an older age, especially in high-resource settings, an increasing number of pregnancies are complicated by chronic hypertension. Chronic hypertension, regardless of the underlying cause, is associated with an increased risk of pre-eclampsia and FGR. In this chapter, the various types of hypertension and their management are discussed.

CLASSIFICATION OF HYPERTENSION IN PREGNANCY

There is a widely agreed classification system for hypertension in pregnancy. Simply put, there are

131

10.1201/9781003196112-9

three conditions that account for the overwhelming majority of cases of hypertension in pregnancy:

1. non-proteinuric pregnancy-induced hypertension
2. pre-eclampsia
3. chronic hypertension

Non-proteinuric pregnancy-induced hypertension (otherwise known as gestational hypertension) is hypertension that arises for the first time in the second half of pregnancy and in the absence of proteinuria. It is not associated with adverse pregnancy outcome, and modest increases in blood pressure in this setting do not require treatment. However, up to one-third of cases of gestational hypertension will progress to pre-eclampsia.

Hypertension in the first half of pregnancy most likely indicates the presence of chronic hypertension. As is the case in the non-pregnant population, most cases of chronic hypertension (~90%) are essential hypertension but it is important to remember that this is a diagnosis of exclusion. Secondary causes of hypertension presenting for the first time in the first half of pregnancy should be excluded. Chronic hypertension, of whatever type, can predispose to the later development of superimposed pre-eclampsia. Even in the absence of superimposed pre-eclampsia, chronic hypertension is associated with increased maternal and fetal morbidity, and pregnancies complicated by chronic hypertension should therefore be regarded as high risk. The physiological fall in blood pressure that occurs in the first trimester secondary to peripheral vasodilatation can mask chronic hypertension. For example, a blood pressure of 138/88 mmHg in the first trimester, while still technically within normal limits, raises the suspicion of an underlying hypertensive tendency.

PRE-ECLAMPSIA

INCIDENCE

Pre-eclampsia complicates approximately 2–3% of pregnancies in the UK, but there is significant global variation. In the most recent UK and Ireland Confidential Enquiry into Maternal Deaths (2017–2019), there were six deaths due to pre-eclampsia, which represents a significant fall from a decade previously when 19 deaths occurred in 2006–2008 triennium because of pre-eclampsia. However, globally, around 70,000 pregnant women die annually of pre-eclampsia, making it a leading cause of maternal death in low-resource settings.

> ### BOX 9.1: Definition of pre-eclampsia
>
> Pre-eclampsia is defined as new-onset gestational hypertension (systolic blood pressure ≥140 mmHg and/or diastolic blood pressure ≥90 mmHg) associated with new onset of at least one of the following:
>
> - proteinuria
> - maternal organ dysfunction (liver, neurological, haematological or renal involvement)
> - uteroplacental dysfunction at or after 20 weeks' gestation
>
> It is important to note that pre-eclampsia may present for the first time in the intra-partum period or in the puerperium.

DIAGNOSIS OF PRE-ECLAMPSIA

MEASUREMENT OF BLOOD PRESSURE

To confirm the presence of hypertension, blood pressure should be measured on at least two occasions 4 hours apart using an appropriately sized cuff and validated device for use in pregnancy. Blood pressure should be measured at every antenatal appointment (see **Chapter 1**). For pregnant women at high risk, guidelines recommend monitoring blood pressure at increased frequency.

PROTEINURIA

Proteinuria is screened for by dipstick testing and confirmed by additional laboratory tests using 24-hour urine collections or, more recently, spot samples of urine. An automated reagent-strip reading device rather than visual analysis should be used for dipstick screening. Previously, a 24-hour urine collection was considered the gold standard for confirmation of proteinuria, but it has several problems: it is time consuming and inconvenient for pregnant women

Table 9.1 Testing for proteinuria

Test/result	Interpretation
Dipstick urinalysis	Instant result but quantitatively inaccurate
Trace	Seldom significant
1+	Possible significant proteinuria, warrants quantifying
≥2+	Probable significant proteinuria, warrants quantifying
Protein:creatinine ratio (results semi-quantitative)	Fast (within 1 hour)
>30 mg/mol	Probable significant proteinuria
24-hour collection	Slow
300 mg/24 hours	Confirmed significant proteinuria

and samples are often incomplete. By definition, it leads to a 24-hour delay in confirming the diagnosis. Therefore, the use of either spot urine albumin to creatinine (A:Cr) or protein to creatinine (P:Cr) ratios are now recommended to quantify proteinuria. Both P:Cr and A:Cr testing are shown to significantly correlate with proteinuria as detected by 24-hour urine. Diagnostic thresholds of 30 mg/mmol and 8 mg/mmol have been determined to provide high sensitivity and specificity, respectively (see **Table 9.1**).

ADDITIONAL LABORATORY TESTS

International guidelines recommend that pregnant women suspected of having pre-eclampsia are investigated with laboratory tests measuring haemoglobin, platelet count, serum creatinine, liver enzymes and serum uric acid to determine the presence of maternal organ dysfunction and the diagnosis of pre-eclampsia. New guidelines also recommend the use of placental growth factor (PlGF) or soluble fms-like tyrosine kinase (sFlt-1):PlGF ratio testing for pre-eclampsia in specific circumstances. sFlt-1 is an anti-angiogenic protein that acts as an antagonist to the angiogenic proteins PlGF and vascular endothelial growth factor (VEGF). By inhibiting VEGF and PlGF, sFlt-1 alters downstream signalling pathways, which results in vasoconstriction and endothelial dysfunction. Recent large trials have shown that low PlGF has a high sensitivity and negative predictive value in diagnosing pre-eclampsia needing delivery within 14 days, and a sFlt-1:PlGF ratio of <38 can rule out pre-eclampsia within the next 7 days. The National Institute for Health and Care Excellence (NICE) therefore recommends the use of PlGF or sFlt-1:PlGF ratio to help rule out pre-eclampsia in pregnant women between 20 and 34 + 6 weeks' gestation who present with suspected pre-eclampsia.

FETAL ASSESSMENT

Uteroplacental dysfunction can be evaluated with ultrasound assessment of fetal growth and umbilical artery Doppler velocimetry to assess blood flow redistribution in placental insufficiency (see **Chapter 4**).

RISK FACTORS

Pre-eclampsia is more common in first pregnancies. The reason for this has been the subject of intense speculation in recent decades. One theory suggests that the normal fetal–maternal transfusion that occurs during pregnancy and particularly during delivery exposes the pregnant woman to products of the fetal (and hence paternal) genome, protecting them in subsequent pregnancies. In line with this, the protective effect of first pregnancy seems to be

---

BOX 9.2: Risk factors for pre-eclampsia

Major risk factors
- Pre-eclampsia in any previous pregnancy
- Chronic kidney disease
- Autoimmune disease such as systemic lupus erythematosus or antiphospholipid syndrome
- Chronic hypertension
- Type 1 or 2 diabetes

Moderate risk factors
- First pregnancy
- Aged 40 years or older
- Pregnancy interval of more than 10 years
- Body mass index (BMI) of 35 kg/m² or more at first visit
- Family history of pre-eclampsia
- Multi-fetal pregnancy

(Adapted from NICE (2019). *Hypertension in Pregnancy: Diagnosis and Management*. NICE guideline [NG133]).

lost if a woman has a subsequent pregnancy with a new partner. Conversely, a previous history of pre-eclampsia is a major risk factor for pre-eclampsia in subsequent pregnancies. This may, in part, be due to a genetic predisposition to pre-eclampsia, as there is a three- to fourfold increase in the incidence of pre-eclampsia in the first-degree relatives of affected individuals. Finally, there are a number of general medical conditions and pregnancy-specific factors that predispose to the development of pre-eclampsia.

PATHOPHYSIOLOGY

Pre-eclampsia is unusual in medicine in that it is defined by the symptoms and signs it presents with. This has arisen largely because, until very recently, the underlying pathophysiology of this disorder was poorly understood. Pre-eclampsia occurs only in pregnancy, but it has been described in pregnancies lacking a fetus (molar pregnancies) and in the absence of a uterus (abdominal pregnancies), suggesting that it is the presence of trophoblast tissue that provides the stimulus for the disorder. General thinking suggests that the development of pre-eclampsia is a two-stage process, which originates in early pregnancy (**Figure 9.1**). In the first stage, trophoblast invasion is patchy and the spiral arteries retain their muscular walls. This is thought to prevent the development of a high-flow, low-impedance uteroplacental circulation and leads to uteroplacental ischaemia (**Figure 9.2**). The reason why trophoblasts invade less effectively in these pregnancies is not known but may reflect an abnormal adaptation of the maternal immune system.

In the second stage, uteroplacental ischaemia results in oxidative and inflammatory stress, with

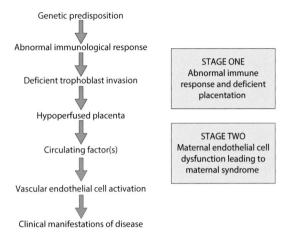

Figure 9.2 The proposed aetiology of pre-eclampsia.

the involvement of secondary mediators leading to endothelial dysfunction, vasospasm and activation of the coagulation system (**Figure 9.1**). As the target cell of the disease process, the vascular endothelial cell, is so ubiquitous, pre-eclampsia is a truly multisystem disorder, affecting multiple organ systems, often concurrently.

CARDIOVASCULAR SYSTEM

Normal pregnancy is characterized by marked peripheral vasodilatation resulting in a fall in total peripheral resistance despite an increase in plasma volume and cardiac rate. Pre-eclampsia is characterized by marked peripheral vasoconstriction, resulting in hypertension. The intravascular high pressure and loss of endothelial cell integrity results in greater vascular permeability and contributes to the formation of generalized oedema.

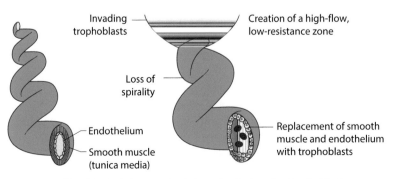

Figure 9.1 Physiological change of spiral arteries by invading trophoblasts.

RENAL SYSTEM

In the kidney, a highly characteristic lesion called glomeruloendotheliosis is seen. This is relatively specific for pre-eclampsia (it is not seen with other hypertensive disorders) and is associated with impaired glomerular filtration and selective loss of intermediate weight proteins, such as albumin and transferrin, leading to proteinuria. This in turn causes a reduction in plasma oncotic pressure and exacerbates the development of oedema.

HAEMATOLOGICAL SYSTEM

In the event of endothelial damage, platelets adhere to the damaged area. Furthermore, diffuse vascular damage is associated with the laying down of fibrin. Pre-eclampsia in association with increased fibrin deposition and a reduction in the platelet count may accompany and occasionally predate the onset of disease.

LIVER

In the liver, subendothelial fibrin deposition is associated with elevation of liver enzymes. This can be associated with haemolysis and a low platelet count due to platelet consumption (and subsequent widespread activation of the coagulation system). The presence of these findings is called haemolysis, elevation of liver enzymes and low platelets (HELLP) syndrome. HELLP syndrome is a particularly severe

BOX 9.3: HELLP syndrome

- HELLP syndrome is an acronym for haemolysis, elevation of liver enzymes and low platelets.
- Pregnant women with HELLP syndrome typically present with epigastric pain, nausea and vomiting.
- Hypertension may be mild or even absent.
- HELLP syndrome is associated with a range of serious complications including acute renal failure, placental abruption and stillbirth.
- The management of HELLP syndrome involves stabilizing the pregnant patient, correcting any coagulation deficits and assessing the fetus for delivery.

form of pre-eclampsia, occurring in just 2–4% of pregnant women with the disease. It is associated with a high fetal loss rate (of up to 60%) (see the box 'HELLP syndrome').

NEUROLOGICAL SYSTEM

The development of convulsions in a pregnant woman with pre-eclampsia, in the absence of any other known or likely cause, is defined as eclampsia. Vasospasm and cerebral oedema have both been implicated in the pathogenesis of eclampsia. Retinal haemorrhages, exudates and papilloedema are characteristic of hypertensive encephalopathy and are rare in pre-eclampsia, suggesting that hypertension alone is not responsible for the cerebral pathology.

PLACENTAL INSUFFICIENCY AND FETAL GROWTH RESTRICTION

The underlying pathophysiology of pre-eclampsia predisposes to FGR, which frequently, but not invariably, occurs in pregnancies with pre-eclampsia. The presence of placental insufficiency after 20 weeks' gestation is one of the defining features of pre-eclampsia. However, it is important to note the severe FGR may occur in the absence of maternal hypertension or any other features of pre-eclampsia and, similarly, severe pre-eclampsia can occur without evidence of FGR.

CLINICAL PRESENTATION

The classic symptoms of pre-eclampsia include a frontal headache, visual disturbance and epigastric pain. However, the majority of pregnant women with pre-eclampsia are asymptomatic or merely complain of general vague 'flu-like' symptoms.

Clinical examination should include a complete obstetric and neurological examination (see **Chapter 1**). Hypertension is usually the first sign but occasionally is absent or transient until the late stages of the disease. Dependent oedema of the feet is very common in healthy pregnant women. However, rapidly progressive oedema of the face and hands may suggest pre-eclampsia. Epigastric tenderness is a worrying sign and suggests liver involvement.

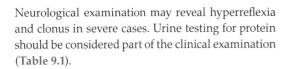

Neurological examination may reveal hyperreflexia and clonus in severe cases. Urine testing for protein should be considered part of the clinical examination (**Table 9.1**).

MANAGEMENT AND TREATMENT

There is no cure for pre-eclampsia other than to end the pregnancy by delivering the baby (and placenta). This can be a significant problem if pre-eclampsia occurs early in pregnancy, particularly at gestations less than 34 weeks. Therefore, management strategies are aimed at minimizing risk to the pregnant woman in order to permit continued fetal growth. In severe cases this is often not possible.

The principles of management of pre-eclampsia are:

- early recognition of the symptomless syndrome
- awareness of the serious nature of the condition in its severest form
- adherence to agreed guidelines for admission to hospital, investigation and the use of antihypertensive and anticonvulsant therapy
- well-timed delivery to pre-empt serious maternal or fetal complications
- postnatal follow-up and counselling for future pregnancies

A diagnosis of pre-eclampsia usually requires admission (**Table 9.2**). Patients with mild hypertension,

Table 9.2 The management of pregnancy complicated by pre-eclampsia, depending on the degree of hypertension

Management	Hypertension: Blood pressure of 140/90–159/109 mmHg	Severe hypertension: Blood pressure of 160/110 mmHg or more
Admission to hospital	Admit if any clinical concerns for the well-being of the pregnant woman or baby or if there is a high risk of adverse events	Admit, but if blood pressure falls below 160/110 mmHg, then manage as for hypertension
Antihypertensive pharmacological treatment	Offer pharmacological treatment if blood pressure remains above 140/90 mmHg	Offer pharmacological treatment to all pregnant women
Target blood pressure once on antihypertensive treatment	Aim for blood pressure of 135/85 mmHg or less	Aim for blood pressure of 135/85 mmHg or less
Blood pressure measurement	At least every 48 hours, and more frequently if the pregnant woman is admitted to hospital	Every 15–30 minutes until blood pressure is less than 160/110 mmHg, then at least four times daily while the pregnant woman is an inpatient, depending on clinical circumstances
Dipstick proteinuria testing	Only repeat if clinically indicated, for example if new symptoms and signs develop or if there is uncertainty over diagnosis	Only repeat if clinically indicated, for example if new symptoms and signs develop or if there is uncertainty over diagnosis
Blood tests	Measure full blood count, liver function and renal function twice a week	Measure full blood count, liver function and renal function three times a week
Fetal assessment	Offer fetal heart auscultation at every antenatal appointment Carry out ultrasound assessment of the fetus at diagnosis and, if normal, repeat every 2 weeks Carry out cardiotocography at diagnosis and then only if clinically indicated	Offer fetal heart auscultation at every antenatal appointment Carry out ultrasound assessment of the fetus at diagnosis and, if normal, repeat every 2 weeks Carry out cardiotocography at diagnosis and then only if clinically indicated

Source: Adapted from NICE (2019). *Hypertension in Pregnancy: Diagnosis and Management.* NICE guideline [NG133]. Last updated: 17 April 2023.

minimal protein and normal haematological and biochemical parameters may be monitored as out-patients, but will require frequent attendance for fetal and maternal assessment. Pregnant women with severe hypertension, significant proteinuria or abnormal haematological or biochemical parameters require admission and inpatient management.

INVESTIGATIONS

To monitor maternal complications, the following investigations are required:

- full blood count (with particular emphasis on falling platelet count and rising haematocrit)
- if platelet values are normal, additional clotting studies are not indicated
- serum renal profile (including serum uric acid levels)
- serum liver profile
- frequent repeat proteinuria quantification is probably unhelpful once a diagnosis of pre-eclampsia has been made

To monitor fetal complications, the following investigations are required:

- ultrasound assessment of:
  - fetal size
  - amniotic fluid volume
  - maternal and fetal Doppler assessments
- antenatal cardiotocography, used in conjunction with ultrasound surveillance – provides a useful but by no means infallible indication of fetal well-being; a loss of baseline variability or decelerations may indicate fetal hypoxia.

TREATMENT OF HYPERTENSION

The most common cause of death in women who die of pre-eclampsia in the UK is cerebral bleeding secondary to uncontrolled systolic blood pressure. Therefore, the aim of antihypertensive therapy is to lower the blood pressure and reduce the risk of maternal cerebrovascular accident without reducing uterine blood flow and compromising the fetus. There are a variety of antihypertensives used in the management of pre-eclampsia.

Labetalol is an alpha-blocking and beta-blocking agent. It has a good safety record in pregnancy and can be given orally and intravenously. It is the first drug of choice in most national guidelines including the current NICE guideline *Hypertension in Pregnancy: Diagnosis and Management*. Nifedipine is a calcium-channel blocker with a rapid onset of action. It can, however, cause severe headache that may mimic worsening disease. Methyldopa is a centrally acting antihypertensive agent. It has a long-established safety record in pregnancy. However, it can only be given orally, it takes upwards of 24 hours to take effect and it has a range of unpleasant side effects including sedation and depression. These properties limit its usefulness. In severe cases of fulminating disease, an intravenous infusion of hydralazine or labetalol can be titrated rapidly against changes in the blood pressure.

TREATMENT AND PREVENTION OF ECLAMPSIA

The drug of choice for the treatment of eclampsia is magnesium sulphate. This is given intravenously and has been shown to reduce the incidence of further convulsions in pregnant women with eclampsia. Magnesium sulphate should also be used in patients with severe pre-eclampsia to prevent the onset of convulsions. The management of eclampsia is described in further detail in **Chapter 14**.

SCREENING AND PREVENTION

The accurate prediction of pregnant women at risk of developing pre-eclampsia will facilitate targeting of increased antenatal surveillance while allowing those at low risk to participate in community-based antenatal care. In addition, a predictive test would in turn facilitate the development of novel therapeutic preventative interventions.

Unfortunately, there is currently no early pregnancy screening test for pre-eclampsia. Despite intensive research in this area, no single blood biomarker has emerged that either alone or in combination with other biomarkers or clinical data possesses sufficient sensitivity and specificity to be clinically useful.

The ability of Doppler ultrasound uterine artery waveform analysis to identify pregnant women at risk of pre-eclampsia (and other adverse pregnancy outcomes) has been investigated with varying success. In pregnancies with incomplete trophoblast remodelling of the spiral arteries, a characteristic 'notch' can often be seen in the waveform pattern that frequently also demonstrates high resistance (see **Chapter 4** and **Figure 4.20**). This screening test may have a role in women who have already been identified as being at risk of the disease because of their medical or past obstetric history. However, it is not of value in screening low-risk pregnancies.

Established preventative interventions include low-dose aspirin (typically 75–150 mg daily), which modestly reduces the risk of pre-eclampsia in high-risk pregnant women; calcium supplementation may also reduce risk, but only in individuals with low dietary intake.

ADDITIONAL POINTS IN MANAGEMENT

Iatrogenic premature delivery of the fetus is often required in severe pre-eclampsia. If the pregnant woman is sufficiently stable, she should be transferred to a centre with adequate facilities to care for the baby, and prior to 34 weeks' gestation steroids should be given intramuscularly to the pregnant woman to reduce the chance of neonatal respiratory distress syndrome. Delivery before term is often by caesarean section. Such patients are at particularly high risk for thromboembolism and should be given prophylactic subcutaneous heparin and issued with anti-thromboembolic stockings. In the case of spontaneous or induced labour and if clotting studies are normal, epidural anaesthesia is indicated, as it helps control blood pressure. Ergometrine is avoided in the management of the third stage, as it can significantly increase blood pressure.

Postnatally, blood pressure and proteinuria will resolve. However, in a minority of cases, one or both persist beyond 6 weeks postpartum and this suggests the presence of underlying chronic hypertension or renal disease. Additionally, a careful search should be made postnatally for underlying medical disorders in anyone who presents with severe pre-eclampsia before 34 weeks' gestation.

> ### ⊙⟲ KEY LEARNING POINTS
>
> - Pre-eclampsia is a multisystem disorder that likely originates in the placenta and is a significant cause of maternal and perinatal morbidity and mortality.
> - There is no cure other than delivery; the aim of management is to stabilize the maternal blood pressure and prevent seizures and cerebral bleeding.

CHRONIC HYPERTENSION

Essential hypertension is the underlying cause of chronic hypertension in 90% of cases. However, before a diagnosis is made, other causes need to be excluded. Appropriate investigations include serum creatinine, electrolytes, urine analysis (blood, protein and glucose), protein quantification and renal ultrasound. Autoantibody screen and cardiac investigations including electrocardiography and echocardiography should be considered when there is clinical suspicion (history, examination or investigation results) of a secondary cause. Renal causes account for over 80% of cases of secondary hypertension (see **Chapter 10**).

> ### BOX 9.4: Causes of chronic hypertension
>
> - Idiopathic
> - Essential hypertension
> - Vascular disorders
> - Renal artery stenosis
> - Coarctation of the aorta
> - Renal disease
> - Polycystic disease
> - Diabetic nephropathy
> - Chronic glomerulonephritis
> - Nephrotic and nephritic syndrome
> - Collagen vascular disease
> - Systemic sclerosis
> - Systemic lupus erythematosus
> - Rheumatoid disease
> - Endocrine disease
> - Phaeochromocytoma
> - Conn syndrome
> - Cushing syndrome
> - Diabetes mellitus

The maternal risks of pre-existing hypertension include pre-eclampsia, abruption, heart failure and intracerebral haemorrhage. Pre-eclampsia develops in around one-third of pregnant women with pre-existing hypertension and is more likely to affect those with severe hypertension and/or renal disease.

MANAGEMENT

In mild cases (<150/100 mmHg) there is no immediate indication to treat; however, the pregnancy should be monitored carefully to detect changes in blood pressure or features of pre-eclampsia (usually indicated by new proteinuria), as well as FGR by serial ultrasound scans. Antihypertensive medication taken before pregnancy can often be discontinued in the first half of pregnancy, as there is a physiological reduction in blood pressure. Angiotensin-converting enzyme (ACE) inhibitors, angiotensin-receptor blockers and atenolol should be discontinued because of concerns of teratogenicity and negative effects on fetal growth.

If the blood pressure is consistently >150/100 mmHg, antihypertensive medication should be offered to reduce the risk of severe hypertension and the attendant risks of intracerebral haemorrhage, although treatment does not prevent placental abruption or superimposed pre-eclampsia, nor does it influence perinatal outcome. Preferred antihypertensive agents include labetolol, nifedipine and methyldopa (centrally acting agent). The aim of antihypertensive medication is to maintain the blood pressure below 160 mmHg systolic and 80–100 mmHg diastolic.

The obstetric management of pre-existing hypertension involves close monitoring for the development of superimposed pre-eclampsia and FGR. In pregnant women requiring antihypertensive medication, delivery is usually offered around 39 weeks, but may need to be earlier if complications have developed.

Following delivery, the maternal blood pressure often decreases, but careful surveillance is required, as it tends to increase again on the third or fourth post-partum day. Breastfeeding is encouraged and medication should be changed to those drugs that are considered safe.

BOX 9.5: Risk factors for developing superimposed pre-eclampsia

- Renal disease
- Maternal age >40 years
- Pre-existing diabetes
- Multiple pregnancy
- Connective tissue disease (e.g. antiphospholipid syndrome)
- Coarctation of the aorta
- Blood pressure ≥160/100 mmHg in early pregnancy
- Pre-pregnancy BMI >35
- Previous pre-eclampsia

⚷ KEY LEARNING POINTS

- Chronic hypertension is associated with a range of adverse maternal and perinatal outcomes and it should be regarded as a high-risk pregnancy.
- Chronic hypertension may present for the first time in pregnancy and it may initially be masked by the profound vasodilatation and decrease in peripheral vascular resistance seen in the first trimester of pregnancy.

FETAL GROWTH RESTRICTION

DEFINITION AND INCIDENCE

FGR is defined as a failure of a fetus to achieve its genetic growth potential. This usually results in a fetus that is small for gestational age (SGA). SGA means that the weight of the fetus is less than the 10th centile for its gestation. Other cut-off points (e.g. the 3rd centile) can be used. The terms SGA and FGR are not synonymous. It is important to remember that most SGA fetuses are constitutionally small and are not compromised. FGR indicates that there is a pathological process operating to restrict the growth rate of the fetus. Consequently, some FGR fetuses may not actually be SGA, but nevertheless will have failed to fulfil their growth potential.

There are a wide variety of reasons why a baby may be born small, including congenital anomalies, fetal infections and chromosomal abnormalities (these are discussed in more detail in **Chapter 5**).

However, most babies that are born small are either constitutionally small (i.e. healthy but born to small parents and fulfilling their genetic growth potential) or are small secondary to abnormal placenta function and have FGR.

FGR is a major cause of neonatal and infant morbidity and mortality. There is a significant cost associated with providing adequate facilities to look after these babies. In addition, there is an increasing body of evidence that certain adult diseases (such as diabetes and hypertension) are more common in adults who were born with FGR.

AETIOLOGY

The common causes of FGR are listed in **Table 9.3**. They are grouped into two main categories: factors that directly affect the intrinsic growth potential of the fetus and external influences that reduce the support for fetal growth. Chromosome abnormalities, genetic syndromes and fetal infections can alter intrinsic fetal growth potential. External influences that affect fetal growth can be subdivided into maternal systemic factors and placental insufficiency.

Table 9.3 Causes of fetal growth restriction

Type	Causes
Reduced fetal growth potential	Aneuploidies (e.g. trisomy 18)
	Single gene defects (e.g. Seckel syndrome)
	Structural abnormalities (e.g. renal agenesis)
	Intrauterine infections (e.g. cytomegalovirus, toxoplasmosis)
Reduced fetal growth support	
Maternal factors	Undernutrition (e.g. poverty, eating disorders)
	Maternal hypoxia (e.g. living at altitude, cyanotic heart disease)
	Drugs (e.g. alcohol, cigarettes, cocaine)
Placental factors	Reduced uteroplacental perfusion (e.g. inadequate trophoblast invasion, sickle cell disease, multiple gestation)
	Reduced fetoplacental perfusion (e.g. single umbilical artery, twin–twin transfusion syndrome)

Maternal undernutrition is globally the major cause of FGR. Low maternal oxygen saturation, which can occur with cyanotic heart disease or at high altitude, will reduce fetal oxygen levels and fetal metabolism. Smoking, by increasing the amount of carboxyhaemoglobin in the maternal circulation, effectively reduces the amount of oxygen available to the fetus, thus causing FGR. A wide variety of drugs other than tobacco can affect fetal growth, including alcohol and cocaine, probably through multiple mechanisms affecting fetal enzyme systems, placental blood flow and maternal substrate levels.

In developed countries, the most common cause of FGR is poor placental function secondary to inadequate trophoblast invasion of the spiral arteries. This results in reduced perfusion of the intracotyledon space, which in turn leads to abnormal development of the terminal villi and impaired transfer of oxygen and nutrients to the fetus. The placental pathology of this is similar to that seen in pre-eclampsia and accounts for why pre-eclampsia and FGR commonly present together. Less frequently, reduced perfusion can occur from other conditions such as maternal sickle cell disease and antiphospholipid syndrome (see **Chapter 10**). Multiple pregnancy usually results in a sharing of the uterine vascularity, which causes a relative reduction in the blood flow to each placenta. On the fetal side of the placental circulation, abnormalities of the umbilical cord, such as a single umbilical artery, are associated with FGR as are the intraplacental vascular connections found in monochorionic twinning.

PATHOPHYSIOLOGY

FGR is frequently classified as symmetrical or asymmetrical. Symmetrically small fetuses are normally associated with factors that directly impair fetal growth such as chromosomal disorders and fetal infections. Asymmetrical growth restriction is classically associated with uteroplacental insufficiency, which leads to reduced oxygen transfer to the fetus and impaired excretion of carbon dioxide by the placenta. A fall in fetal oxygen and a rise in fetal carbon dioxide in the fetal blood induces a chemoreceptor response in the fetal carotid bodies with resulting vasodilatation in the fetal brain, myocardium and adrenal glands, and vasoconstriction in the kidneys, splanchnic vessels, limbs and subcutaneous tissues. The liver circulation is also severely reduced. Normally, 50% of the well-oxygenated blood in the umbilical vein passes to the right atrium through the ductus venosus, eventually to reach the fetal brain, with the remainder going to the portal circulation in the liver. When there is fetal hypoxia, more of the well-oxygenated blood from the umbilical vein is diverted through the ductus venosus, which means that the liver receives less. The result of all these circulatory changes is an asymmetrical fetus with relative brain sparing, reduced abdominal girth and skin thickness. The vasoconstriction in the fetal kidneys results in impaired urine production and oligohydramnios. Fetal hypoxaemia also leads to severe metabolic changes in the fetus reflecting intrauterine starvation. Antenatal fetal blood sampling has shown reduced levels of nutrients such as glucose and amino acids (especially essential amino acids) and of hormones such as thyroxine and insulin. There are increased levels of corticosteroids and catecholamines, which reflect the increased perfusion of the adrenal gland. Haematological changes also reflect chronic hypoxia, with increased levels of erythropoietin and nucleated red blood cells.

Chronic fetal hypoxia in FGR may eventually lead to fetal acidaemia, both respiratory and metabolic, which if prolonged can lead to intrauterine death if the fetus is not removed from its hostile environment. FGR fetuses are especially at risk from profound asphyxia in labour due to further compromise of the uteroplacental circulation by uterine contractions.

MANAGEMENT

The assessment of fetal well-being is described in detail in **Chapter 4**. In brief, the detection of an SGA infant contains two elements: first, the accurate assessment of gestational age and, second, the recognition of fetal smallness.

Early measurement of the fetal crown–rump length before 13 weeks + 6 days' gestation or a head circumference between 13 + 6 and 20 weeks' gestation remains the method of choice for confirming gestational age. Thereafter, the most precise way of assessing fetal growth is by ultrasound biometry (biparietal diameter, head circumference, abdominal circumference and femur length) serially at set time intervals

(usually of 4 weeks and no less than 2 weeks). As resources in most units do not permit comprehensive serial ultrasound in all pregnancies, serial ultrasound biometry is usually performed in 'at risk' pregnancies (see **Box 9.6**, 'Pregnancies at risk of FGR').

BOX 9.6: Pregnancies at risk of FGR

- Multiple pregnancies (see **Chapter 7**)
- History of FGR in previous pregnancy
- Current heavy smokers
- Current drug users
- Women with underlying medical disorders:
  - hypertension
  - diabetes
  - cyanotic heart disease
  - antiphospholipid syndrome
- Pregnancies where the symphysis–fundal height is less than expected

When a diagnosis of SGA has been made, the next step is to clarify whether the baby is normal and simply constitutionally small or whether it is FGR. A comprehensive ultrasound examination of the fetal anatomy should be made, looking for fetal abnormalities that may explain the size. Even if the anatomy appears normal, the presence of symmetrical growth restriction in the presence of a normal amniotic fluid volume raises the suspicion of a fetal genetic defect and the parents should be counselled accordingly. Amniocentesis and rapid fetal karyotype should be offered. Features suspicious of uteroplacental insufficiency are an asymmetrically growth restricted fetus with a relatively small abdominal circumference, oligohydramnios and a high umbilical artery resistance (see **Chapter 4**, **Figures 4.14–4.16**).

At present, there are no widely accepted treatments available for FGR related to uteroplacental insufficiency. Obvious contributing factors such as smoking, alcohol and drug abuse should be stopped and the health of the woman should be optimized. Low-dose aspirin may have a role in the prevention of FGR in high-risk pregnancies but is not effective in the treatment of established cases.

When growth restriction is severe and the fetus is too immature to be delivered safely, bed rest in hospital is usually advised in an effort to maximize placental blood flow, although the evidence supporting this practice is limited. The aim of these interventions is to gain as much maturity as possible before delivering the fetus, thereby reducing the morbidity associated with prematurity. However, timing the delivery in such a way that maximizes gestation without risking the baby dying in utero demands intensive fetal surveillance. The most widely accepted methods of monitoring the fetus are discussed in detail in **Chapter 4** and are summarized briefly in **Box 9.7**, 'Surveillance of the FGR fetus'.

BOX 9.7: Surveillance of the FGR fetus

- Serial biometry and amniotic fluid volume measurement performed at no less than 2-weekly intervals
- In the FGR fetus, dynamic tests of fetal well-being include:
  - umbilical artery Doppler wave form analysis
  - absence or reversed flow of blood in the umbilical artery during fetal diastole – requires delivery in the near future
  - in extremely preterm or pre-viable infants with absent or reversed end diastolic flow in the umbilical artery, other fetal arterial and venous Doppler studies, although their use has not yet been proven by large prospective trials
- Fetal CTG

PROGNOSIS

The prognosis of FGR is highly dependent upon the cause, severity and gestation at delivery. When FGR is related to a congenital infection or chromosomal abnormality, subsequent development of the child will be determined by the precise abnormality.

Among babies with FGR secondary to uteroplacental insufficiency, some babies will suffer morbidity or mortality as a result of prematurity. For the survivors, the long-term prognosis is good, with low incidences of mental and physical disability, and most infants demonstrate 'catch-up growth' after delivery when feeding is established. A link between FGR and the adult onset of hypertension and diabetes has been established. It remains to be seen whether other associations will be found in the future.

KEY LEARNING POINTS

- SGA refers to those fetuses whose estimated weight is less than the 10th centile for their gestational age. Most SGA fetuses are healthy.
- FGR refers to any fetus failing to achieve its growth potential. Not all SGA fetuses are FGR and some FGR fetuses are not SGA.
- FGR carries an increased risk of intra-partum asphyxia and stillbirth and a possible long-term risk of hypertension and other cardiovascular diseases.
- There is no effective treatment and the management involves appropriate monitoring and timely delivery.

FURTHER READING

Knight M, Bunch K, Tuffnell D, Patel R, Shakespeare J, Kotnis R, Kenyon S, Kurinczuk JJ (eds.); MBRRACE-UK (2021). *Saving Lives, Improving Mothers' Care - Lessons learned to inform maternity care from the UK and Ireland Confidential Enquiries into Maternal Deaths and Morbidity 2017-19.* National Perinatal Epidemiology Unit, University of Oxford.

Magee LA, Brown MA, Hall DR, Gupte S, Hennessy A, Karumanchi SA, Kenny LC, McCarthy F, Myers J, Poon LC, Rana S, Saito S, Staff AC, Tsigas E, von Dadelszen P (2022). The 2021 International Society for the Study of Hypertension in Pregnancy classification, diagnosis & management recommendations for international practice. *Pregnancy Hypertension*, 27: 148–169. https:doi.org/10.1016/j.preghy.2021.09.008.

NICE (2019). *Hypertension in Pregnancy: Diagnosis and Management.* NICE guideline [NG 133]. Last updated: 17 April 2023. https://www.nice.org.uk/guidance/ng133/resources/hypertension-in-pregnancy-diagnosis-and-management-pdf-66141717671365.

SELF-ASSESSMENT

For interactive SBAs and EMQs relating to this chapter, visit www.routledge.com/cw/mccarthy.

CASE HISTORY 1

MB is a 34-year-old White primigravid teacher. She presents in the hospital antenatal clinic for the first time at 11 weeks' gestation. She is noted to be a non-smoker. There is no relevant past medical history, but her family history reveals that her mother has had hypertension since her late 40s. MB is 1.56 m tall and weighs 83 kg. Her booking blood pressure was 110/74 mmHg and urinalysis was normal.

The antenatal period was uneventful until 37 weeks. At 37 weeks' gestation, a community midwife noted that MB's blood pressure had risen to 150/100 mmHg and that there was 1+ of protein in the urine. MB was referred to the hospital as an emergency admission.

On arrival at the hospital, MB's blood pressure was 160/110 mmHg and there was 3+ of protein in the urine. She was complaining of some upper abdominal pain and there was hyperreflexia. The fetal heart rate was normal. What are the risks in this case?

ANSWER

MB is hypertensive and has marked proteinuria, having previously been normotensive. The diagnosis is pre-eclampsia. The level of the blood pressure denotes severe disease. The pregnancy is at term.

MB is at risk of developing a worsening condition. A further rise in her blood pressure will put her at risk of intracranial haemorrhage. She may have an eclamptic fit, develop a coagulopathy and HELLP syndrome, and possibly experience renal failure. There is a further risk of placental abruption and severe haemorrhage. The fetus is at risk secondary to the mother's condition.

Plan of action

- The patient does not require resuscitation.
- The fetus does not require emergency delivery.
- Call for help.
- Establish an intravenous line with a wide-bore cannula.
- Take blood for clotting studies, full blood count and blood biochemistry and save serum.
- Prevent an eclamptic fit from occurring: give magnesium sulphate intravenously 4 g bolus over 20 minutes. Continue with 1 g/hour.
- At these doses, monitoring blood levels is not necessary unless the urine output falls to less than 20 mL/hour (magnesium sulphate is excreted via the kidneys).

- Lower the blood pressure. The aim is to achieve a diastolic blood pressure of 90–100 mmHg and the systolic blood pressure should be treated if above 160 mmHg. Check the blood pressure every 5 minutes. Oral labetalol or nifedipine can be used to treat blood pressure. If unsuccessful, intravenous hydralazine or labetalol, as a bolus followed by an infusion, will be needed.
- Measure input and output of fluids.
- Put a Foley catheter into the bladder.
- Restrict input from all sources to 80 mL/hour (or 1 mL/kg/hour).
- If the clotting becomes deranged (platelets <50 × 10^9/L), contact a consultant haematologist for advice.

Management of the case

In this case, the blood pressure fell to 145/96 mmHg on treatment with labetalol. Treatment with magnesium sulphate was started and the urine output averaged 35 mL/hour. Clotting studies, full blood count and biochemistry remained normal. The CTG showed a normal fetal heart pattern.

Once stabilization had been achieved, delivery was planned. Because the clotting studies were normal, an epidural was put in place. Vaginal examination showed that the cervix was favourable, with the fetus presenting by the head. Therefore, induction of labour was commenced, and after a rapid labour a 3.2-kg boy was delivered, with normal Apgar scores. The estimated blood loss was 600 mL.

After delivery, MB was monitored in the delivery suite for 36 hours. The magnesium sulphate infusion was continued for 24 hours after delivery. Oral labetalol was commenced, and the infusion was discontinued. There was initial concern with regard to the urine output, which remained at 25 mL/hour for the first 6 hours after delivery. The position was watched, but no active steps were taken to redress the issue and, between 6 and 12 hours after delivery, the patient began to have a marked diuresis. Seven days after delivery, MB's blood pressure had returned to normal without medication.

Conclusion

This case demonstrates appropriate management of pre-eclampsia at term. Major problems were prevented by swift action. MB is at risk of pre-eclampsia in her next pregnancy, although it is likely to be less severe. She is also at risk of developing hypertension and other forms of cardiovascular disease later in life.

CASE HISTORY 2

LK is a 25-year-old Black primigravid woman who works as a fitness instructor. She was seen in the hospital antenatal clinic for the first time at 13 weeks' gestation. She is a non-smoker. There is no relevant past medical history and no relevant family history. LK is 1.6 m tall and weighs 55 kg. Her booking blood pressure was 100/60 mmHg and urinalysis was normal.

The antenatal period was uneventful until 28 + 5 weeks, when the community midwife noted that LK's symphysial–fundal height was 24 cm and her blood pressure was 140/90 mmHg. There was no protein in the urine. LK was referred to the hospital and attended the fetal assessment unit the following day.

At the hospital, LK's blood pressure was 150/96 mmHg. Urinalysis was negative for protein. An ultrasound scan revealed the presence of a fetus with biometry all less than the 10th centile for gestational age, a significantly reduced amniotic fluid index and raised umbilical artery resistance on Doppler wave form analysis. Laboratory investigations were performed. The PlGF was low and her platelet count was 90 × 10⁹/L.

What is the likely diagnosis and how should the patient be managed?

ANSWER

LK had an SGA baby with ultrasound features suggestive of FGR. Her blood pressure was mildly elevated and, although she did not have proteinuria, the presence of uteroplacental dysfunction indicates the diagnosis is pre-eclampsia. A low PlGF indicated that LK was highly likely to require delivery in the next 14 days. A low platelet count indicated that the maternal vascular endothelium was compromised.

Plan of action

- The patient does not require resuscitation.
- The fetus does not require emergency delivery.
- However, the low PlGF indicates a high probability that delivery will be required within the next 14 days.
- Therefore, steroids should be given to promote fetal lung maturity in anticipation of premature delivery.
- A low platelet count is indicative of maternal vascular endothelial involvement and blood tests should be repeated at regular intervals, initially every 24 hours.

- The fetus has FGR with abnormal umbilical artery Doppler and therefore needs increased surveillance.
- LK has high blood pressure, which requires increased surveillance and may require treatment.
- Therefore, inpatient observation is indicated.
- Deteriorating liver and haematological indices indicate worsening disease and the possible onset of HELLP syndrome. This mandates delivery and therefore magnesium sulphate should be given for neuroprotection at this gestation.
- The neonatology team should be informed as the fetus will require admission to the neonatal intensive care unit.

Management of the case

LK was admitted to the antenatal ward for observation. Steroids were administered to promote fetal lung maturity in anticipation of a premature delivery. LK did not require antihypertensive treatment, as her blood pressure was never more than 140/90 mmHg following admission. However, 48 hours later, LK's platelet count had fallen to 50 x10⁻⁹/L and her liver function tests were abnormal. A decision was made to deliver in the light of the diagnosis of pre-eclampsia and deteriorating liver and haematological indices. Magnesium sulphate was given for neuroprotection and LK was delivered by caesarean section of a male infant weighing 975 g at 29 weeks' gestation. He was admitted to the neonatal intensive care unit for ongoing management and was ultimately discharged 6 weeks later having made excellent progress. LK made a rapid recovery post-delivery. Her blood tests normalized within 24 hours and she never required antihypertensive treatment.

Conclusion

This case demonstrates preterm presentation of pre-eclampsia, characterized by uteroplacental dysfunction and severe FGR. LK was delivered promptly in the light of deteriorating liver and haematological indices, thus avoiding severe maternal complications of this disease including HELLP syndrome. This required premature delivery by caesarean section but antenatal treatment with steroids and magnesium sulphate helped to minimize the risks of premature delivery to the fetus. LK is at high risk of pre-eclampsia in her next pregnancy. She is also at risk of developing hypertension and other forms of cardiovascular disease later in life.

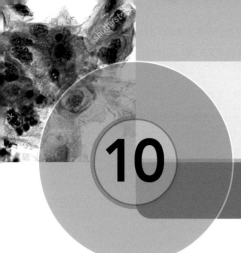

Medical complications of pregnancy

10

PHILIPPA J MARSDEN

Learning Objectives
- Understand the importance of medical conditions in pregnancy in relation to maternal and infant health.
- Appreciate the importance of preconception counselling and its impact on improving pregnancy outcomes.
- Understand the impact of common medical conditions such as hypertension, kidney disease, cardiac disease, epilepsy and diabetes on pregnancy.
- Appreciate the contribution of maternal medical disease to mortality and the need for a multidisciplinary approach to care.

INTRODUCTION

Pregnancy in women with pre-existing medical diseases is becoming increasingly common as the treatment of many chronic conditions improves. Those with underlying medical conditions are at increased risk of developing complications in pregnancy, with an associated increase in maternal and fetal morbidity and mortality, and this is discussed in the next section. In this chapter, the risks and management – including the importance of pre-pregnancy counselling and care during pregnancy by a multidisciplinary team (MDT) of doctors and

health professionals with experience of managing the disorder in question during pregnancy – of the more common pre-existing medical disorders that are seen in pregnancy are discussed.

MATERNAL DEATHS AND MEDICAL DISORDERS

Confidential enquiries into maternal deaths (defined as the death of a woman during pregnancy and up to 6 weeks after birth) have been undertaken within the UK since 1952. Initially, the reports were triennial

10.1201/9781003196112-10

but, since 2009, there has been an annual report from Mothers and Babies, Reducing Risk through Audits and Confidential Enquiries across the UK (MBRRACE-UK) specifically aimed at reducing maternal mortality and morbidity. MBRRACE-UK publishes recommendations to inform future maternity care based on lessons learnt from the enquiry.

For many years, direct maternal deaths, which includes deaths from obstetric complications of pregnancy (e.g. haemorrhage, pre-eclampsia and venous thromboembolism), predominated over indirect maternal deaths, which include deaths that result from pre-existing disease, primarily medical conditions. Direct deaths have decreased over the years as maternity care has improved, with new guidelines, treatments and prophylactic measures being introduced for common obstetric complications. However, indirect deaths have, in recent years, plateaued, and are now more common than direct deaths. This is thought to be multifactorial but is likely to be because (1) more women with complex medical conditions are surviving to adulthood and therefore becoming pregnant, (2) women are starting their families at an older age and (3) obesity has dramatically increased. The most common cause of maternal death is currently deaths associated with cardiac disease, with deaths from neurological causes being the third most common.

Many of the deaths in the MBRRACE-UK reports involve common medical disorders, but at times the level of complexity and/or severity was not recognized. There are examples of pregnant women who died despite excellent multidisciplinary care, but in almost a quarter of these cases improvements to their care may have made a difference to their outcome. There are also examples in which the medical complexity of the pregnant woman was compounded by mental health conditions, difficult social circumstances or learning difficulties. These pregnant women should be regarded as extremely vulnerable, as their ability to comply with treatment may be compromised.

PRE-CONCEPTION COUNSELLING

Women with pre-existing medical problems can often pose complex management issues in pregnancy. Ideally, these individuals should be seen for preconception care with a multidisciplinary approach. Unfortunately, while such counselling is available and does occur, many pregnancies are unplanned. It is therefore vital to be aware of the most common medical disorders that occur in the reproductive-age group and to have an appreciation of the associated risks and the appropriate management.

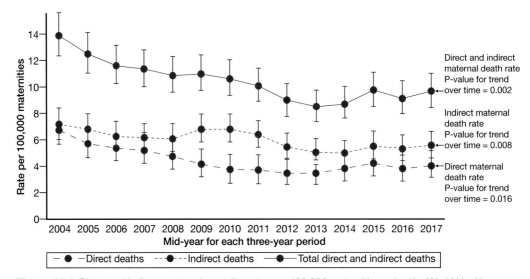

Figure 10.1 Direct and indirect maternal mortality rates per 100,000 maternities using the World Health Organization International Classification of Diseases Maternal Mortality (ICD-MM) tool and previous UK classification systems; 3-year rolling average rates (2004–2017).

- Will I have a normal healthy baby?
- Will pregnancy make my disease worse?
- Will my disease be worse after pregnancy?
- Will my pregnancy be complicated because of my disease?
- How will the care in my pregnancy be different because of my disease?
- Is there a risk of my children inheriting my condition?
- What treatment is safe during pregnancy?
- Can I have an epidural?
- Should I be delivered by caesarean section?
- Is breastfeeding advisable?

RENAL DISEASE

Renal plasma flow increases very early in pregnancy and by the second trimester has increased by 60–80%. Other changes include sodium and water retention; therefore, 80% of pregnant women have oedema by the end of pregnancy and a significant dilatation of the urinary collecting system.

Women with chronic kidney disease (CKD) are less able to make the renal adaptations necessary for a healthy pregnancy. Therefore, pregnancy in women with renal disease requires increased maternal and fetal surveillance. Pre-pregnancy counselling is recommended in all women with CKD, and they should be made aware of the risks to the fetus and to their long-term renal function before conception.

The pre-pregnancy counselling discussion should include the following factors:

- reliable, safe contraception until the patient is advised that renal disease is optimized for pregnancy
- fertility issues, if indicated
- genetic counselling, if it is an inherited disorder
- any risks to the mother and fetus during pregnancy
- a review of medication, namely for the treatment of blood pressure and an adjustment of antihypertensives; in addition, changing to a medication that is safe in pregnancy may need to be considered

- the need for low-dose aspirin to reduce the risk of pre-eclampsia
- the need for anticoagulation once pregnant in women with significant proteinuria
- the likelihood of prolonged admission or early delivery
- the possibility of accelerated decline in maternal renal function
- the need for post-partum follow-up

CHRONIC KIDNEY DISEASE

CKD is classified into five stages based on the level of renal function (Table 10.1). Stages 1 and 2 affect around 3% of the reproductive-age (20–39) population and, while stages 3–5 affect 1 in 150 people in this age group, pregnancy in these women is less common. Some women are found to have CKD for the first time in their pregnancy, and pregnancy can unmask previously unrecognized renal disease.

EFFECT OF PREGNANCY ON CHRONIC KIDNEY DISEASE

Women with CKD stages 1–2 have mild renal dysfunction and usually have an uneventful pregnancy and good renal outcome. Pregnancy with a serum creatinine level <125 µmol/L, minimal proteinuria (i.e. albumin/creatinine ratio of less than 3 mg/mmol) and absent or well-controlled hypertension pre-pregnancy has been shown to have little or no adverse effect on long-term maternal renal function. Women with moderate to severe disease (stages 3–5) are at highest risk of complications during pregnancy and of an accelerated

Table 10.1 Stages of chronic kidney disease

Stage	Description	Estimated GFR (mL/min)
1	Kidney damage with normal/raised GFR	>90
2	Kidney damage with mildly low GFR	60–89
3a	Moderately low GFR	44–59
3b	Moderately low GFR	30–44
4	Severely low GFR	15–29
5	Kidney failure	<15 or dialysis

GFR, glomerular filtration rate.

decline in their renal function. Clinical complications including hypertension, proteinuria and recurrent urinary infections independently and additively enhance the risk of a poor pregnancy outcome.

The diagnosis of pre-eclampsia is often difficult due to the presence of pre-existing hypertension and/or proteinuria. If pre-eclampsia develops, maternal renal function often deteriorates further, but any other additional complications, such as postpartum haemorrhage or the use of non-steroidal anti-inflammatory drugs (NSAIDs), can critically threaten maternal renal function.

EFFECT OF CHRONIC KIDNEY DISEASE ON PREGNANCY OUTCOME

Pregnancies in individuals with CKD have increased risks of preterm delivery, delivery by caesarean section and fetal growth restriction (FGR), dependent on the degree of renal impairment. The risk of adverse pregnancy outcome correlates with the degree of renal dysfunction (Table 10.2).

DIALYSIS

The incidence of pregnant women on dialysis (stage 5 CKD) is increasing. Dialysis must be adjusted to allow for the physiological changes of pregnancy (plasma volume, fluid retention, electrolytes), and haemodialysis is usually more effective then peritoneal dialysis

Table 10.2 Estimated effects of renal function on pregnancy outcome and maternal renal function

	Mean pre-pregnancy serum creatinine value (mg/dL)		
	<125	125–180	>180
Fetal growth restriction (%)	25	40	65
Preterm delivery (%)	30	60	>90
Pre-eclampsia (%)	22	40	60
Loss of >25% renal function post-partum (%)	0	20	50
End-stage renal failure after 1 year (%)	0	2	35

Source: Data adapted from Williams and Davidson (2008). Chronic kidney disease in pregnancy. *BMJ*, 326: 211–15.

in achieving this. Complications include preterm delivery, polyhydramnios (30–60%), pre-eclampsia (40–80%) and caesarean delivery (50%).

PREGNANCY IN WOMEN WITH RENAL TRANSPLANTS

Conception is rare in women with end-stage kidney disease. However, fertility returns rapidly after renal transplantation and it is estimated that 2–10% of female recipients conceive. Of pregnancies progressing beyond the third trimester, the majority (>90%) result in a successful pregnancy outcome.

All pregnancies in transplant recipients are high risk and should be managed by an MDT. Better maternal outcomes have been found with lower doses of immunosuppressive therapy, a longer time since transplantation and better graft function with the absence of chronic rejection. There is an increased risk of complications in pregnant women with renal transplants, often related to residual underlying disease; complications include preterm delivery, pre-eclampsia and urinary tract infection. It is considered safe to aim for a vaginal birth. With respect to caesarean section, there is a small risk of damage to the transplant during the operation, which is increased during an emergency caesarean delivery.

ENDOCRINE DISORDERS

Endocrine disorders frequently complicate pregnancy, with the most common disorders being pre-existing diabetes and thyroid dysfunction. Affected individuals should be under the care of a health professional – either their general practitioner (GP) or a specialist – and pre-conception counselling is recommended opportunistically at each encounter. Nevertheless, many pregnancies are unplanned, and those individuals with the most complex lives are at the highest risk of morbidity and mortality. In the 2023 MBRRACE-UK report, it was reported that thirty-three women died from endocrine causes, fourteen during pregnancy and within 6 weeks of birth. Causes of maternal death in recent reports include diabetes, particularly diabetic ketoacidosis and hypoglycaemia, Addison disease, Conn syndrome, phaechromocytoma and hyperemesis. Some of these women had new onset of an endocrine disorder that went unrecognised during or after pregnancy. Many of these women also had complex lives with a history of substance misuse and domestic abuse causing difficulties with treatment adherence.

DIABETES MELLITUS

Pregnancy is a physiological state of glucose intolerance and insulin resistance; therefore, glucose handling is significantly altered in pregnancy. Pregnant women without diabetes have a doubling of insulin production from the pancreas, which explains the dramatic increase in insulin requirements in women with pre-existing diabetes. Fasting levels of plasma glucose are lower in pregnancy. This is often difficult to achieve and maintain in individuals with pre-existing diabetes, with poor glycaemic control having a detrimental effect on the fetus. The renal threshold for glucose falls in pregnancy and glycosuria is common, which is why glycosuria is not a reliable test for diabetes in pregnancy.

Diabetes may complicate a pregnancy either because a woman has pre-existing (type 1 or type 2) diabetes mellitus before pregnancy or because diabetes develops during the course of the pregnancy, known as gestational diabetes mellitus (GDM).

PRE-PREGNANCY COUNSELLING

The aim of pre-pregnancy counselling for women with pre-existing diabetes is to achieve the best possible glycaemic control before pregnancy and to provide education about the implications of pregnancy. Preparation for pregnancy is best if the healthcare providers delivering care to the pregnant woman or person outside of pregnancy are able to provide information to help them optimize their diabetes and other medications before they embark on a pregnancy. Advice includes:

- optimization of glycaemic control to achieve a glycated haemoglobin (HbA1c) level of <48 mmol/mol without inducing hypoglycaemia
- high-dose folic acid (5 mg daily) to reduce the risk of neural tube defects
- planning adjustments, and considering stopping, other medications such as statins and angiotensin-converting enzyme (ACE) inhibitors before pregnancy

Poor glycaemic control is associated with a significantly increased risk of congenital malformations, particularly neural tube defects and cardiac anomalies. The most critical period for the embryo is the period of organogenesis, which occurs in the first 42 days of pregnancy, often before the pregnancy is medically confirmed. The level of HbA1c in early pregnancy correlates with the risk of early fetal loss. The UK National Institute for Health and Care Excellence (NICE) guidelines (2020) strongly advise that women with diabetes whose HbA1c is >86 mmol/mol should not become pregnant, as above that level there is a high incidence of congenital malformation and fetal loss during pregnancy. Pre-pregnancy care with optimization of glycaemic control is associated with reduced rates of all maternal and fetal complications. In the pre-conception period, blood sugar monitoring and diabetes therapy should be intensified, and reliable contraception is advised until glucose control is good. The pre-pregnancy target is pre-meal glucose levels of 4–7 mmol/L.

Diabetic vascular complications are common in women of reproductive age and in those with significant retinopathy, nephropathy and/or neuropathy benefit from MDT review prior to pregnancy. It is important that a plan for medication adjustment is made and that individuals are counselled regarding the additional potential complications associated with diabetic microvascular disease. This is particularly important for women with nephropathy, which is associated with a significantly increased risk of complications necessitating preterm delivery. There is also a risk that retinopathy can progress in pregnancy and during the post-partum period.

MATERNAL AND FETAL COMPLICATIONS OF DIABETES AND PREGNANCY

Congenital malformation is a significant cause of mortality and morbidity in women with pre-existing diabetes, due to the adverse effect of high glucose levels on the developing fetus in the first trimester. Congenital malformations occur in 7 in 100 pregnancies with diabetes. This represents a fourfold higher risk than in pregnancies without diabetes, with cardiac and neural tube defects being the most common malformations.

The fetus produces high levels of insulin during the third trimester in response to high glucose levels, and the resulting fetal hyperinsulinaemia explains the associated neonatal morbidity, including fetal macrosomia and neonatal complications such as hypoglycaemia, jaundice, respiratory distress syndrome and polycythaemia.

Fetal macrosomia increases the risk of a traumatic birth and shoulder dystocia. Accelerated growth patterns are typically seen in the late second and third trimesters and are attributable to poorly controlled diabetes in the majority of cases. Stillbirth, particularly in the third trimester, is five times higher in pregnancies complicated by diabetes than in the general population. Concerns regarding fetal wellbeing, particularly in the presence of fetal macrosomia, frequently prompts early term delivery in women with diabetes, which in turn increases the likelihood of neonatal unit admission and reduces breastfeeding rates.

The risk of pre-eclampsia is increased threefold in women with diabetes, and particularly in those with underlying microvascular disease. All individuals with diabetes should be offered low-dose aspirin (150 mg) from 12 weeks' until 36 weeks' gestation to reduce the risk of pre-eclampsia. Pregnant women with diabetic retinopathy are at risk of progression of the disease and should be kept under careful surveillance (retinal screening at booking, at 16–20 weeks' and at 28 weeks' gestation). Other possible complications include an increased incidence of infection, severe hyperglycaemia, hypoglycaemia and diabetic ketoacidosis. Complications that may arise also include an increased rate of caesarean and instrumental deliveries.

MANAGEMENT OF TYPES 1 AND 2 DIABETES IN PREGNANCY

Women with diabetes should be managed throughout their pregnancy in joint obstetric/diabetes antenatal clinics, where they are seen either once a week or once every 2 weeks by an MDT involving diabetic specialist midwives and nurses, a dietician, an obstetrician and a physician. The aim is to support the pregnant woman and her family during the pregnancy to safely optimize glycaemic control and to improve outcomes for the mother and baby. Women with diabetes should be seen as early as possible by the specialist team, ideally by 10 weeks, but earlier if possible, in view of the high percentage of unplanned pregnancies, even among those with pre-existing diabetes. Blood glucose monitoring is encouraged seven times a day (before and 1-hour after meals) with a target of <5.3 mmol/L and a 1-hour postprandial level target of <7.8 mmol/L. Pregnant women will require additional support and education regarding diet, the use of oral hypoglycaemic agents such as metformin (where appropriate), insulin adjustments for hyperglycaemia and the management of hypoglycaemia, particularly in individuals with reduced hypoglycaemic awareness, a condition that is common in pregnancy. Insulin resistance increases dramatically over the course of pregnancy and, therefore, women with pre-existing diabetes are usually required to increase their dose of insulin or metformin during the second half of pregnancy.

A plan for the pregnancy should be set out in early pregnancy and should include renal and retinal screening, fetal surveillance and a plan for delivery. Women with diabetes should be offered a fetal anomaly scan at 19–20 weeks to detect congenital malformations, and this should include a detailed assessment of the cardiac outflow tracts. Serial growth scans in the third trimester are recommended to assess fetal growth and diagnose macrosomia and polyhydramnios. Timing and mode of delivery should be determined on an individual basis but, in general, provided the pregnancy has gone well and there are no other contraindications, pregnant women with diabetes should be able to aim for a vaginal birth between 37 and 39 weeks. However, the development of macrosomia or maternal complications such as pre-eclampsia, together with the rate of failed induction, is such that the caesarean section rate among diabetic women is as high as 50%. For pregnant women requiring insulin, there should be close monitoring of maternal blood glucose levels in established labour, and an insulin/glucose infusion to reduce the risk of neonatal hypoglycaemia should be considered. Insulin requirements return to pre-pregnancy levels immediately following delivery and insulin doses should be adjusted accordingly. Women should be informed of the increased risk of hypoglycaemia in the postnatal period, particularly if they are breastfeeding.

GESTATIONAL DIABETES

GDM complicates 10–15% of pregnancies depending on the diagnostic criteria used. Screening for GDM is important, as the diagnosis and treatment of GDM

BOX 10.3: Effects of pregnancy on diabetes

- Nausea and vomiting, particularly in early pregnancy
- Greater importance of tight glucose control
- Increase in insulin dose requirements in the second half of pregnancy
- Increased risk of severe hypoglycaemia with unawareness
- Increase in risk of diabetic ketoacidosis
- Risk of deterioration of pre-existing retinopathy
- Risk of deterioration of established nephropathy

BOX 10.4: Effects of diabetes on pregnancy

- Increased risk of miscarriage
- Risk of congenital malformation
- Risk of macrosomia
- Increased risk of pre-eclampsia
- Increased risk of stillbirth
- Increased risk of infection
- Increased operative delivery rate
- Increased risk of shoulder dystocia
- Increased risk of neonatal complications such as respiratory distress syndrome, hypoglycaemia, jaundice and polycythaemia

---

has been shown to improve outcomes for the mother and baby, including reducing the risk of fetal macrosomia, trauma during birth (for both the mother and the baby), induction of labour and/or caesarean section, neonatal hypoglycaemia and perinatal death. Women who develop GDM are also at increased risk of type 2 diabetes, and education about diet and lifestyle during pregnancy can have important implications for future health.

NICE guidelines (2020) recommend a diagnosis of GDM based on a fasting glucose level of ≥5.6 mmol/L and/or a 2-hour (post-75 g glucose load) of 7.8 mmol/L. Screening involves a glucose tolerance test at 24–28 weeks in the presence of any of the following risk factors:

- previous GDM – this group of pregnant women should also have a glucose tolerance test or self-monitoring of glucose as early as possible in pregnancy, to detect previously undiagnosed type 2 diabetes
- body mass index (BMI) above 30 kg/m^2
- previous macrosomic baby weighing 4.5 kg or more
- an ethnicity with a high prevalence of diabetes
- a family history of diabetes (a first-degree relative with diabetes)

The principles of management during pregnancy are the same as for women with pre-existing diabetes. Pregnant women who have a fasting plasma glucose level below 7 mmol/L at diagnosis should be offered a trial of diet and exercise change. However, if targets are not met with 1–2 weeks, metformin and/or insulin should be offered.

One of the most important components of the management of women who develop GDM is the exclusion of type 2 diabetes after pregnancy. Screening with a fasting glucose should be offered at 6–13 weeks after childbirth, or an HBA1c if after 13 weeks.

THYROID DISEASE

Thyroid disease is common in those of childbearing age. Many of the symptoms of thyroid disease, such as heat intolerance, constipation, fatigue, palpitations and weight gain, resemble those of normal pregnancy and therefore new presentations of thyroid disease can be difficult to detect during pregnancy. Physiological changes of pregnancy, including plasma volume expansion, increased thyroid-binding globulin production and relative iodine deficiency, mean that thyroid hormone reference ranges for the non-pregnant population are not useful in pregnancy. Free thyroxine (fT4), free triiodothyronine (fT3) and thyroid-stimulating hormone (TSH) should be analysed when assessing thyroid function in pregnancy; total T3 and T4 should not be used. There is a fall in TSH and a rise in fT4 concentrations in the first trimester of normal pregnancy, followed by a fall in fT4 concentration with advancing gestation.

HYPOTHYROIDISM

Hypothyroidism is common and found in around 1% of pregnant women. Worldwide, the commonest cause of hypothyroidism is iodine deficiency, but this is rarely seen in the developed world, where autoimmune Hashimoto thyroiditis is more common. Women diagnosed with hypothyroidism should continue thyroid replacement therapy during pregnancy, and biochemical euthyroidism is the aim, that is, maintaining the TSH at the lower end of the normal range. Thyroid function tests should be performed at booking and at 28 weeks, or more often if dose adjustments are required. Suboptimal replacement therapy with levothyroxine has been associated with developmental delay and pregnancy loss in some studies; however, corrected hypothyroidism does not seem to influence pregnancy outcome or complications.

HYPERTHYROIDISM

Autoimmune thyrotoxicosis (Graves' disease) affects around 2 per 1,000 pregnancies and is usually diagnosed before pregnancy. Other causes of hyperthyroidism (5% overall) include toxic adenoma, subacute thyroiditis and toxic multinodular goitre. Symptoms include tremor, sweating, insomnia, hyperactivity and anxiety. Signs include goitre, Graves' ophthalmopathy, tachycardia, hypertension with a wide pulse pressure, weight loss and pretibial myxoedema. Treatment during pregnancy should be drug therapy with the aim of maintaining maternal fT3 and fT4 levels in the high/normal range. Radioactive iodine is contraindicated because it completely obliterates

the fetal thyroid gland. Treatment options include carbimazole or propylthiouracil using the lowest acceptable dose, as high doses cross the placenta and may cause fetal hypothyroidism.

Uncontrolled thyrotoxicosis is associated with increased risks of miscarriage, preterm delivery and FGR. Thyroid function therefore needs to be closely monitored, and many women can reduce their dose of medication, with almost one-third able to stop treatment in pregnancy. As TSH receptor-stimulating antibodies cross the placenta, women with positive antibody titres during pregnancy should be referred for fetal surveillance during pregnancy, and after birth the baby should be reviewed by the neonatology team to exclude thyroid dysfunction.

PITUITARY TUMOURS IN PREGNANCY

Hyperprolactinaemia is an important cause of infertility and amenorrhoea, and is most often due to a benign pituitary microadenoma. The pituitary gland enlarges by 50% during pregnancy, but it is rare for microadenomas to cause problems. Serial prolactin levels are unhelpful for monitoring tumour growth in pregnancy. Bromocriptine and cabergoline are usually stopped in pregnancy, and visual fields and relevant symptoms such as frontal headache are monitored. If there is any suspicion of tumour growth during pregnancy, appropriate neuroimaging should be arranged. Women with macroadenomas (>1 cm) should be managed by an MDT during pregnancy (obstetrician/endocrinologist).

ADRENAL DISEASE

Adrenal disorders are covered here because, although they are uncommon in pregnancy, they can mimic common pregnancy symptoms and are also important to remember as a differential diagnosis in gestational hypertension that proves difficult to control. MBRRACE-UK report recommended that, when presented with a pregnant woman with complex symptoms, the emphasis should be on making a diagnosis, not simply excluding a diagnosis. Individuals on long-term steroids may need additional steroids (e.g. intravenous hydrocortisone) in labour, as adrenal function will be suppressed by the endogenous steroids.

CUSHING SYNDROME

Cushing syndrome is rare in pregnancy, as most affected women are infertile. It is characterized by increased glucocorticoid production, usually due to hypersecretion of adrenocorticotrophic hormone from a pituitary tumour. However, in pregnancy, adrenal causes (tumours) are more common. Diagnosis is difficult because many of the symptoms (e.g. striae, weight gain, weakness, glucose intolerance and hypertension) mimic normal pregnancy changes. If suspected, plasma cortisol levels should be measured (although levels increase in pregnancy) and adrenal imaging with ultrasound, computed tomography (CT) scan or magnetic resonance imaging (MRI) should be used. There is a high incidence of pre-eclampsia, preterm delivery and stillbirth among those with Cushing syndrome.

CONN SYNDROME

Conn syndrome is caused by an adrenal tumour producing excess aldosterone. While rare in pregnancy, it is considered one of the more common causes of secondary hypertension and therefore it is important to remember as a cause of gestational hypertension. Conn syndrome usually presents with hypertension and hypokalaemia and is diagnosed by high aldosterone and low renin and enlargement of adrenals with CT scan or ultrasound.

ADDISON DISEASE

Addison disease (adrenal insufficiency) is an autoimmune condition associated with clinical symptoms of exhaustion, nausea, hypotension, hypoglycaemia and weight loss. In previously diagnosed and adequately treated patients, the pregnancy usually continues normally. Replacement steroids should be continued in pregnancy and increased at times of stress such as hyperemesis and delivery. A new diagnosis is difficult to make in pregnancy because the cortisol levels, instead of being characteristically very low, may be in the low–normal range due to the physiological increase in cortisol-binding globulin in pregnancy. Occasionally, the disease may present as a crisis, and treatment consists of glucocorticoid and fluid replacement.

PHAEOCHROMOCYTOMA

Phaeochromocytoma is a very rare catecholamine-producing tumour usually arising within the adrenal medulla. In pregnancy, affected individuals may present with a hypertensive crisis, and the symptoms may be similar to those of pre-eclampsia or gestational hypertension. It should therefore be considered as a differential diagnosis when a pregnant woman presents with new-onset severe hypertension. A characteristic feature of a phaeochromocytoma is that the hypertension is paroxysmal, whereas in pre-eclampsia the hypertension is sustained. The diagnosis is confirmed by measurement of catecholamines in a 24-hour urine collection and in plasma, as well as by adrenal imaging.

HEART DISEASE

Peripheral dilatation and subsequent fall in systemic vascular resistance leads to an increase in plasma volume and a 40% increase in cardiac output in pregnancy. This is achieved primarily by an increase in stroke/volume but also by an increase in heart rate. The increase in plasma volume is greater than the increase in cardiac output, with a resulting lowering of blood pressure in pregnancy. The changes start early in pregnancy with a maximum cardiac output at about 28 weeks. Labour is associated with a further increase in cardiac output (15% in the first stage and 50% in the second stage). Immediately after birth, contraction of the uterus causes the transfer of a significant volume of blood from the uterus into the systemic circulation. This explains why pregnancy increases the risk of pulmonary oedema and cardiac compromise for women with cardiac conditions, the degree of risk depending on the underlying heart condition, with the greatest risk being in the second stage and immediately after birth.

MATERNAL MORTALITY/MORBIDITY FROM CARDIAC CAUSES

Cardiac disease remains the most common cause of indirect maternal death and the most common cause of maternal death overall. There has been no statistically significant change in the maternal mortality

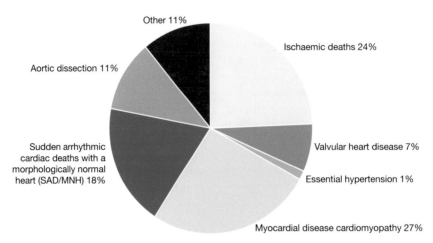

Figure 10.2 Causes of cardiovascular deaths in the UK and Ireland, 2015–2017.

rate from cardiovascular disease in the UK over the last 30 years. Almost a quarter of the individuals (22%) who died from cardiovascular causes in recent MBRRACE-UK reports were recognized to have a pre-existing cardiac problem, although some had clear symptoms and signs of cardiac disease, which were not recognised. Maternal mortality rates from cardiovascular disease increase with age, with women aged 35–39 years at a three times higher risk of death than women aged 20–24 years.

Despite cardiovascular disease being the leading cause of maternal death in both the UK and Ireland for almost 20 years, it is commonly not considered when pregnant women present with typical symptoms. Considering a cardiac cause for symptoms is very important; see the following 'Red flags' box for important indicators of cardiovascular disease.

RED FLAGS

- Sudden onset of pain radiating to arm, shoulder, back or jaw
- Breathlessness with chest pain, haemoptysis or syncope
- Orthopnoea
- Syncope during exercise
- Persistent tachycardia
- Repeated presentation with pain and/or pain requiring opiates
- Pain severe enough to prevent the new parent from caring for their baby

Electrocardiography, the measurement of troponin levels and echocardiography are recommended when a pregnant woman has chest pain and unexplained or new cardiovascular signs or symptoms.

PRE-EXISTING CARDIAC CONDITIONS

PRE-PREGNANCY COUNSELLING

Most women with heart disease will be aware of their condition prior to becoming pregnant. These individuals should be fully assessed by an MDT, including an obstetrician and cardiologist specializing in looking after pregnant women with cardiac problems. This should preferably occur before embarking on a pregnancy and the maternal and fetal risks should be carefully explained. An echocardiogram should be arranged and a plan to optimize medication should be made.

ANTENATAL MANAGEMENT

Experienced cardiologists/physicians and obstetricians should manage pregnant women with significant heart disease in a joint obstetric/cardiac clinic. Continuity of care makes the detection of subtle changes in maternal well-being more likely. In trying to distinguish between 'normal' symptoms of pregnancy and impending cardiac failure, it is important to ask the pregnant woman if she has noted

- Risk of maternal death
- Possible reduction of maternal life expectancy
- Effects of pregnancy on cardiac disease
- Mortality associated with high-risk conditions
- Risk of fetus developing congenital heart disease
- Risk of preterm labour and FGR
- Need for frequent hospital attendance and possible admission
- Intensive maternal and fetal monitoring during labour
- Other options – contraception, adoption, surrogacy
- Timing of pregnancy – often, early delivery will be advised

any breathlessness (particularly at night or when lying flat), any change in her heart rate or rhythm, any increased tiredness or a reduction in exercise tolerance (Table 10.3). Routine physical examination should include pulse rate, blood pressure, jugular venous pressure, heart sounds, ankle and sacral oedema, and the presence of basal crepitations.

Table 10.3 Stages of heart failure – New York Heart Association (NYHA) classification

Class	Patient symptoms
1: Mild	No limitation of physical activity. Ordinary physical activity does not precipitate fatigue, palpitations, dyspnoea or angina
2: Mild	Slight limitation of physical activity. Comfortable at rest, but ordinary physical activity results in fatigue, palpitation or dyspnoea
3: Moderate	Marked limitation of physical activity. Comfortable at rest, but less than ordinary activity causes fatigue, palpitation or dyspnoea
4: Severe	Unable to carry out any physical activity without discomfort. Symptoms of cardiac insufficiency at rest. If any physical activity is undertaken, discomfort is increased

Most women will remain well during the antenatal period, and outpatient management is usually possible, although they should be advised to have a low threshold for reducing their normal physical activities (see Table 10.3). Echocardiography is non-invasive and is useful for assessing heart function and valves over time, and an echocardiogram at the booking visit and at around 28 weeks' gestation is usual. Any signs of deteriorating cardiac status should be carefully investigated and treated.

Anticoagulation is essential in patients with congenital heart disease who have pulmonary hypertension (PH) or artificial valve replacements, and in those in or at risk of atrial fibrillation. Low-molecular-weight heparin is used as an alternative to warfarin or to the direct factor Xa inhibitors (such as rivaroxaban), neither of which are recommended in pregnancy.

MANAGEMENT OF LABOUR AND DELIVERY

In most cases, the aim of management is to await the onset of spontaneous labour, but the induction of labour should be considered for obstetric indications

BOX 10.6: High-risk cardiac conditions

- Systemic ventricular dysfunction (ejection fraction <30%, New York Heart Association classes III–IV)
- Pulmonary hypertension
- Cyanotic congenital heart disease
- Aortic pathology (dilated aortic root >4 cm, Marfan syndrome)
- Ischaemic heart disease
- Left heart obstructive lesions (aortic, mitral stenosis)
- Prosthetic heart valves (metal)
- Cardiomyopathy

BOX 10.7: Fetal risks of maternal cardiac disease

- Recurrence (congenital heart disease)
- Maternal cyanosis (fetal hypoxia)
- Iatrogenic prematurity
- FGR
- Effects of maternal drugs (teratogenesis, FGR, fetal loss)

and in very high-risk individuals to ensure that delivery occurs at a predictable time when all of the relevant staff are present or available. Epidural anaesthesia is often recommended, as this reduces pain-related stress and, thereby, some of the demand on cardiac function. However, regional anaesthesia is not without some risk to both the mother and the baby in some cardiac conditions, principally because of the potential complication of maternal hypotension. The input of a senior anaesthetist to formulate and document an anaesthetic management plan and minimize the procedure-related risks is essential. Prophylactic antibiotics should be given to anyone with a structural heart defect to reduce the risk of bacterial endocarditis.

Assuming normal progress in labour, the second stage may be kept short, with an elective forceps or ventouse delivery to reduce maternal effort and the requirement for increased cardiac output. Caesarean section should be performed when the maternal condition is considered too unstable to tolerate the physiological demands of labour. Post-partum haemorrhage, in particular, can lead to major

cardiovascular instability. Ergometrine may be associated with intense vasoconstriction, hypertension and heart failure, and therefore active management of the third stage is usually with Syntocinon™ (synthetic oxytocin) alone, which should be given slowly to patients with significant heart disease. High-level maternal surveillance is required until the main haemodynamic changes following delivery have passed.

SPECIFIC CONDITIONS

ISCHAEMIC HEART DISEASE

The risk of myocardial infarction (MI) during pregnancy is estimated to be 1 in 10,000, with a peak incidence in the third trimester, although the incidence appears to be increasing. Risk factors include multiparity, age >40 years, increased BMI, smoking, hypertension/pre-eclampsia and multiple pregnancy. The maternal mortality from an acute MI is approximately 20%. Neonatal and fetal morbidity/mortality are also markedly increased.

The underlying pathology is atherosclerotic in under half of cases, with coronary artery dissection being the primary cause in the post-partum period. The diagnosis of MI in pregnant women is often missed, and prompt diagnosis and therapy are necessary to reduce the high associated maternal and perinatal mortality. Thrombolytic therapy can be used in pregnancy, as the risks of fetal and maternal haemorrhage are small and treatment can save the life of the mother.

MITRAL AND AORTIC STENOSIS

Obstructive lesions of the left heart are well-recognized risk factors for maternal morbidity and mortality, as they result in an inability to increase cardiac output to meet the demands of pregnancy. Aortic stenosis (AS) is usually congenital and mitral stenosis is usually rheumatic in origin. For those with known mitral stenosis, 40% experience worsening symptoms during pregnancy, with the average time of onset of pulmonary oedema being 30 weeks. Maternal mortality is reported to be 2%, and the risk of an adverse fetal outcome is directly related to the severity of mitral stenosis. Pregnancy is usually well tolerated in women with isolated, mild and moderate AS, with normal exercise capacity and good ventricular function.

BOX 10.8: Management of labour in women with heart disease

- Avoid induction of labour if possible
- Use prophylactic antibiotics
- Ensure fluid balance
- Avoid the supine position
- Discuss regional/epidural anaesthesia/analgesia with senior anaesthetist
- Keep the second stage short
- Use Syntocinon™ judiciously

BOX 10.9: Risk factors for the development of heart failure in pregnancy

- Respiratory or urinary infections
- Anaemia
- Obesity
- Corticosteroids
- Multiple gestation
- Hypertension
- Arrhythmias
- Pain-related stress
- Fluid overload

However, the risk of maternal death in those with severe AS is reported to be 17%, with fetal mortality 30%. Treatment in pregnancy for both AS and mitral stenosis is bed rest and medical treatment.

MARFAN SYNDROME

Marfan syndrome is a rare, autosomal dominant, connective tissue abnormality that may lead to mitral valve prolapse, aortic regurgitation and aortic rupture or dissection. Aortic dissection classically presents with severe sudden-onset pain in the chest, back, neck or abdomen. The pain may be tearing in nature, and typically between the shoulder blades. Pregnancy increases the risk of aortic rupture or dissection and has been associated with maternal mortality of up to 50% when there is marked aortic root dilatation. Uterine inversion and post-partum haemorrhage are more common in women with Marfan syndrome.

PULMONARY HYPERTENSION

PH is characterized by an increase in the pulmonary vascular resistance resulting in an increased workload placed on the right side of the heart. The demands of increasing blood volume and cardiac output may not be met by an already compromised right ventricle and pregnancy is associated with a high risk of maternal death.

Women with PH should have pre-conception counselling and should be advised about the very significant risks of pregnancy, including the high risk of maternal death, with a recommendation for reliable contraception such as vasectomy, sterilization or long-acting contraception such as the Mirena® intra-uterine device or implant. Termination of pregnancy should be discussed with women who conceive with PH or who are diagnosed with PH in pregnancy, as the mortality of the condition is high, at 30–50%.

The main symptoms are fatigue, breathlessness and syncope, and clinical signs are those of right heart failure. Close monitoring by an MDT is crucial.

PERI-PARTUM CARDIOMYOPATHY

This is a rare condition and is the development of heart failure without an obvious cause late in the third trimester and in the first few months after birth.

Risk factors include multiple pregnancy, advanced maternal age, multiparity, hypertension and Afro-Caribbean origin. It is important to remember as a possible cause if a pregnant woman presents with shortness of breath, particularly at night or when lying flat. If a pulmonary embolism has been excluded, an echocardiogram should be performed.

RESPIRATORY DISEASE

There is a significant increase in oxygen demand in normal pregnancy due to the increase in both metabolic rate and the consumption of oxygen. There is a 40–50% increase in ventilation, primarily related to an increase in tidal volume, rather than an increase in respiratory rate. Breathlessness is common in pregnancy, particularly in the third trimester, and is often a subjective feeling of breathlessness. However, breathlessness may be caused by a range of pathologies (including anaemia, asthma, respiratory infection, pulmonary embolism and heart failure) and must be investigated if there is any concern.

The MBRRACE-UK 2023 report, which reported on maternal deaths between 2019 and 2021, reported twelve maternal deaths from respiratory disorders: the commonest causes being from asthma and cystic fibrosis. The number of women dying from cystic fibrosis in pregnancy is increasing, which probably reflects the improvements in care for this condition resulting in larger numbers of affected individuals surviving into adulthood and choosing to embark upon pregnancy.

RESPIRATORY INFECTION

Respiratory infection is more likely to cause severe illness in pregnant people than in the general population due to the changes to the immune system, heart, and lungs during pregnancy. Outbreaks of influenza H1N1, influenza A and, more recently, the global coronavirus disease 19 (COVID-19) pandemic have been associated with a significant number of maternal deaths attributed to respiratory infection. Viral pneumonia follows a more complicated course in pregnancy, and affected individuals often decompensate more quickly. Influenza and COVID-19 are covered in detail in **Chapter 11**.

BOX 10.10: Pneumonia: Warning signs

- Respiratory rate >30 breaths/minute
- Hypoxaemia; pO_2 <7.9 kPa on room air
- Acidosis; pH <7.3
- Hypotension
- Disseminated intravascular coagulation
- Elevated blood urea
- Evidence of multiple organ failure

BOX 10.11: Key messages

- Women should be advised of the importance of maintaining good control of their asthma during pregnancy to avoid problems for both them and their baby.
- Women with asthma should be counselled regarding the importance and safety of continuing their asthma medications during pregnancy to ensure good asthma control.

Bacterial pneumonia should be treated using the same antibiotics as outside pregnancy, with penicillin or cephalosporins usually the first choice, and erythromycin used if atypical organisms are suspected.

ASTHMA IN PREGNANCY

The worldwide prevalence of asthma is increasing, with 2–4% of pregnant women affected, making it the most common chronic condition in pregnancy. Asthma is not consistently affected by pregnancy, although exacerbations of asthma are more likely to occur in individuals with severe asthma than in those with mild asthma, and most episodes occur later in pregnancy, with respiratory viral infections being the most frequent trigger, followed by poor adherence to inhaled or oral corticosteroid therapy.

There is evidence that proactive management of asthma-related symptoms and attacks during pregnancy reduces maternal and fetal morbidity. An association between gestational hypertension and asthma has been shown, but asthma does not appear to be a risk factor for pre-eclampsia.

Labour and delivery are usually unaffected by asthma, and attacks are uncommon in labour.

Parenteral steroid cover may be needed for those who are on regular corticosteroids, regular medications should be continued throughout labour and bronchoconstrictors such as ergometrine or prostaglandin F2α should be avoided in individuals with severe asthma. Adequate hydration is important in labour, and regional anaesthesia is favoured over general anaesthesia to decrease the risk of bronchospasm, to provide adequate pain relief and to reduce oxygen consumption and minute ventilation.

Many women with asthma are concerned about the effect of drugs on the fetus, and this can lead to inappropriate cessation of treatment in early pregnancy. Women should be reassured that inhaled beta-sympathomimetics, long-acting β2 agonists such as salmeterol and corticosteroids are safe in pregnancy with no association with fetal malformations or perinatal morbidity in large studies and reviews. Very low levels of oral corticosteroids cross the placenta, and the safety data are also reassuring. The data are also reassuring on the safety of the leukotriene antagonist montelukast during pregnancy. Overall, it is safer to take asthma drugs in pregnancy than to leave asthma uncontrolled.

BOX 10.12: Key messages for asthma and pregnancy

- Pregnancy is a time to improve asthma care.
- Poorly controlled asthma confers an increased risk to the mother and fetus.
- Smoking cessation should be encouraged.
- There is no contraindication to most first-line treatments for asthma when used in pregnancy.
- Overall, it is safer to take asthma drugs in pregnancy than to leave asthma uncontrolled. Oral corticosteroids can be used in pregnancy.
- Patient education regarding the condition and the adequate use of medications should be ensured.
- Optimal control and response to therapy should be ensured throughout pregnancy.
- Exacerbations should be managed aggressively and delays in treatment should be avoided.
- Acute attacks should be managed the same as in a non-pregnant individual.
- An MDT approach should be offered.

CYSTIC FIBROSIS

Cystic fibrosis (CF) is the most common inherited life-threatening disease. It is an inherited autosomal recessive condition, with a carrier frequency of around 1 in 25 in the general population. The thick mucus that is produced leads to infections and chronic inflammation, particularly affecting the lungs, gut and pancreas. Life expectancy is increasing and, therefore, more women are surviving to an age at which pregnancy is possible. Pre-conception counselling by a specialist MDT is important. This will include the impact of CF on the pregnancy, but will also include genetic counselling and the offer of checking the CF carrier status of the father so that the risk of the fetus being affected or being a carrier can be determined. This will help to inform discussions about whether a pregnant woman and her partner may wish to opt for prenatal diagnosis, either by testing during pregnancy or by pre-implantation genetic diagnosis. In the latter, the couple undergoes assisted conception, the embryos are tested for CF and healthy embryos are inserted in the uterus.

Individuals with CF who have higher forced expiratory volume in 1 second (FEV$_1$) and higher body weights have been shown to be more likely to become pregnant. The live birth rate ranges from 70% to 90%, and the rate of spontaneous miscarriage is no different from the general population. However, the prematurity rate is around 25% due to a higher rate of spontaneous preterm labour and early planned delivery when maternal health deteriorates. Maternal prognosis is poor if there is pulmonary hypertension, infection with *Burkholderia cepacia*, if FEV$_1$ is <50% that predicted or if there is chronic hypoxia. While pregnancy does not significantly shorten survival in women with CF, the long-term prognosis still needs to be considered, as individuals with CF still have a much shortened life expectancy, particularly those with poor lung function at the start of pregnancy.

Pregnant women with CF should be jointly managed by an obstetrician and a respiratory physician with expertise in CF, ideally in a specialist centre. Most individuals will have a daily physiotherapy regimen and will require prolonged antibiotic therapy and hospital admission during infective exacerbations. Close attention should be paid to maternal nutritional status and weight gain during pregnancy, with screening for GDM also indicated. Fetal growth and well-being should be monitored by serial ultrasound scans, as there is an association with FGR. Ideally, a vaginal delivery should be the aim in the absence of any other obstetric indications for caesarean section.

NEUROLOGICAL DISORDERS

EPILEPSY

Epilepsy is the most common serious neurological condition in pregnancy. Approximately 30% of those with epilepsy are women in their childbearing years, which means that 1 in 200–250 pregnancies occur in women with a history of epilepsy. Anti-epileptic medication increases the risk to the baby and, although the majority of women with epilepsy (about two-thirds) will not have an increase in seizure frequency during pregnancy, there is a 10-fold increase in mortality among pregnant women with epilepsy, which is directly related to poorly controlled epilepsy.

Maternal deaths in individuals with epilepsy have increased in recent years, now accounting for one in five indirect maternal deaths in recent MBRRACE-UK reports. The majority of those who died as a result of epilepsy had not had pre-conception counselling and many had stopped their medication. Contributing factors included women being concerned about taking medication in pregnancy or being unable to tolerate medication in early pregnancy, as well as the falling levels of some AEDs in pregnancy due to the physiological and pharmacokinetic changes in pregnancy. In the MBRRACE-UK 2023 report, 14 of the 17 women died as a result of SUDEP. It is important that individuals with epilepsy and health professionals are aware of the risk factors for SUDEP in pregnancy (see **Box 10.13**, 'SUDEP known risk factors').

The management of epilepsy and pregnancy can be challenging owing to the need to balance the risk of AEDs to the fetus and the risk of seizures to the mother. The principles of epilepsy management are that while the risks to pregnancy from seizures outweigh those from anticonvulsant medication, seizures should still be controlled with the minimum possible dose of the optimal drug.

Box 10.13: Key messages for epilepsy

- Having epilepsy carries significant risks to the mother and the baby.
- Pre-conception counselling is important to reduce those risks.
- Sodium valproate and Topiramate are not recommended in those of childbearing age unless there is a Pregnancy Prevention Programme (PPP) in place.
- Early referral in pregnancy to an obstetric/ epilepsy specialist team is recommended, urgently if the pregnancy is unplanned, to optimize anti-epileptic drug (AED) regimens.
- It is never recommended to stop or change AEDs abruptly without an informed discussion.
- Pregnant women with epilepsy should have regular planned antenatal care with a designated obstetric/epilepsy care team.
- Women with epilepsy should be informed that the introduction of safety precautions may significantly reduce the risk of accidents and minimize anxiety.
- It is important that women with epilepsy are aware of the increased risk of sudden unexpected death in epilepsy (SUDEP) in pregnancy and have a risk assessment and plan of care before, during and after pregnancy.
- Women should be regularly assessed for risk factors for seizures and adherence to AEDs with rapid referral for neurology review if women have worsening epilepsy symptoms.
- Nocturnal seizures should be regarded as a 'red flag' indicating that women with epilepsy need urgent referral to an epilepsy service.
- Women should have access to their designated epilepsy care team within a maximum of 2 weeks.
- Postnatal review is recommended to ensure AED doses are appropriately adjusted.

Source: MBRRACE-UK, NICE, RCOG.

PRE-PREGNANCY COUNSELLING IN EPILEPSY

The majority (96%) of women with epilepsy have a good outcome, and those who have been seizure-free for >12 months are likely to remain seizure-free if they are compliant with treatment. Pregnant women and children should be referred to an epilepsy specialist if they are taking valproate, if they are taking more than one AED (polytherapy), or if they have been seizure-free for more than 2 years and wish to discuss the option of stopping AEDs. There should also be a discussion about the impact of AEDs on contraception. Since up to half of pregnancies are unplanned, pre-conception counselling should be part of any consultation with a woman with epilepsy of childbearing age. A summary of pre-pregnancy advice is detailed in **Box 10.14**.

Women with epilepsy should be provided with verbal and written information on the risks of self-discontinuation of AEDs. This discussion should include the risk of SUDEP and the effects of seizures on the fetus. It should be stressed that it is never recommended to stop or change AEDs abruptly without an informed discussion.

The majority of AEDs cross the placenta and are potentially teratogenic and, therefore, the principal concern for the fetus is the increased risk of congenital malformations, with the risk to the fetus being highest in the first trimester during organogenesis.

BOX 10.14: SUDEP known risk factors

Seizure-related factors
- Uncontrolled seizures
- Tonic–clonic seizures
- Nocturnal seizures
- Epilepsy starting before the age of 16 years
- Increasing frequency of seizures

Treatment factors
- Infrequent epilepsy reviews and engagement with an epilepsy clinician
- Ineffective AED treatment
- Frequent medication changes
- Sub-therapeutic doses of AEDs

Individual factors
- Living alone or sleeping alone
- Not taking medication as prescribed
- Sleep deprivation
- Stress
- Alcohol or substance misuse
- Learning disability

Source: MBRRACE-UK 2020; adapted from https://sudep.org.

- Individuals with epilepsy should be offered effective contraception to avoid unplanned pregnancies.
- The importance of compliance with medication should be stressed.
- Folic acid 5 mg should be taken for a minimum of 3 months before conception.
- The specific risk of congenital malformation should be explained for the AED that the woman is taking.
- The risk of recurrent seizures should be explained and a discussion should be had about SUDEP.
- Seek epilepsy specialist advice for the following:
  - altering medication according to seizure frequency – the lowest effective dose of the most appropriate AED should be used
  - if the woman is having recurrent seizures or is on polytherapy or sodium valproate

The major fetal abnormalities associated with AEDs are neural tube defects, facial clefts, and cardiac and urogenital defects. Polytherapy increases the risk of major congenital abnormality by about 3% for each additional AED. Many of these abnormalities are detectable by ultrasound and therefore all pregnant women should be offered detailed anomaly scanning. There is also an association between AEDs and FGR, particularly with polytherapy. Women on multiple drug therapy should, wherever possible, be converted to monotherapy before pregnancy, and all women with epilepsy should be advised to start taking a folic acid 5 mg daily supplement prior to conception to reduce the risk of neural tube defects and continue this through pregnancy.

Of all the AEDs, lamotrigine and levetiracetam have the lowest incidence of fetal malformations, whereas sodium valproate is associated with a particularly high risk of congenital malformations (10%). Children exposed to valproate in utero also have a higher risk of neurodevelopmental delay, including learning difficulties and autistic spectrum disorder. Sodium valproate must not be used unless epilepsy cannot be controlled with other AEDs. A Pregnancy Prevention Programme (PPP), designed to make sure these women are fully aware of the risks and the need to avoid becoming pregnant, should be in place for any woman or girl on Valproate able to have children.

Despite the risks of continuing anticonvulsants in pregnancy, failure to do so may lead to an increased frequency of epileptic seizures that may result in both maternal and fetal hypoxia. It is clear that, while polytherapy and valproate exposure should be minimized, women should be maintained on the lowest effective dose of an AED. Minimizing exposure through the use of an ineffective AED or dose will benefit neither the pregnant woman nor the fetus. However, any increases in dose need to be made in response to the clinical picture.

PREGNANCY, LABOUR AND POSTNATAL APPROACH

A multidisciplinary approach to the care of pregnant women with epilepsy is paramount, with the MDT including an obstetrician with expertise of epilepsy and pregnancy, a neurologist with an interest in epilepsy and pregnancy, epilepsy specialist nurses, a midwife and the pregnant woman's GP. If the woman is not taking folic acid 5 mg, this should be started as soon as pregnancy is suspected and this dose should be continued throughout pregnancy. Pregnant women with epilepsy taking AEDs who have well-controlled epilepsy and have had pre-conceptual advice should be seen in a hospital antenatal clinic (a specialist MDT is recommended by MBRRACE-UK and the Royal College of Obstetricians and Gynaecologists) at the time of their dating scan. Women who become unexpectedly pregnant whose epilepsy is not well controlled or who are on polytherapy or valproate should be seen as soon as possible in the first trimester, before the dating scan, and should either be seen in a specialist MDT antenatal clinic or be referred to an epilepsy specialist on an urgent basis.

Many factors contribute to altered drug metabolism in pregnancy and result in a fall in anticonvulsant drug levels. This combined with sleep deprivation or stress and poor compliance with medication can all lead to an increase in fit frequency in pregnancy. In particular, lamotrigine and levetiracetam levels fall significantly and early in pregnancy, resulting in seizure activity, often necessitating an increased dose. This is very significant, as the incidence of SUDEP is higher in individuals taking lamotrigine than in those taking other AEDs.

BOX 10.16: Causes of seizures in pregnancy

- Epilepsy
- Eclampsia
- Cerebral vascular accident
- Space-occupying lesions (e.g. tumour, tuberculoma)
- Encephalitis or meningitis
- Cerebral venous thrombosis
- Drug and alcohol withdrawal
- Hypoglycaemia
- Rarely, cerebral malaria, toxoplasmosis or thrombotic thrombocytopenic purpura

In view of the association with FGR, serial growth scans should be arranged in the third trimester. In the antenatal period, women with epilepsy should be regularly assessed for the following: risk factors for seizures, such as sleep deprivation and stress; adherence to AEDs; and seizure type and frequency. The most likely cause of a seizure in pregnancy is an epileptic seizure; however, there are also important causes to be aware of during pregnancy, for example eclampsia or intracranial pathology (see **Box 10.15**, 'Causes of seizures in pregnancy').

The risk of seizures in labour and in the postnatal period is low, but seizures are more likely with poorly controlled epilepsy and are aggravated by pain, stress, dehydration and sleep deprivation. Most women with epilepsy can aim for a vaginal birth unless there are obstetric indications. In addition, epilepsy alone is not usually an indication for induction of labour or caesarean section, unless there is an accelerated seizure frequency in pregnancy. Anti-epileptic medication should be continued during labour.

There should be a discussion, during pregnancy, about the impact of AEDs on breastfeeding and contraception. The concentration of most AEDs in breast milk is negligible and breastfeeding should be encouraged, although feeding is best avoided for a few hours after taking medication. Information on safe handling of the neonate should be given to all epileptic mothers. Effective contraception is extremely important with regard to stabilization of epilepsy and planning of future pregnancies to optimize outcomes.

MULTIPLE SCLEROSIS

Multiple sclerosis (MS) is a relapsing and remitting disease that causes disability through demyelination of nerves, leading to weakness, lack of coordination, numbness in the hands or feet, blurred vision, tremor, spasticity and voiding dysfunction. One in 1,000 pregnancies is estimated to occur in women with MS. The onset of MS during pregnancy is unusual, with optic neuritis reported as the predominant symptom, usually post-partum. Pregnant women with MS are no more likely to experience complications in their pregnancy than those unaffected, nor are there increased risks of preterm delivery, FGR or congenital malformation. The course of MS during pregnancy changes, with a lower relapse rate antenatally and a significantly higher rate of relapse during the first 3 months post-partum. Pregnancy has no adverse effect on the progression of long-term disability and, in fact, pregnancy after MS onset may be associated with a lower risk of progression of the condition.

Having MS should not make birth more complicated, and the mode of delivery should be decided using obstetric indications. Regional anaesthesia is not contraindicated and no effect on the subsequent risk of relapse has been found.

HEADACHES AND PREGNANCY

Headaches are common in pregnancy and usually are benign, self-limiting and either tension headaches or migraine. However, pregnant women are at risk of catastrophic intracranial pathology, and failure to consider a more serious cause can lead to significant morbidity and mortality. Alongside epilepsy, stroke represents the other major neurological cause of maternal death in the UK. In the MBRRACE-UK 2023 report, in 2019–2021 there were 13 women who died from stroke during or up to 6 weeks after pregnancy: six died from subarachnoid haemorrhage, one died from intracerebral haemorrhage and two died from thrombotic strokes. A further nine women died between 6 weeks and 1 year after the end of pregnancy (subarachnoid haemorrhage and intracerebral haemorrhage being the commonest causes). Headache is also the most common prodromal symptom with eclampsia and may be the only presenting symptom of cerebral venous thrombosis, which is more common in pregnancy. A number of maternal deaths are reported each year due to eclampsia and cerebral venous thrombosis.

It is therefore important to be aware of 'red flags' when a pregnant woman presents with a headache that may indicate a more serious cause (see the following 'Red flags' box). A detailed and thorough neurological examination is crucial and should include fundoscopy. It is vital that there is an MDT approach and that senior obstetric, physician, anaesthetic and radiological opinions are sought at an early stage. High blood pressure should be promptly managed and appropriate investigations, including imaging, should be arranged urgently. It is also important to recognize that pregnancy should not alter the standard of care for stroke. Pregnancy, caesarean section or the immediate post-partum state are not absolute contraindications to thrombolysis (intravenous or intra-arterial), clot retrieval or craniotomy.

More benign headaches can usually be managed in pregnancy with simple analgesia and antiemetics. Migraine is influenced by cyclical changes in the sex hormones, and attacks often occur during the menstrual period, attributed to a fall in oestrogen levels. Migraine can improve in pregnancy, but 20% of pregnant women will experience migraine-like headaches, many of whom do not get migraines outside pregnancy. Obstetric complications are not increased in migraine sufferers. Migraine during pregnancy should also be treated with simple analgesia (codeine may make migraine worse) and, where possible, avoidance of factors that trigger the attack. Low-dose aspirin, beta-blockers and amitriptyline may be used as migraine prophylaxis.

RED FLAGS

Red flags in the history and examination of a pregnant woman presenting with headache:

- Sudden-onset headache/thunderclap or worst headache ever
- Headache that takes longer than usual to resolve or persists for more than 48 hours
- Has associated symptoms – fever, seizures, focal neurology, photophobia, diplopia
- Excessive use of opioids

HAEMATOLOGICAL ABNORMALITIES

HAEMOGLOBINOPATHIES

SICKLE CELL DISEASE

Sickle cell disease (SCD) is the most common inherited condition in the world and mostly affects people whose family origins are in the Middle East, Sub-Saharan Africa, parts of India and parts of the Mediterranean. It is an autosomally inherited genetic condition in which abnormal haemoglobin contains beta-globin chains with an amino acid substitution that results in the red blood cells becoming sickle shaped, which can then occlude small blood vessels. There is often severe anaemia, chronic hyperbilirubinaemia, a predisposition to infection and CKD. Pulmonary hypertension is found in up to 30% of patients and is associated with a high mortality rate. Advances in the treatment of SCD have resulted in the average lifespan in the Western world extending past 50 years, which means many more women with the condition are now becoming pregnant.

Pregnancy is associated with an increased incidence of sickle cell crises, which may result in episodes of severe pain, typically affecting the bones or chest. Acute chest syndrome may result from an initial uncomplicated crisis and is responsible for around 25% of all deaths in SCD. Crises in pregnancy may be precipitated by hypoxia, stress, infection and haemorrhage. Affected individuals are also at an increased risk of miscarriage, pre-eclampsia, placental dysfunction resulting in FGR and premature labour, with three times the risk of eclampsia compared with those without SCD. Thromboembolic events including cerebral vein thrombosis and deep venous thrombosis are implicated in the higher rates of maternal deaths reported in SCD.

BOX 10.17: Clinically significant variants of haemoglobin

- Sickle cell trait (HbAS)
- Sickle cell disease (HbSS)
- Sickle cell/haemoglobin C disease (HbSC)
- Sickle cell/beta thalassaemia

Like other medical disorders, ideal management begins with pre-pregnancy optimization of maternal health and education about the risks in pregnancy. If the partner also has SCD or is a carrier, specialist counselling is advisable to decide whether the couple wish to find out whether their baby has SCD. This could involve pre-implantation genetic diagnosis as part of an in vitro fertilization (IVF) cycle or prenatal diagnosis during pregnancy.

Pregnant women with SCD should be managed by a specialist MDT consisting of an obstetrician and a haematology team specialising in SCD and should be seen regularly throughout pregnancy, with regular growth scans of the baby. High-dose folate supplements (5 mg daily) are recommended and low-dose aspirin (150 mg daily) is advised from 12 to 36 weeks. Hydroxycarbamide is usually stopped in early pregnancy, but pregnant women with SCD are advised to continue antibiotic prophylaxis. There is a low threshold for antenatal thromboprophylaxis, and all affected individuals are advised to take daily heparin injections after birth for 6 weeks. Blood transfusions are not often given in pregnancy but can be if necessary. People with SCD often have antibodies due to multiple previous transfusions and therefore blood needs to be carefully cross-matched.

Sickle cell carriers have a 1:4 risk of having a baby with SCD if their partner also has sickle cell trait. Carriers are usually fit and well, but are at an increased risk of urinary tract infection, and rarely suffer from crises.

THALASSAEMIA

Thalassaemia is a common genetic blood disorder causing a reduced production of normal haemoglobin. Depending on which globin chain is affected, alpha- or beta-thalssaemia results. In alpha-thalassaemia minor, there is a deletion of one of the two normal alpha genes required for haemoglobin production. Although the affected individual is chronically anaemic, this condition rarely produces obstetric complications except in cases of severe blood loss. It is important to discuss genetic counselling and offer screening of the partner for thalassaemia. If the partner is also affected, there is a 1:4 chance of the fetus having alpha-thalassaemia major, which is lethal. In this situation, either pre-implantation genetic diagnosis as part of an IVF cycle or prenatal diagnosis would be offered.

The beta-thalassaemias result from defects in the normal production of the beta chains. Beta-thalassaemia minor/trait is more commonly found in people from the eastern Mediterranean, but may also occur sporadically in other communities. Consequently, all pregnant women should be offered electrophoresis as part of the antenatal screening process. Partners should also be offered screening. If both partners have beta-thalassaemia minor, there is a 1:4 chance the fetus could have beta-thalassaemia major, which is associated with profound anaemia from birth and again genetic counselling would be advised. Beta-thalassaemia minor is usually not a problem antenatally, although women tend to be mildly anaemic. Iron and folate supplements should be given.

Women with beta thalassaemia major should be cared for by a specialist obstetric and haematology team. They may need regular blood transfusions during pregnancy, which can lead to too much iron in their body (iron overload), which can cause problems with organs such as the liver, heart, lungs, pancreas and pituitary gland. To prevent this, iron chelation can be given by injection in the second half of pregnancy.

THROMBOCYTOPENIA

Thrombocytopenia is defined as a platelet count <150 × 10⁹/L. Gestational thrombocytopenia is common and is found in 7–8% of the pregnant population. A modest drop in the platelet count to 100–150 × 10⁹/L

Idiopathic

- Increased consumption or destruction
- Autoimmune
- Antiphospholipid syndrome
- Pre-eclampsia
- Haemolysis, elevated liver enzymes and low platelets (HELLP) syndrome
- Disseminated intravascular coagulation
- Thrombotic thrombocytopenic purpura
- Hypersplenism

Decreased production

- Sepsis
- Human immunodeficiency virus (HIV) infection
- Malignant marrow infiltration

is very unlikely to be associated with complications and bleeding is rarely a complication unless the count is $<50 \times 10^9$/L. However, the diagnosis of gestational thrombocytopenia is a diagnosis of exclusion and can be made only when autoimmune and other causes have been excluded. It usually occurs in later pregnancy, with no prior history of thrombocytopenia outside pregnancy and a normal platelet count recorded at the start of pregnancy. No intervention is required other than monitoring of the platelet count during and after pregnancy. There is no association with fetal thrombocytopenia and spontaneous resolution occurs after delivery.

AUTOIMMUNE THROMBOCYTOPENIA

In immune thrombocytopenic purpura, autoantibodies are produced against platelet surface antigens, leading to platelet destruction. The incidence in pregnancy is around 1 in 5,000. The maternal platelet count may fall at any stage of pregnancy and can reach levels of $<50 \times 10^9$/L, but maternal bleeding during pregnancy or at birth is unlikely if the platelet count is $>50 \times 10^9$/L. There is a 5–10% chance of associated fetal thrombocytopenia ($<50 \times 10^9$/L), which cannot be predicted using maternal counts or antibody tests.

Pregnant women with immune thrombocytopenic purpura who become pregnant should be cared

for by a specialist obstetric/haematology team. If the platelet count is very low, treatment with corticosteroids or intravenous immunoglobulin (Ig)G may be considered. Vaginal delivery should be facilitated, and epidural/spinal anaesthesia should be avoided if the platelet count is $<80 \times 10^9$/L. Fetal blood sampling in labour and instrumental delivery are best avoided because of the risk of fetal thrombocytopenia causing neonatal haemorrhage/haematomas. A cord blood sample must be collected to exclude neonatal thrombocytopenia.

BLEEDING DISORDERS

INHERITED COAGULATION DISORDERS

Von Willebrand disease, carriers of haemophilia A and B, and factor XI deficiency account for over 90% of all women with inherited bleeding disorders. Haemophilia A (FVIII deficiency) and haemophilia B (FIX deficiency) are X-linked defects with prevalences of 1 in 10,000 and 1 in 100,000, respectively, in the population. Carriers of haemophilia A or B usually have clotting factor activity about 50% of normal, but while factor VIIIC levels increase in pregnancy, factor IXC levels increase only slightly. Von Willebrand disease is the most common inherited bleeding disorder, with an estimated prevalence of 1%. It results from either a qualitative or quantitative defect in von Willebrand factor (VWF). The inheritance of von Willebrand disease is usually autosomal dominant and, while increases in factor VIIIC and VWF antigen activity usually occur during normal pregnancy, they cannot be relied on

Inherited

- Vascular abnormalities
- Platelet disorders
- Coagulation disorders

Acquired

- Thrombocytopenia
- Disseminated intravascular coagulation
- Acquired coagulation disorders
- Marrow disorders

to buffer the effects of the disease, particularly in severe cases.

Where possible, carriers of haemophilia and women with von Willebrand disease should be identified and counselled prior to pregnancy. Baseline coagulation factor assays should be performed as soon as pregnancy is confirmed and should be repeated in the third trimester. In haemophilia carriers, tests to confirm fetal sex should be offered, either by ultrasound or through sampling fetal deoxyribonucleic acid (DNA) in maternal blood, as this influences the use of interventions in labour.

Individuals with bleeding disorders are at significant risk of primary and secondary post-partum haemorrhage, and this risk can be minimized by appropriate prophylactic treatment. Planning for delivery requires multidisciplinary input, including a specialist obstetric/haematology team, and is guided by the third-trimester clotting factor levels, taking into account the precise nature of the bleeding tendency. Those deemed to be at significant risk should have a care plan written that may include the use of factor concentrate, tranexamic acid or desmopressin (DDAVP®) to cover labour and delivery.

In haemophilia carriers, epidurals may be permitted if the clotting factor is considered to be satisfactory. Invasive fetal monitoring, ventouse and rotational forceps should be avoided if there is a possibility that the fetus may be affected, and cord blood samples should be collected for coagulation tests.

GASTROINTESTINAL DISORDERS

Pregnant women with pre-existing gastrointestinal disease may or not be under consultant care. Pre-conception counselling, as with other medical conditions, is important to review medication and consider the impact of the disease on the pregnancy and the baby, and the impact of pregnancy on the disease. Opportunistic discussions about contraception and pregnancy should be had wherever possible.

Gastrointestinal disorders can be associated with significant maternal and perinatal mortality/morbidity. In the MBRRACE-UK report (2023), there were 14 women who died from gastrointestinal disorders, six of whom died between 6 weeks and 1 year after the end of pregnancy. Causes of morbidity and death from gastrointestinal disorders include pancreatitis, bowel perforations, ulcers and hepatitis and volvulus. There was a delay in diagnosis in many of these women, and the need to investigate women who present recurrently with pain, breathlessness and, more recently, mental health concerns is paramount.

COELIAC DISEASE

Coeliac disease is a gluten-sensitive enteropathy with a prevalence of around 0.3–1% in the general population. It has been estimated that up to 1 in 70 pregnant women are affected by coeliac disease, but that many are undiagnosed. Untreated coeliac disease is associated with high rates of spontaneous miscarriage and other adverse pregnancy outcomes such as FGR. Once a gluten-free diet is established, women with coeliac disease can expect a healthy pregnancy outcome. Awareness that they are predisposed to other autoimmune diseases is the only other consideration.

INFLAMMATORY BOWEL DISEASE

The majority of patients with inflammatory bowel disease (IBD), which includes ulcerative colitis and Crohn disease, are diagnosed during their reproductive years (incidence 3 per 1,000 pregnancies). Pregnancy does not usually alter the course of IBD, but new-onset IBD, uncontrolled disease activity at conception and previous bowel resection increases the risk of an adverse pregnancy outcome. Similarly, disease flare during pregnancy is more likely if the disease is active at the time of conception. Pregnant women with either ulcerative colitis or Crohn disease have been shown to have similar rates of disease exacerbation, although flares in the first trimester and post-partum are more common in disease.

Supplementation with high-dose folic acid (5 mg daily) is recommended, and supplementation with other vitamins is indicated according to measured deficiencies. Women with IBD have increased rates of delivery by caesarean section, preterm birth and FGR. Caesarean section is indicated for the usual obstetric indications, if there is active perianal disease in Crohn disease and usually if there is an ileo-anal pouch.

The use of medication during conception and pregnancy is a cause of concern for many patients with IBD. Methotrexate is contraindicated, but the majority of other medications used to induce or maintain remission, including 5-aminosalicylates (including sulphasalazine, azathioprine, ciclosporin and corticosteroids), are considered safe in pregnancy and during breastfeeding. Experience with anti-inflammatory monoclonal antibodies is growing and increasing evidence suggests agents such as infliximab are low risk in the first two trimesters of pregnancy. A relapse of IBD in pregnancy may be treated with corticosteroids: oral, intravenous or enemas.

PEPTIC ULCER DISEASE

Peptic ulceration is less common in pregnancy, and pre-existing ulceration tends to improve during pregnancy, probably due to altered oestrogen levels and the improved maternal diet. Complications such as haemorrhage or perforation are rare. Treatment with antacids and common anti-ulcer medication (e.g. ranitidine, omeprazole) is safe. Pregnancy is not a contraindication to endoscopy.

GALLSTONES

The prevalence of gallstones in pregnancy is around 19% in the multiparous population and 8% in the nulliparous. However, acute cholecystitis is much less common, occurring in around 0.1% of pregnancies. The aetiology of increased biliary sludge and gallstones in pregnancy is multifactorial. Increased oestrogen levels lead to increased cholesterol secretion and supersaturation of bile, and increased progesterone levels cause a decrease in small intestinal motility. Conservative medical management is recommended initially, especially during the first and third trimesters, in which surgical intervention may confer a risk of miscarriage or premature labour, respectively. Medical management involves intravenous fluids, correction of electrolytes, bowel rest, pain management and broad-spectrum antibiotics. However, relapse rates (40–90%) are high during pregnancy and surgical intervention may be warranted, preferentially performed (open or laparoscopic cholecystectomy) in the second trimester.

PANCREATITIS

Pancreatitis is uncommon in pregnancy. The clinical presentation combines nausea and vomiting with severe epigastric pain, and attacks usually occur in the third trimester of pregnancy. The most common cause of pancreatitis in pregnancy is gallstones, followed by alcohol, with hypertriglyceridaemia and hyperparathyroidism much rarer causes. Acute pancreatitis in pregnancy can be life threatening and is associated with a significant preterm birth rate and high fetal mortality. It is therefore an important differential diagnosis in pregnant women with upper abdominal pain who are clinically unwell and an amylase test is an important investigation. Management is usually supportive, with a small percentage of women developing chemical peritonitis associated with cardiac, renal and gastrointestinal complications, necessitating intensive care. The decision to deliver the baby should be considered if the clinical condition deteriorates, must be an MDT approach and must take into account the gestation of the pregnancy.

RED FLAGS

Repeated presentation in pregnancy or postnatally with pain and/or pain requiring opiates should be considered a 'red flag' and warrants a thorough assessment to establish the cause.

CONNECTIVE TISSUE DISEASE

SYSTEMIC LUPUS ERYTHEMATOSUS

Systemic lupus erythematosus (SLE) is a chronic autoimmune inflammatory disease. SLE affects approximately 1 in 1,000 people in the UK and is six times more common in women than in men. It is also six times more common in people of Black Caribbean ethnicity. It may cause disease in any organ system, but it principally affects the joints (90%), skin (80%), lungs, nervous system, kidneys and heart. The diagnosis is suggested by the finding of a positive assay for antinuclear antibodies, while the presence of antibodies to double-stranded DNA is the most specific for SLE. Pre-conception counselling is important in individuals with SLE.

BOX 10.21: American College of Rheumatology criteria for the classification of SLE

- Malar rash
- Discoid rash
- Photosensitivity
- Oral ulcers
- Non-erosive arthritis
- Pleuritis or pericarditis
- Renal disorder
- Neurological disorder
- Haematological disorder
- Immunological disorder
- Positive antinuclear antibodies

BOX 10.22: Classification criteria for APS

Clinical

- Thrombosis: venous or arterial
- Pregnancy morbidity:
  - fetal death at >10 weeks
  - preterm birth at <35 weeks due to severe pre-eclampsia or growth restriction
  - three or more unexplained miscarriages at ≤10 weeks

Laboratory

- Anticardiolipin antibodies: IgG and/or IgM and/or beta-2 glycoprotein: significant on two occasions, 12 weeks apart
- Lupus anticoagulant: two occasions, 12 weeks apart

SLE is characterized by periods of disease activity, flares and remissions. Pregnancy increases the risk of flares, and flares are more common in the late second and third trimesters. Active disease at the time of conception or new-onset SLE in pregnancy increase the chance of a flare. SLE is associated with significant risks of miscarriage, fetal death, pre-eclampsia, preterm delivery and FGR. Those with lupus nephritis are at greatest risk of these adverse outcomes, although pregnancy does not seem to alter renal function in the long term. Pregnancy outcome is also adversely affected by pre-existing hypertension and the presence of antiphospholipid antibodies.

Owing to these significant risks, pregnant women with SLE require intensive monitoring for both maternal and fetal indications and should be prescribed low-dose aspirin to start by 12 weeks' gestation. Baseline renal studies, including a 24-hour urine collection for protein, should be performed. Blood pressure should be monitored closely because of the increased risk of pre-eclampsia. Serial ultrasonography is performed to assess fetal growth and well-being with umbilical artery Doppler. If antenatal treatment is required for SLE, steroids, azathioprine, sulfasalazine and hydroxychloroquine may be given safely. NSAIDs should be avoided before 12 weeks and after 20 weeks of pregnancy.

Among mothers with SLE, 30% also have anti-Ro/La antibodies, which cross the placenta and can cause the clinical syndromes neonatal lupus and congenital heart block. The risk of neonatal lupus is around 5%, rising to 25% if a previous child was affected. The risk of congenital heart block is around 2% and usually appears in utero at 18–20 weeks' gestation, is permanent and difficult to treat and is associated with a 20% rate of perinatal mortality.

ANTIPHOSPHOLIPID SYNDROME

The term antiphospholipid syndrome (APS) is used to describe the association of anticardiolipin antibodies and/or lupus anticoagulant with the typical clinical features of arterial or venous thrombosis, fetal loss after 10 weeks' gestation, three or more miscarriages at less than 10 weeks' gestation or delivery before 35 weeks' gestation due to FGR or pre-eclampsia. Importantly, a diagnosis of APS requires that the positive antibody titres must be present on two occasions, 3 months apart. APS may be primary or found in association with SLE.

In women with APS who have suffered repeated pregnancy loss or severe obstetric complications, the combined use of low-dose aspirin and low-molecular-weight heparin has been shown to reduce the pregnancy loss rate.

RHEUMATOID ARTHRITIS

Rheumatoid arthritis (RA) is a chronic inflammatory autoimmune disease that affects more women than men, and around 1 in 1,000 pregnancies is affected. Most individuals with RA (75%) experience improvement during pregnancy but, of those who improve, 90% suffer a flare post-partum. Unlike other connective tissue diseases, no adverse effects of RA on pregnancy are reported, and there are no increases in pregnancy loss rates. The main concern for patients with RA is the safety of medication used to control the disease. If paracetamol-based analgesics are insufficient, corticosteroids are preferred to NSAIDs, although the latter can be used between 12 and 20 weeks if needed. Azathioprine and hydroxychloroquine can be used in pregnancy. The mode of delivery is determined by the usual obstetric indications, except when severe RA limits hip abduction and vaginal delivery is not possible.

SKIN DISEASE

PHYSIOLOGY

Many physiological changes affect the skin during pregnancy. Increased pigmentation, especially on the face, areolae, axillae and abdominal midline, is common. Spider naevi affect the face, arms and upper torso, and broad pink linear striae (striae gravidarum) frequently appear over the lower abdomen and thighs. Pruritus without rash affects up to 20% of normal pregnancies, but bile acids should always be performed to exclude intrahepatic cholestasis of pregnancy (see **Chapter 6**).

PRE-EXISTING SKIN DISEASE

Atopic eczema is a common pruritic skin condition affecting 1–5% of the general population. Although it usually improves in pregnancy, it is the most common pregnancy rash. It can be treated with emollients, bath additives and topical steroids if necessary. Hand and nipple eczema are particularly common post-partum.

Psoriasis affects 2% of the population and, during pregnancy, it remains unchanged in around 40% of patients, improves in another 40% and worsens in around 20%. Topical steroids can still be used, while methotrexate is contraindicated.

Acne usually improves in pregnancy but can flare in the third trimester and acne rosacea often

worsens. Oral or topical erythromycin can be used, but tetracyclines and retinoids are contraindicated.

SPECIFIC DERMATOSES OF PREGNANCY

POLYMORPHIC ERUPTION OF PREGNANCY

Polymorphic eruption of pregnancy is the most common pregnancy-specific dermatosis. It is a self-limiting pruritic inflammatory disorder that usually presents in the third trimester and/or immediately post-partum. The estimated incidence is about 1 in 200 pregnancies and it is more common in primigravida and twin pregnancies. Polymorphic eruption of pregnancy often begins on the lower abdomen, involving pregnancy striae, and extends to the thighs, buttocks, legs and arms, while sparing the umbilicus and rarely involving the face, hands and feet. In 70% of patients, the lesions become confluent and widespread, resembling a toxic erythema. Symptomatic treatment is usually sufficient with antihistamines and emollients, but topical steroids may be required. Pregnancies appear to be otherwise unaffected, with no tendency to recur.

PRURIGO OF PREGNANCY

Prurigo of pregnancy is a common pruritic disorder that occurs in 1 in 300 pregnancies and presents as excoriated papules on extensor limbs, the abdomen and the shoulders. It is more common in individuals with a history of atopy. Prurigo usually starts at around 25–30 weeks of pregnancy and resolves after delivery with no effect on the mother or baby. Treatment is symptomatic with topical steroids and emollients.

PRURITIC FOLLICULITIS OF PREGNANCY

Pruritic folliculitis is a pruritic follicular eruption with papules and pustules that mainly affect the trunk, but can involve the limbs. It is similar in appearance to acne lesions and is sometimes considered a type of hormonally induced acne. Its onset is usually in the second and third trimester and it resolves weeks after delivery. Topical steroid treatment is effective.

PEMPHIGOID GESTATIONIS

Pemphigoid gestationis is a rare pruritic autoimmune bullous disorder with an incidence of around 1 in 10,000–60,000 pregnancies. It most commonly presents in the late second or third trimester with lesions beginning around the umbilicus and progressing to widespread clustered blisters, spreading to the limbs, palms and soles but sparing the face. It is intensely pruritic and very distressing. Diagnosis is made by the clinical appearance and by direct immunofluorescence. Once established, the disease runs a complex course with exacerbations and remissions, and flares post-partum in 75% of cases. Management aims to relieve pruritus and prevent new blister formation, and is achieved through the use of potent topical steroids and/or oral prednisolone. There is some association with preterm delivery and small-for-gestational-age births, but no increase in pregnancy loss has been reported. Pemphigoid gestationis recurs in most subsequent pregnancies and may recur on the combined oral contraceptive pill.

KEY LEARNING POINTS

- Women with medical conditions that adversely affect pregnancy outcome should be offered pre-pregnancy counselling by an appropriately experienced MDT of healthcare professionals.
- Women with medical problems that preclude safe pregnancy should be offered safe, effective and appropriate contraception.
- Asthma is the most common chronic disease encountered in pregnancy.
- Pulmonary hypertension is associated with a risk of maternal mortality of up to 50% in pregnancy.
- Individuals who become pregnant with serum creatinine values above 124 µmol/L have an increased risk of accelerated decline in renal function and poor outcome of pregnancy.
- Pre-existing diabetes increases maternal and fetal obstetric morbidity.
- The incidence of fetal macrosomia in diabetes can be reduced through good blood glucose control.
- The risk of perinatal and maternal morbidity is increased in pregnancies complicated by SCD.
- The main issues for pregnant women with epilepsy relate to the teratogenic risk of anticonvulsant medication drugs and the risk of SUDEP if epilepsy is poorly controlled.
- It is important to be aware of red flags that suggest serious illness so that a diagnosis can be made and promptly managed.

FURTHER READING

James DK, Steer PJ, Weiner CP, Gonik B (2018). *High Risk Pregnancy: Management Options*, 5th edn.
Nelson-Piercy C (2020). *Handbook of Obstetric Medicine*, 6th edn.
Williams D, Davison J (2008). Chronic kidney disease in pregnancy. *BMJ*, 336 (7637): 211–215.
MBRRACE-UK. https://www.npeu.ox.ac.uk/mbrrace-uk.

SELF-ASSESSMENT

For interactive SBAs and EMQs relating to this chapter, visit www.routledge.com/cw/mccarthy.

CASE HISTORY 1

A 36-year-old woman with a history of type 1 diabetes is referred to the diabetes pregnancy service, as she is considering a pregnancy. She has mild retinopathy, has not had any previous pregnancies and does not currently take any regular medication in addition to her insulin. Her most recent HbA1c is 65 mmol/mol.

A What medication should she start prior to trying for a pregnancy?

B Is her diabetes satisfactorily controlled and should she be encouraged to delay pregnancy?

C What important pregnancy complications should be discussed with her prior to her embarking on a pregnancy?

ANSWERS

A Folic acid should be recommended to all women planning a pregnancy, but a higher dose should be prescribed to those with diabetes in view of the increased risk of neural tube defects. They should be advised to take 5 mg daily for 3 months prior to pregnancy.

B Her diabetes is not satisfactorily controlled, as her HbA1c is above the target range (42 mmol/mol). She should be encouraged to test her blood sugars pre- and post-meals and make adjustments to her insulin, aiming to maintain her blood sugars between 4 and 7 mmol/L.

C Prior to pregnancy, it is useful to inform women of the need for the additional surveillance required in pregnancies complicated by maternal diabetes. The increased risk of miscarriage, congenital anomalies and pregnancy complications such as pre-eclampsia, fetal macrosomia, stillbirth and neonatal complications should be discussed. It should be emphasized that good glycaemic control significantly reduces the risk of all of these complications.

CASE HISTORY 2

Mrs L, a 42-year-old woman, presents to your clinic at 32 weeks' gestation. Her platelets have been recorded as 40 × 10⁹/L. No previous full blood count has been performed. List the differential diagnosis for thrombocytopenia in pregnancy.

ANSWER

The causes of thrombocytopenia include increased consumption or destruction, autoimmune, APS, pre-eclampsia, HELLP syndrome, disseminated intravascular coagulation, thrombotic thrombocytopenic purpura and hypersplenism. It can also occur due to decreased production due to sepsis, HIV infection and malignant marrow infiltration. Gestational thrombocytopenia and pre-eclampsia are the commonest causes of low platelets in pregnancy.

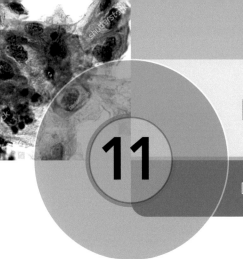

Perinatal infections

DAVID LISSAUER

Learning Objectives
- Know about the common infections that may affect the pregnant woman, fetus and neonate.
- Be aware of the infections included in routine pregnancy screening.
- Know about the principles of management of perinatal infection.

INTRODUCTION

This chapter covers the main infections affecting the pregnant woman, fetus and neonate immediately after birth. An overview of perinatal infections is shown in **Figure 11.1**.

The pregnant woman may encounter the same range of infections as all adults, but the illness may be more severe because of the physical and immunological changes that occur during pregnancy. Bacterial sepsis is a major problem; although uncommon in the UK and other high-income countries, it can cause severe illness requiring intensive care and it places both the mother and the fetus at risk of death. Viral infections can also cause severe illness, as encountered with coronavirus disease 2019 (COVID-19) during the pandemic. Congenital infection may occur from transplacental spread and may be detected on antenatal screening or at birth or months or years later. Neonatal infection is usually acquired from organisms encountered from ascending infection shortly before birth or during delivery, or by nosocomial spread or in breast milk.

MATERNAL INFECTIONS AND SEPSIS

The most common infections experienced in pregnancy are genital tract and urinary tract infections and skin or wound infections, especially after caesarean section or perineal wounds. Genital tract infections include chorioamnionitis – an intra-amniotic infection that occurs prior to birth and involves infection of any combination of the amniotic fluid, placenta, fetus or fetal membranes – and endometritis, namely intrauterine infection after birth, miscarriage or termination of pregnancy. Common maternal infections and their clinical features are shown in **Table 11.1**.

If a maternal infection is associated with organ dysfunction and becomes life threatening, it is termed maternal sepsis. Maternal sepsis is one of the most important causes of maternal mortality worldwide, including in high-income countries. In the UK, infections are the second most common cause of pregnant women being admitted to intensive

173

10.1201/9781003196112-11

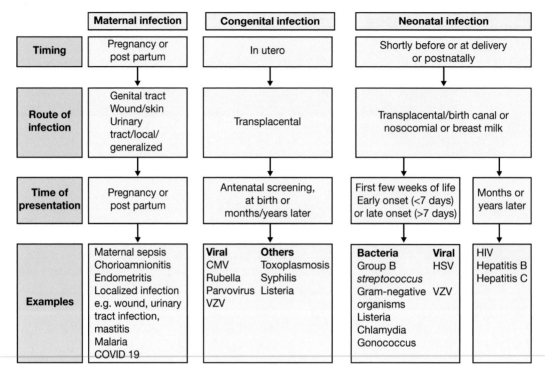

Figure 11.1 An overview of perinatal infections. (CMV, cytomegalovirus; COVID-19, coronavirus disease 2019; HIV, human immunodeficiency virus; HSV, herpes simplex virus; VZV, varicella zoster virus.)

Table 11.1 Common maternal infections and their clinical features

Infection	Clinical features
Chorioamnionitis	Abdominal pain, offensive vaginal discharge or lochia, uterine tenderness, fetal tachycardia >160 beats per minute, fever
Endometritis	Abdominal pain, vaginal bleeding, offensive discharge, uterine tenderness, delayed uterine involution, fever
Infected wound (perineal or abdominal)	Discharge from wound, pain, erythema and swelling around wound
Urinary tract infection	Dysuria, increased frequency, urgency, abdominal/flank/back pain, rigors, fever, nausea and vomiting
Breast abscess/mastitis	Breast pain and tenderness, erythema, painful induration, nipple discharge
Respiratory tract infection	Productive cough, sore throat, shortness of breath/difficulty breathing, chest pain, fever
Toxic shock syndrome (streptococcal and staphylococcal)	Nausea, vomiting, diarrhoea, watery vaginal discharge, generalized maculopapular rash, conjunctival suffusion
Meningitis	Headache, rash, photophobia, neck stiffness, confusion, fever, nausea and vomiting

care. Globally, in 2020, maternal sepsis accounted for 10% of the 280,000 maternal deaths, making it a major cause of maternal mortality alongside post-partum haemorrhage and eclampsia.

AETIOLOGY AND EPIDEMIOLOGY

Some infections occur more commonly in the pregnant population (e.g. mastitis and malaria) and others are more severe during pregnancy (e.g. influenza

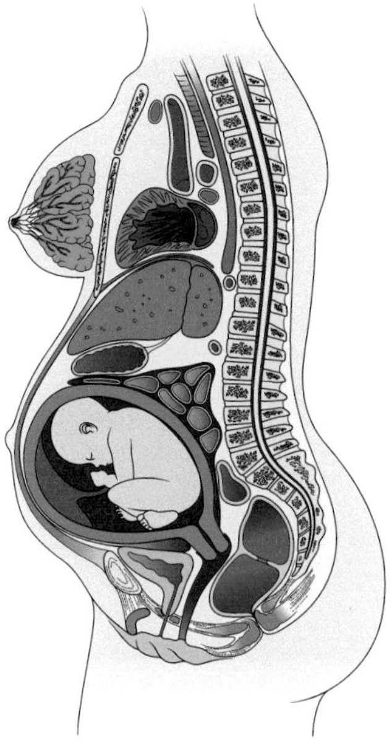

Figure 11.2 Factors causing an increased risk of maternal infections.

Table 11.2 Risk factors for developing maternal sepsis during pregnancy or post-partum

Maternal risk factors	Obstetric risk factors
Social factors (poverty, lack of access to care)	Cervical cerclage
Obesity	Prolonged rupture of membranes
Diabetes in pregnancy	Amniocentesis and other invasive procedures
Iron deficiency anaemia	
Maternal age >35 years	
Impaired immunity/ immunosuppressant medication	Vaginal trauma
	Caesarean birth
Ethnicity (Black and South East Asian)	Retained pregnancy tissue
Renal/cardiac/liver disease	Multiple gestation
History of pelvic infection	

and varicella zoster). This is because, during pregnancy, there are physical and immunological changes to accommodate the developing fetus (**Figure 11.2**). While anyone can be affected by infections during or after pregnancy, there are some important risk factors (**Table 11.2**).

Maternal infections and sepsis are caused by a wide range of organisms, but the most common are *Escherichia coli*, beta-haemolytic streptococci of Lancefield group A (group A strep) and mixed infections. Infections with coliform bacteria are particularly common in urinary sepsis or in pregnant women with premature rupture of the membranes. Wound infections are associated with staphylococcal infection, including methicillin-resistant *Staphylococcus aureus* (MRSA). Like in all populations, antimicrobial resistance is increasing and makes management more difficult.

PREVENTION

Preventing infections includes meticulous attention to hand hygiene and other infection prevention and control practices, such as aseptic technique during sterile procedures. Vaccination against important infections such as influenza and COVID-19 should be encouraged. There are also a number of obstetric situations and procedures in which the risks of infection are sufficiently high that antibiotic prophylaxis is recommended.

MANAGEMENT

All providers looking after women who are pregnant or post-partum need to be very vigilant to spot infections early and treat them appropriately. This can be

BOX 11.1: Situations in which antibiotic prophylaxis is and is not recommended

Recommended

- Third- or fourth-degree perineal tears (these involve the anal sphincter muscle or rectal mucosa)
- Caesarean section (given before skin incision)
- Preterm prelabour rupture of membranes
- Operative vaginal birth
- Manual removal of the placenta
- Known group B *Streptococcus* (GBS) colonization or previous affected infant (given in labour)

Not recommended

- Uncomplicated vaginal birth
- Meconium-stained liquor
- After episiotomy

challenging, as some of the physiological changes of pregnancy make the clinical features more difficult to recognize. For example, increased frequency of urination is both a common feature of normal pregnancy and a feature of urinary tract infections. Some normal investigation ranges must be interpreted in the context of pregnancy (e.g. blood lactate is often raised during labour due to the physical exertion and altered ranges for serum creatinine mean that renal dysfunction could be missed if unadjusted normal ranges are used).

Women from ethnic minorities and other marginalized groups are at particular risk and they must be encouraged to seek advice without delay if they are concerned about symptoms of infection. Providers must ensure that they do not dismiss concerns raised by individuals in these groups and must also be aware that some features of infection may present differently, such as the differing appearance of skin rashes on different skin types.

Women with infections in pregnancy need to be meticulously monitored. They can often compensate physiologically for an extended period and then deteriorate rapidly. This means that careful attention needs to be paid to changes in vital signs and these need to be interpreted in the context of the expected physiological changes of pregnancy. For example, early warning scoring systems adjusted for pregnancy-specific ranges should be used. Early escalation to senior clinicians is recommended in individuals whose clinical condition appears to be deteriorating.

Antimicrobial choices need to take account of not only the clinical presentation and likely source but also the prevalent organisms and their antimicrobial resistance patterns. Consideration is also needed for the safety of any treatments for the fetus or the infant during breastfeeding. Identification of the organism should be attempted so the antibiotic choice can be tailored accordingly. This requires collection of correct specimens for microbiological examination such as blood cultures, urine samples and wound or pus swabs.

Maternal sepsis is a life-threatening emergency and rapid treatment is required. The use of a sepsis bundle can help ensure pregnant women reliably and rapidly get the key treatments they need. Crucial aspects of this are ensuring an immediate and senior clinical review, delivery of appropriate antibiotics within 1 hour, intravenous fluids and oxygen if indicated, detailed monitoring to ensure response to treatment and escalation of care if needed.

COVID-19 AND INFLUENZA

The UK Obstetric Surveillance Survey (UKOSS) looks at less common obstetric conditions that have a significant burden on perinatal and maternal mortality and morbidity. UKOSS reviewed the impact of COVID-19 infection on pregnancy outcomes and at the risk factors associated with severe COVID-19 in pregnant women in the UK between March 2020 and October 2021. During this time, 65% of pregnant women admitted to hospital had mild infection, 21% had moderate infection and 14% had severe infection. In total, 22 individuals in this cohort died (all with severe COVID-19), 59 babies were stillborn and 10 infants died in the neonatal period.

Compared with pregnant women who had mild or moderate infection, those with severe COVID-19 infection:

- were more likely to give birth early (before 32 weeks of pregnancy): 22.6% versus 2.7%
- had a 50-fold higher risk of their birth being induced or by caesarean section, specifically due to their COVID-19 infection
- were more likely to give birth by pre-labour caesarean section (76% versus 30%)

- had a higher proportion of stillborn babies (3.3% versus 1.2%)
- had a 12-fold increased risk of their babies being admitted to a neonatal intensive care unit, in part due to an increase in preterm birth

Until the end of 2023, newer variants, such as the Omicron variant, have been associated with less severe maternal and fetal effects, with no evidence of the placentitis that was often observed in the Delta variant, particularly in the unvaccinated population. In addition, pregnant women who are 30 years of age or over, are overweight, are of a minority ethnicity, have gestational diabetes or have pre-existing hypertension have a greater risk of contracting severe COVID-19.

Evidence from the last influenza pandemic (2009/ H1N1) also showed that pregnant women were particularly vulnerable to severe infection resulting in increases in both maternal and perinatal mortality. The UK Confidential Enquiries into Maternal Deaths and Morbidity (2009–2012) showed that, during that time, 1 in 11 pregnant women who died had influenza. Factors associated with admission to hospital included obesity, asthma, multiparity, multiple pregnancy, being of Black or of another minority group ethnicity and smoking.

All pregnant women in the UK are encouraged to have seasonal flu and COVID-19 vaccines and the importance of this in preventing serious morbidity and mortality cannot be overemphasized. Prompt treatment with antiviral agents; a multidisciplinary team approach with early involvement of respiratory physicians, infectious disease specialists and senior obstetricians; and consideration of intensive care at an early stage are essential.

MALARIA

INFECTIVE ORGANISMS

Although malaria can be caused by four species of malarial parasite (*Plasmodium falciparum, P. vivax, P. ovale* and *P. malariae*), the one that carries the worst prognosis for the mother and fetus, and the organism of greatest importance on a worldwide scale, is *P. falciparum*. This is a protozoan parasite transmitted by the female anopheline mosquito.

INCIDENCE

Incidence varies depending on geographical location, but malaria is endemic in sub-Saharan Africa, South Asia and some parts of South America. It is estimated that one billion people worldwide carry parasites at any time, and 620,000 died from malaria in 2020. Pregnant women have an increased risk of malarial infection compared with the non-pregnant population. The incidence of parasitaemia has been found to be higher in the primiparous population (66%) than in the multiparous population (21–29%).

In endemic areas, where many people are semi-immune, malarial parasites are often found in large numbers sequestrated in the placenta, even when blood films are negative. This may lead to the diagnosis being missed, unless there is a high index of suspicion and the placenta is examined appropriately.

CLINICAL FEATURES

Maternal effects include a cyclical spiking pyrexia, which may be associated with miscarriage and preterm labour. Severe anaemia may develop rapidly, but many pregnant women from endemic areas may also have other risk factors for severe anaemia. Hypoglycaemia is common and may be severe in pregnancy. Pulmonary oedema, due to abnormal capillary permeability, results in high mortality (approximately 50%). Haemolysis causes jaundice and renal failure.

Fetal effects include premature delivery and fetal growth restriction (FGR). Placental sequestration of parasites is associated with abnormal uteroplacental Doppler wave forms and is also implicated in the higher rate of transmission of human immunodeficiency virus (HIV). Coinfection with HIV is common in many of the areas where malaria is endemic, and vertical transmission of both malaria and HIV to the fetus is more common if the two infections coexist.

MANAGEMENT

If malaria is suspected, prompt symptomatic and supportive treatment with appropriate antimalarial therapy is indicated. The choice of antimalarial will vary, depending on local patterns of disease and drug resistance, and expert advice should be sought. In endemic areas, preventative strategies include the use of insecticide-treated bed nets and intermittent preventative treatment during pregnancy.

If pregnant women from non-endemic areas are planning to travel to endemic areas, they should do so only if absolutely necessary during pregnancy. Insecticide sprays, mosquito nets, appropriate clothing to reduce the risk of mosquito bites and drug prophylaxis can all be used. Expert advice on which antimalarial is appropriate for the area should be obtained. The potential risks of teratogenicity must be balanced against the serious risk of contracting malaria.

CONGENITAL INFECTIONS

CYTOMEGALOVIRUS

Cytomegalovirus (CMV) is the most common congenital infection in the UK, affecting 0.5–1 in every 1,000 live births.

INFECTIVE ORGANISM

CMV is a deoxyribonucleic acid (DNA) herpes virus. It is transmitted by respiratory droplet transmission and is excreted in the urine.

PREVALENCE

CMV infection is common in the UK; about 60% of women are CMV seropositive when they become pregnant, so 40% are susceptible, although there is also a risk of reactivation or reinfection. It is estimated that 1–2% of individuals seroconvert during pregnancy. Of these, it is estimated that 5–10% of their babies will be severely affected at birth. Although 90% appear asymptomatic at birth, 10–15% of them are at risk of sensorineural hearing loss (which may be progressive) and developmental delay.

Primary infection is more likely to cause symptomatic congenital CMV (40% transmission rate) and long-term sequelae than reactivation or reinfection (1%). However, the high incidence of CMV seropositivity among the pregnant population worldwide (>90%) means that more infants with congenital infection are born following reactivation or reinfection than from primary infection.

CLINICAL FEATURES

Primary infection in the mother usually produces no symptoms or mild non-specific flu-like symptoms. The diagnosis is often made after abnormalities are identified in the severely affected fetus on ultrasound scanning. The main features are growth restriction, microcephaly, intracranial calcification (**Figure 11.3**), ventriculomegaly, ascites (see **Figure 11.5**) and hydrops. The neonate may be anaemic and thrombocytopaenic, with hepatosplenomegaly, jaundice and a purpuric rash.

MANAGEMENT

A serological diagnosis of primary CMV can be made by demonstrating the development of CMV antibodies in a seronegative individual, who initially develops CMV immunoglobulin (Ig)M antibody and subsequently IgG antibody. Virology laboratories usually keep the blood sample taken in early pregnancy, so, if infection is suspected, a sample taken at the time of presentation can be compared with the initial booking sample to determine if seroconversion has occurred. As IgM can be secreted for several months, it is not sufficient to simply demonstrate IgM in a sample at the time of presentation; it has to be a new finding in someone who was negative for IgM at the time of booking.

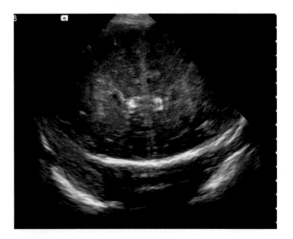

Figure 11.3 Ultrasound of a fetal brain demonstrating intracranial calcification secondary to cytomegalovirus infection. (Courtesy of Dr Ed Johnstone, St Mary's Hospital, Manchester.)

If it is suspected that the fetus may be infected, as the virus is excreted in fetal urine, amniotic fluid can be tested for the virus by polymerase chain reaction (PCR). There may be a role in some cases for treatment of an infected fetus with antivirals.

If severe abnormalities from congenital CMV infection are detected on ultrasound, termination of pregnancy should be considered. More difficult is when CMV infection is identified but the fetus appears normal on ultrasound, as there remains a 10–20% risk of hearing loss and neurodisability. There is some evidence that antiviral treatment of infants with central nervous system involvement improves hearing and neurodevelopmental outcomes.

SYPHILIS

Syphilis is a sexually acquired infection caused by *Treponema pallidum*, which in pregnancy is associated with FGR, non-immune fetal hydrops, congenital syphilis (cerebral calcification and other cerebral and gastrointestinal anomalies and bone lesions), stillbirth, preterm birth and neonatal death. In the infant it can cause anaemia, jaundice, hepatosplenomegaly, rhinitis, eye abnormalities, a rash on the hands and feet and neurodisability.

Its incidence during pregnancy in the UK is low and has reduced over the last decade. There is a highly effective screening programme with more than 99% of the eligible population screened. Of 676,000 pregnant women screened in 2018 in England, 1,028 were screen positive, of whom 470 required treatment, and only three cases of congenital syphilis were reported. However, syphilis remains a problem worldwide, with more than one million pregnant women estimated to be infected globally in 2020, making it an important cause of stillbirth worldwide. The global incidence of congenital syphilis in 2020 was estimated at 425 cases per 100,000 livebirths.

CLINICAL FEATURES

Primary syphilis may present as a painless genital ulcer 3–6 weeks after the infection is acquired, which is called a chancre (condylomata lata) (**Figure 11.4**). However, this may be on the cervix and so may go unnoticed.

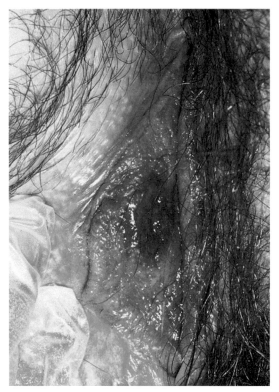

Figure 11.4 Primary syphilitic chancre. (Courtesy of Dr Raymond Maw, Royal Victoria Hospital, Belfast.)

Secondary manifestations occur 6 weeks to 6 months after infection and present as a maculopapular rash or lesions affecting the mucous membranes. Ultimately, 20% of untreated patients will develop symptomatic cardiovascular tertiary syphilis and 5–10% will develop symptomatic neurosyphilis.

In pregnant women with early, untreated (primary or secondary) syphilis, 70–100% of infants will be infected and approximately 25% will be stillborn. The risk of congenital transmission declines with increasing duration of maternal syphilis prior to pregnancy.

SCREENING

As treatment is highly effective, routine antenatal screening is recommended for all pregnant women and the uptake for national screening in the UK is very high (>95%). Treponemal tests detect specific treponemal antibodies and include enzyme immunoassays (EIAs), *T. pallidum* haemagglutination assay and the fluorescent treponemal antibody-absorbed test. EIAs detect IgG and IgM and are rapidly replacing the non-specific treponemal antibody tests, the venereal diseases research laboratory (VDRL) test and rapid plasma reagin tests. EIAs are over 98% sensitive and over 99% specific, in contrast with the non-treponemal tests, which may result in false-negatives, particularly in very early or late syphilis, in patients with reinfection or in those who are HIV positive. The VDRL test may be false-positive in patients with lupus. Overall, there is a significant false-positive rate from screening tests; pregnant women should therefore be referred for expert assessment and diagnosis in a genitourinary medicine (GUM) clinic.

None of these serological tests will detect syphilis in its incubation stage, which may last for an average of 25 days. Congenital infections including syphilis may be suspected from abnormalities on antenatal ultrasound.

MANAGEMENT

The initial step is to confirm the diagnosis and to test for any other sexually transmitted diseases. Once a diagnosis of syphilis is confirmed, the GUM clinic will institute appropriate contact tracing of sexual partners. Older children may also need to be screened for congenital infection. Treatment is indicated for acute infection, for inadequately treated infection or if treatment prior to pregnancy is uncertain.

Parenteral penicillin has a 98% success rate for preventing congenital syphilis if given before 36 weeks' gestation. A Jarish–Herxheimer reaction may occur with treatment as a result of the release of pro-inflammatory cytokines in response to dying organisms. This presents as a worsening of symptoms and fever for 12–24 hours after commencement of treatment. It may be associated with uterine contractions and fetal distress. Some clinicians therefore admit pregnant women at the time of commencement of treatment for monitoring.

If the pregnant woman is not treated during pregnancy, the baby should be treated after delivery. An infected baby may be born without signs or symptoms of disease but if untreated may develop seizures and developmental impairment. Infants of treated mothers should be assessed at birth.

TOXOPLASMOSIS

INFECTIVE ORGANISM

Toxoplasma gondii is a protozoan parasite found in cat faeces, soil, uncooked meat and unwashed salads or raw vegetables. Infection occurs by ingestion of the parasite from undercooked meat or from unwashed hands or food.

PREVALENCE

Around 350 cases of toxoplasmosis are reported in England and Wales each year, but the actual number of infections could be as high as 350,000 and estimates suggest up to one-third of the population will be infected by toxoplasmosis at some point in their life. However, congenital toxoplasmosis is rare in the UK, with estimates suggesting only 1 in every 10,000–30,000 live births.

SCREENING

Only about 10 severely affected babies are diagnosed per year in the UK and, for this reason, the UK National Screening Committee recommends that screening for toxoplasmosis should not be offered routinely. There is a lack of evidence that antenatal screening and treatment reduces mother-to-child transmission or the complications associated with *T. gondii* infection. In the UK, pregnant women should be advised about appropriate preventative measures, such as avoiding eating undercooked meat and wearing gloves and washing hands when handling cat litter or gardening.

Even in France, where the infection rate during pregnancy is higher and the pregnant population is screened monthly, the benefits of such a programme appear to be limited.

CLINICAL FEATURES

The initial infection is usually asymptomatic or may be a glandular fever-like illness. Parasitaemia usually occurs within 3 weeks of infection. Therefore, congenital infection is only a significant risk if the mother acquires the infection during or immediately before pregnancy.

Infection during the first trimester of pregnancy is most likely to cause severe fetal damage (85%), but only 10% of infections are transmitted to the fetus at this gestation. In the third trimester, 85% of infections are transmitted, but the risk of fetal damage decreases to around 10%.

Severely infected infants may have ventriculomegaly or microcephaly, chorioretinitis and cerebral calcification. These features may be detected on ultrasound scan. The majority of infected infants are asymptomatic at birth but develop sequelae several years later.

MANAGEMENT

The diagnosis of primary infection with toxoplasmosis during pregnancy is made by the Sabin–Feldman dye test. Enzyme-linked immunosorbent assays are available for IgM antibody. However, IgM may persist for months or even years, so often serial testing for rising titres is necessary. If suspicion of congenital toxoplasmosis has arisen because of an abnormal ultrasound scan of the fetus, an amniocentesis can be performed. PCR analysis of amniotic fluid is highly accurate for the identification of *T. gondii*.

Spiramycin treatment can be used in pregnancy. This reduces the incidence of transplacental infection but has not been shown to definitively reduce the incidence of clinical congenital disease. If congenital infection is identified on ultrasound, termination of pregnancy can be considered, or treatment with sulphadiazine and pyrimethamine may be given, although evidence of the efficacy of this treatment is lacking.

CHICKENPOX (VARICELLA ZOSTER VIRUS)

INFECTIVE ORGANISM

Chickenpox is caused by the varicella zoster virus (VZV), a herpes virus that is transmitted by droplet spread and direct personal contact.

PREVALENCE

In the UK, over 90% of individuals over 15 years of age are immune to chickenpox. Although contact with chickenpox is common in pregnancy, infection during pregnancy is uncommon, with an estimated prevalence of 3 in every 1,000 pregnancies. Antenatal screening for chickenpox is not currently recommended in the UK, but individuals identified as being seronegative can consider vaccination either pre-pregnancy or in the postnatal period.

CLINICAL FEATURES

Non-immune pregnant women are more vulnerable to chickenpox and may develop a serious pneumonia, hepatitis or encephalitis. The mortality rate is approximately five times higher in the pregnant population than in the non-pregnant population. Pneumonia occurs in about 10% of pregnant women with chickenpox and is more severe at later gestations. It may also cause fetal varicella syndrome (FVS) or varicella infection of the newborn.

MANAGEMENT

Women should be asked whether they have had chickenpox or shingles or 2 recorded doses of varicella vaccine at the initial booking visit. If this is the case, and they are immunocompetent, this is sufficient evidence of immunity. If not, they should be advised to avoid contact with infected individuals during pregnancy, and, if contact occurs, to advise their doctor or midwife as soon as possible. Significant contact is defined as being in the same room as an infected person for 15 or more minutes or face-to-face contact. Individuals are infectious for 48 hours prior to appearance of the rash and until the vesicles crust over (usually 5 days).

Testing for immunity

If a pregnant woman with no history of immunity has been in contact with chickenpox, she should have a blood test for confirmation of VZV immunity by testing for VZV IgG. This can usually be performed within 24–48 hours and the virology laboratory may be able to use serum stored from the early pregnancy booking blood sample.

Management of the non-immune pregnant woman exposed to chickenpox

If immunity is not confirmed and there has been significant exposure, the individual should be offered post-exposure prophylaxis (PEP). As the efficacy of varicella zoster immunoglobulin (VZIG) in preventing chickenpox has been found to be poor, guidelines for the UK from 2023 (UK Health Security Agency) are for antivirals to be used for PEP in susceptible individuals, with VZIG recommended only for neonates.

Management of chickenpox in pregnancy

Women with chickenpox should avoid contact with other pregnant women and neonates until the lesions have crusted over. Current recommendations state that oral aciclovir should be prescribed for pregnant women if they present within 24 hours of the onset of the rash and if they are more than 20 weeks' gestation. Aciclovir should also be considered before 20 weeks' gestation. VZIG has no therapeutic benefit once chickenpox has developed. If the pregnant woman smokes, has chronic lung disease, is taking corticosteroids or is in the second half of pregnancy, a hospital assessment should be considered, even in the absence of complications.

Individuals hospitalized with varicella should be nursed in isolation from babies or potentially susceptible pregnant women or non-immune staff.

Delivery during the viraemic period may be hazardous. The maternal risks are bleeding, thrombocytopaenia, disseminated intravascular coagulopathy and hepatitis. There is a risk of varicella infection of the newborn with significant morbidity and mortality. Supportive treatment and intravenous aciclovir is therefore desirable, allowing resolution of the rash and transfer of protective antibodies from the mother to the fetus. However, delivery may be required to facilitate assisted ventilation in cases in which varicella pneumonia is complicated by respiratory failure.

Fetus

Spontaneous miscarriage does not appear to be increased if chickenpox occurs in the first trimester. FVS is characterized by one or more of the following:

- skin scarring in a dermatomal distribution
- eye defects (microphthalmia, chorioretinitis, cataracts)
- hypoplasia of the limbs
- neurological abnormalities (microcephaly, cortical atrophy, mental restriction and dysfunction of bowel and bladder sphincters)

FVS occurs in only very few infected fetuses (approximately 1%). FVS has been reported as early as 3 weeks' and up to 28 weeks' gestation. The risk appears to be lower in the first trimester (0.55%). No case of FVS has been reported when maternal infection has occurred after 28 weeks.

If chickenpox occurs in pregnancy, referral to a fetal medicine specialist should be considered at 16–20 weeks or 5 weeks after infection for discussion and detailed ultrasound examination, when findings such as limb deformity, microcephaly, hydrocephalus, soft-tissue calcification and FGR can be detected. A time lag of at least 5 weeks after the primary infection is advised, as it takes several weeks for these features to manifest.

Following the primary infection, the virus remains dormant in sensory nerve root ganglia but can be reactivated to cause herpes zoster or shingles, a vesicular erythematous skin rash in a dermatomal distribution. The risk of a pregnant woman acquiring infection from an individual with herpes zoster in non-exposed sites (for example thoracolumbar) is low.

Management around delivery

If infection occurs at term, there is a significant risk of varicella of the newborn. Elective delivery should normally be avoided until 7 days after the onset of maternal rash to allow for the passive transfer of antibodies from the mother to the infant.

If birth occurs within the 7-day period following the onset of the maternal rash or if the mother develops the chickenpox rash within 7 days after birth, prophylactic VZIG and antiviral therapy may be indicated. The infant should be monitored for signs of infection.

Neonatal infection should be treated with aciclovir following discussion with a neonatologist and virologist.

PARVOVIRUS

INFECTIVE ORGANISM

Parvovirus B19 is a relatively common infection in pregnancy and is transmitted through respiratory droplets.

INCIDENCE

About 50% of the pregnant population is susceptible to infection. Infection is most common in those who work with young children, for example teachers. Routine screening in pregnancy is not recommended, as prevention of fetal infection is not possible.

CLINICAL FEATURES

In adults, many (20–25%) are asymptomatic or experience a mild flu-like illness and/or arthropathy. In children, it usually causes a characteristic rash (slapped cheek syndrome). There is a transplacental transmission rate of 17–33% and the fetus is most vulnerable in the second trimester. In most, there is spontaneous resolution with no long-term consequences, but the virus can infect the liver, which is the main source of haematopoiesis in the second trimester. This can lead to an aplastic anaemia, which may result in fetal hydrops. Hydrops is when fluid accumulates in two or more spaces in the fetus, such as pleural effusions, pericardial effusion, ascites (**Figure 11.5**) or skin oedema. This occurs secondary to high-output cardiac failure. Presentation is usually on ultrasound scan. In an anaemic fetus that has not developed hydrops or in a fetus in which this has progressed to cause hydrops, the velocity of blood flow in the fetal middle cerebral artery is high and this can be detected on ultrasound (**Figure 11.6**).

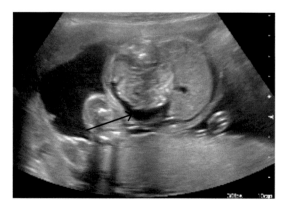

Figure 11.5 Fetal ascites. (Courtesy of Dr Ed Johnstone, St Mary's Hospital, Manchester.)

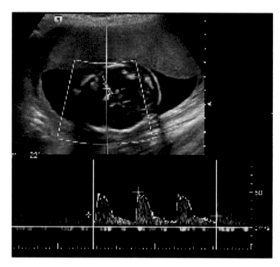

Figure 11.6 Middle cerebral Doppler assessment to test for fetal anaemia. (Courtesy of Dr Ed Johnstone, St Mary's Hospital, Manchester.)

MANAGEMENT

The diagnosis is made by demonstrating seroconversion of the mother, who develops IgM antibodies to parvovirus B19, having previously tested negative. PCR in maternal and fetal blood or amniotic fluid is the most sensitive and accurate diagnostic test.

If a fetus is severely anaemic or has developed hydrops, an in utero blood transfusion may be required. If the fetus survives the anaemia, the outcome is usually normal. Before 20 weeks, intrauterine transfusion is not possible and the fetal loss rate is approximately 10%. Beyond 20 weeks, treatment with transfusion can reduce the fetal loss rate to approximately 1%.

RUBELLA

The importance of maternal infection with rubella lies in its ability to cause congenital rubella syndrome in the fetus. Rubella infection in the mother may cause a maculo-papular rash or is asymptomatic. The risk and extent of fetal damage are mainly determined by the gestational age at maternal infection. Infection before 12 weeks' gestation causes deafness, congenital heart disease, cataracts and other abnormalities in over 80% of cases. About 30% of fetuses of mothers infected at 13 to 16 weeks' gestation have impaired hearing; beyond 18 weeks' gestation, the risk to the fetus is low. Viraemia after birth continues to damage the infant.

In the UK, European Union, North America and other high-income countries where the mumps, measles and rubella vaccine is part of the routine childhood vaccination programme, rubella infection has become extremely rare and congenital rubella syndrome is rarely encountered. This is why routine antenatal screening for immunity to rubella has been discontinued in the UK. By 2020, the rubella vaccine had been incorporated into the national immunization schedule of 194 countries, and 93 (48%) have eliminated rubella transmission. However, it may still be encountered in countries without a sufficiently high immunization rate.

LISTERIA

INFECTIVE ORGANISM

Listeria monocytogenes is an aerobic and facultatively anaerobic motile Gram-positive bacillus. It has an unusual life cycle with obligate intracellular replication. People with reduced cell-mediated immunity, and hence pregnant individuals, are therefore most at risk.

INCIDENCE

The incidence of *L. monocytogenes* infection in pregnant women is around 18 times higher than in the non-pregnant population, but is still rare, with rates of 1 in 8,000. Contaminated food is the usual source of infection. Usual sources are unpasteurized milk, ripened soft cheeses, pâté and ready-to-eat food unless thoroughly reheated, and pregnant women should be given information on risk reduction by dietary modification.

CLINICAL FEATURES

Pregnant women with listeriosis most commonly suffer from a flu-like illness with fever and general malaise. About one-third of cases may be asymptomatic. Transmission to the fetus may occur either via the ascending route through the cervix or transplacentally secondary to maternal bacteraemia. Approximately 20% of affected pregnancies result in miscarriage or stillbirth. Premature delivery may occur in over 50%. Neonates may have respiratory distress, fever, seizures or sepsis and the overall neonatal mortality rate has been estimated at 38%. Meconium staining of the amniotic fluid in a preterm infant may increase clinical suspicion of listeriosis. Neonatal infection is rare.

MANAGEMENT

The diagnosis of listeriosis depends on clinical suspicion and isolation of the organism from blood, vaginal swabs or the placenta. Intravenous antibiotic treatment is indicated for affected adults and neonates.

NEONATAL INFECTION

GROUP B *STREPTOCOCCUS*

INFECTIVE ORGANISM

GBS (*Streptococcus agalactiae*) is a Gram-positive coccus frequently found as a vaginal commensal. It can cause sepsis in the neonate and transmission can occur from the time the membranes are ruptured until delivery.

PREVALENCE

GBS is recognized as the most frequent cause of severe early-onset (less than 7 days of age) infection in newborn infants in high-income countries. Approximately 21% of pregnant women in the UK carry GBS as a commensal in the vagina. The background incidence of early-onset GBS disease in the UK is 0.5 in 1,000 births, which increases to 2.5 in 1,000 in women with GBS carriage confirmed in the current pregnancy.

The mortality from early-onset GBS disease in the UK is 6% in term infants and 18% in preterm infants. Even when treated appropriately, some infants will still die of early-onset disease, particularly when the disease is well established prior to birth.

SCREENING

Universal screening is carried out in the USA, but this practice is not currently recommended in the UK. The optimal screening approach remains unclear and can be either based on risk factors, or a universal screening approach can be used. The best strategy may depend on the prevalence of GBS in the population.

CLINICAL FEATURES

The mother will not have symptoms, as GBS is a common vaginal commensal. An infected neonate may demonstrate signs of neonatal sepsis, including sudden collapse, tachypnoea, nasal flaring, poor tone, etc.

MANAGEMENT

Antenatal

If GBS is detected incidentally, antenatal treatment is not recommended, as it does not reduce the likelihood of GBS colonization at the time of delivery.

Intra-partum antibiotic prophylaxis

It is during labour that infection of the fetus/neonate occurs. Antibiotics (benzylpenicillin) given in labour are estimated to be 60–80% effective in reducing early-onset neonatal GBS infection. Clindamycin was traditionally used as an alternative antibiotic in individuals suspected of having a penicillin allergy, but increasing resistance means alternatives such a cephalosporins or vancomycin (for severe allergy) are increasingly recommended.

The Royal College of Obstetricians and Gynaecologists (RCOG) recommends that intra-partum antibiotic prophylaxis is discussed with pregnant women (see **Box 11.2**, 'Risk factors for GBS prophylaxis') and that the recommendation for using prophylaxis is stronger if more than one risk factor is present.

BOX 11.2: Risk factors for GBS prophylaxis

- Intrapartum fever (>38°C)
- Prolonged rupture of membranes greater than 18 hours
- Prematurity (<37 weeks)
- Previous infant with GBS
- Incidental detection of GBS in current pregnancy
- GBS bacteriuria
- GBS colonization is a previous pregnancy, unless they have a recent negative test this pregnancy

Approximately 15% of all UK pregnancies have one or more of the risk factors and, using this strategy, 25% of pregnant women will receive intra-partum antibiotics with 50–69% reduction in early-onset GBS infection in the neonate. Therefore, 5,882 women need to be treated to prevent one neonatal death.

It is recommended that intravenous penicillin is given as soon as possible after the onset of labour (or after development of a risk factor) and 4-hourly until delivery.

Individuals in whom GBS carriage was detected in a previous pregnancy have around a 50% chance of again having GBS in this pregnancy. They should have the option of prophylaxis discussed with them and may opt for either prophylaxis or repeat testing in late pregnancy. If chorioamnionitis is suspected, broad-spectrum antibiotic therapy including an agent active against GBS should replace GBS-specific antibiotic prophylaxis. Women undergoing planned caesarean delivery in the absence of labour or membrane rupture do not require antibiotic prophylaxis for GBS, regardless of GBS colonization status. The risk of neonatal GBS disease is extremely low in this circumstance.

Neonate

Many infants with early-onset GBS disease have symptoms at or soon after birth. Neonatal sepsis can progress rapidly to death. Whether they received intra-partum antibiotics or not, any newborn infant with clinical signs compatible with infection should be treated promptly with broad-spectrum antibiotics, which provide cover against early-onset GBS disease and other common pathogens. Blood cultures should always be obtained before antibiotic treatment is commenced and cerebrospinal fluid cultures should be considered. Randomized controlled trials have not provided a sufficient evidence base for clear treatment recommendations in well newborn infants whose mothers had risk factors for GBS. Some clinicians will recommend treatment of the infants, while others will prefer to observe them because the balance of risks and benefits of treatment is uncertain. Each hospital will have its own guideline.

Gram-negative infection

In high-income countries, infection from Gram-negative organisms is less common than GBS. Infection is acquired by exposure of the infant shortly before or at delivery. The organisms can cause early- or late-onset neonatal infection, and result in significant morbidity and mortality.

HERPES SIMPLEX VIRUS

INFECTIVE ORGANISM

Herpes simplex virus (HSV) is a double-stranded DNA virus. There are two viral types, HSV-1 and HSV-2. The majority of orolabial infections are caused by HSV-1. These infections are usually acquired during childhood through direct physical contact such as kissing. Genital herpes is a sexually transmitted infection and is most commonly caused by HSV-2 (**Figure 11.7**).

INCIDENCE

Genital herpes is the most common ulcerative sexually transmitted infection in the UK. There has been an increasing prevalence of anogenital herpes in the UK over the last decade with around 20,000 cases per year. Neonatal herpes is a viral infection with a high morbidity and mortality, and is most commonly acquired at or near the time of delivery due to contact with infected secretions. It is rare, with an estimated incidence of 2 per 100,000 live births.

CLINICAL FEATURES

Genital herpes presents as ulcerative lesions on the vulva, vagina or cervix. It may be recurrent, when

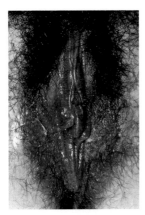

Figure 11.7 Primary genital herpes. (Courtesy of Dr Richard Lau, St George's Hospital, London.)

the lesion is usually less florid. A primary infection may be associated with systemic symptoms and may cause urinary retention.

Neonatal herpes may be caused by HSV-1 or HSV-2, as either viral type can cause genital herpes. Almost all cases of neonatal herpes occur as a result of direct contact with infected maternal secretions, although it can be acquired postnatally from an infected caregiver.

Neonatal herpes is classified into three subgroups: localized (to the skin, eye and/or mouth), local central nervous system disease (encephalitis alone) and disseminated infection (with multiple organ involvement). Factors influencing transmission include the type of maternal infection (primary or recurrent), the presence of transplacental maternal neutralizing antibodies, the duration of rupture of membranes before delivery, the use of fetal scalp electrodes and the mode of delivery. The risks are greatest in the presence of a new infection (primary genital herpes) in the third trimester, particularly within 6 weeks of delivery, as viral shedding may persist and the baby is likely to be born before the development of protective maternal antibodies. Very rarely, congenital herpes may occur as a result of transplacental intrauterine infection.

MANAGEMENT

Symptomatic genital herpes infections are confirmed by direct detection of HSV. A swab for viral detection should be used. Anyone with suspected first-episode genital herpes should be referred to a genitourinary physician, who will confirm the diagnosis by viral culture or PCR, advise on management and arrange a screen for other sexually transmitted infections. The use of aciclovir is recommended and is associated with a reduction in the duration and severity of symptoms and a decrease in the duration of viral shedding. It is well tolerated and considered safe in pregnancy.

It may be difficult to distinguish clinically between recurrent and primary genital HSV infections, as up to 15% of first-episode HSV infections are not true primary infections. For individuals presenting within 6 weeks of expected delivery, type-specific HSV antibody testing is advisable. The presence of antibodies of the same type as the HSV isolated from genital swabs would confirm this episode to be a recurrence rather than a primary infection.

Primary infections

Providing that delivery does not ensue within the next 6 weeks, the pregnancy should be managed expectantly and vaginal delivery anticipated. There is no evidence that HSV acquired in pregnancy is associated with an increased incidence of congenital abnormalities. Following first- or second-trimester acquisition, suppressive aciclovir from 36 weeks of gestation reduces HSV lesions at term and hence the need for delivery by caesarean section.

Caesarean section should be the recommended mode of delivery for all women developing first-episode genital herpes in the third trimester, particularly those developing symptoms within 6 weeks of expected delivery, as the risk of neonatal transmission of HSV is very high, at about 40%. For women who opt for a vaginal birth, rupture of membranes should be avoided and invasive procedures, such as fetal scalp electrodes or fetal scalp pH measurement, should not be used. Intravenous aciclovir given intra-partum to the mother and subsequently to the neonate may be considered.

Recurrent episodes

A recurrent episode of genital herpes occurring during the antenatal period is not an indication for delivery by caesarean section. Women presenting with recurrent genital herpes lesions at the onset of labour should be advised that the risk to the baby of neonatal herpes is very small (1–3%). Daily suppressive aciclovir should be considered from 36 weeks' gestation. Women with recurrent genital herpes lesions and confirmed rupture of membranes at term should be advised to have delivery expedited by the appropriate means. Invasive procedures in labour should be avoided for women with recurrent genital herpes lesions. The neonatologist should be informed of babies born to mothers with recurrent genital herpes lesions at the time of labour.

CHLAMYDIA

INFECTIVE ORGANISM

Chlamydia trachomatis is an obligate intracellular organism.

PREVALENCE

Chlamydia is the most common sexually transmitted organism in the UK and USA. Among the population who are sexually active and under 25 years old, 1 in 8–10 screen positive for chlamydia and there are over 100,000 cases diagnosed in women per year in the UK. In the UK, an opportunistic chlamydia screening programme for those under 25 years has been initiated. While it is not a routine antenatal screening test in the UK, the National Institute for Health and Care Excellence (NICE) recommends that all women booking for antenatal care, who are younger than 25 years, are informed of the national screening programme.

CLINICAL FEATURES

Chlamydia is frequently asymptomatic in the pregnant population. Infection with chlamydia is associated with preterm rupture of membranes, preterm delivery and low birthweight. Transmission to the fetus occurs at the time of delivery and can cause conjunctivitis and pneumonia.

MANAGEMENT

Treatment with azithromycin or erythromycin is recommended. Tetracyclines such as doxycycline should be avoided if possible during pregnancy. Appropriate contact tracing can be arranged via a GUM clinic.

GONORRHOEA

INFECTIVE ORGANISM

Neisseria gonorrhoeae is a Gram-negative diplococcus.

PREVALENCE

The prevalence of gonorrhoea in pregnancy varies with the population studied. In the UK, it is the second most common bacterial sexually transmitted disease, with around 8,000 cases per year in women.

CLINICAL FEATURES

Gonococcal infection in women is frequently asymptomatic, or they may present with a mucopurulent discharge or dysuria. Rarely, disseminated gonor-rhoea may cause low-grade fever, a rash and polyar-thritis. There is an increased risk of coinfection with chlamydia and an increased risk of preterm rupture of membranes and preterm birth. Transmission to the fetus occurs at the time of delivery and can cause ophthalmia neonatorum. Ocular prophylaxis with erythromycin ointment is given to all newborn infants in the USA and a number of countries, but not in the UK.

MANAGEMENT

Bacteriological swabs should be taken and specific swabs/testing for concomitant infection with chla-mydia should also be undertaken. Cephalosporins are effective against gonococcus, but empirical treatment for chlamydia should also be considered. Appropriate contact tracing can be arranged via a GUM clinic.

PERINATAL INFECTIONS CAUSING LONG-TERM DISEASE

HUMAN IMMUNODEFICIENCY VIRUS

INFECTIVE ORGANISM

HIV is a ribonucleic acid (RNA) retrovirus transmit-ted through sexual contact, blood and blood prod-ucts, shared needles usually among intravenous drug users, or vertical (mother-to-child) transmis-sion, which mainly occurs in the late third trimester or during labour, delivery or breastfeeding.

PREVALENCE

In 2019, there were 818 pregnancies in the UK in women living with HIV (about 1 in 1000). Of these, 90% were known to be living with HIV before pregnancy, with the remainder diagnosed during pregnancy. 65% were of Black African women and people. Worldwide, improved access to treatment and prevention of mother-to-child transmission has ensured that the prevalence of HIV is decreasing, but more than 5% of pregnant women in sub-Saharan Africa are still living with HIV.

SCREENING

In the UK, all pregnant women should be offered screening for HIV early in pregnancy, as antenatal interventions have been shown to reduce mother-to-child transmission of HIV infection. A positive HIV antibody test result should be given in person by an appropriately trained health professional; this may be a specialist nurse, midwife, HIV physician or obstetrician. The issue of disclosure of the HIV diagnosis to the partner should be handled with sensitivity and they should be reassured that their confidentiality will be respected.

Some women remain at risk of becoming infected with HIV during their pregnancy. These individuals should be offered repeat testing during pregnancy. Rapid HIV tests should be offered to anyone who presents for labour unbooked.

Pre-exposure prophylaxis is a strategy to prevent HIV in people at high risk of acquiring the disease, such as individuals with partners who have HIV or people who suffer from intimate partner violence. They will need detailed counselling and advice if planning a pregnancy or if they become pregnant, as they will need to balance the risks of acquiring HIV with the potential risks of taking antiviral drugs.

CLINICAL FEATURES

Untreated, infection with HIV begins with an asymp-tomatic stage with gradual compromise of immune function eventually leading to acquired immunode-ficiency syndrome (AIDS). The time between HIV infection and the development of AIDS ranges from a few months to as long as 17 years in untreated patients.

MANAGEMENT

The principal risks of mother-to-child (vertical) transmission are related to maternal plasma viral load, obstetric factors and infant feeding (**Table 11.3**). Interventions to reduce the risk of HIV transmission can reduce the risk of vertical transmission from 25–30% to less than 0.5%. These include:

- antiretroviral therapy, given antenatally, intra-partum and lifelong to the mother to fully suppress plasma viral load

Table 11.3 Risk factors for vertical transmission of human immunodeficiency virus (HIV)

Increased risk of transmission	Reduced risk of transmission
Advanced maternal HIV disease	Low or undetectable viral load at time of delivery
High maternal plasma viral load	Antiretroviral therapy
Low CD4 lymphocyte counts	Delivery by caesarean section
Prolonged rupture of membranes	Exclusive formula feeding
Chorioamnionitis	
Preterm delivery	
Coexisting viral infections (e.g. herpes, hepatitis C)	
Breastfeeding (doubles transmission rate)	

- elective caesarean section in the presence of a detectable viral load at delivery
- post-exposure prophylaxis antiretroviral therapy to the infant for 4 weeks

In high-income countries, mothers are advised to formula feed, although some with an undetectable viral load may choose to breastfeed with close surveillance. In resource-poor settings, mothers are advised to breastfeed on fully suppressed combination antiretroviral therapy. If the mother is not on antiretroviral therapy, the infant should receive daily antiretroviral therapy during the entire period of breastfeeding.

A planned vaginal delivery is an option for individuals who have a viral load below 50 copies/mL at 36 weeks' gestation. Historically, it has been routine obstetric practice to avoid obstetric intervention in this cohort (amniotomy, use of fetal scalp electrodes, fetal blood sampling, instrumental delivery). However, recent evidence shows that pregnant women with an undetectable viral load (<50 copies/mL) are not at an increased risk from these interventions. A caesarean delivery is recommended for individuals with a high viral load (>400 copies/mL). Anyone with a very high viral load (>1,000 copies/mL) at the time of delivery should also be given intravenous azidothymidine if they are undergoing a planned caesarean section or present with spontaneous rupture of membranes.

DIAGNOSIS OF HIV IN INFANTS

Maternal antibodies cross the placenta and are detectable in most neonates of HIV-positive mothers. The HIV antibody test can therefore not be used until after 18 months of age. Direct viral amplification by PCR is therefore required for the diagnosis in infants. Confirmation that the infant is uninfected requires at least two negative tests after cessation of post-exposure prophylaxis or breastfeeding.

⌐☞ KEY LEARNING POINTS

- The prevalence of HIV is around 1 per 1,000 pregnancies in the UK; the majority of infected women are born abroad.
- Antiretroviral therapy is recommended in pregnancy and lifelong, and the choice, dosing and timing of therapy should be planned by an HIV physician.
- Treatment with viral suppression therapy can usually reduce the viral load to undetectable (<50 copies/mL).
- Vaginal delivery is recommended (in the absence of other obstetric contraindications) in individuals with an undetectable viral load at or beyond 36 weeks' gestation.
- Planned caesarean section delivery should be offered to women with a high viral load in late pregnancy.
- Infants born to women with HIV should be given antiretroviral therapy.
- Women living with HIV (regardless of viral load at delivery) in high-income countries are recommended to feed their babies with formula milk.
- In resource-poor countries, breastfeeding on fully suppressive maternal antiretroviral therapy is recommended.

HEPATITIS B

INFECTIVE ORGANISM

The hepatitis B virus (HBV) is a DNA virus that is transmitted mainly in blood, but also in other body fluids such as saliva, semen and vaginal fluid. Drug users who share needles are also at high risk. The most common way chronic infection is acquired is from mother-to-child transmission during labour or at birth from ingestion of maternal blood and from breast milk. It is also spread horizontally within families during childhood.

PREVALENCE

Two billion people worldwide are infected with HBV. More than 350 million have chronic (lifelong) infection. Infants who become infected are usually asymptomatic during childhood, but 30–50% develop chronic HBV liver disease, which may progress to cirrhosis and carries a long-term risk of hepatocellular carcinoma.

In the UK, the prevalence of hepatitis B surface antigen (HBsAg) in pregnancy has been found to range from 0.4% to 1%. Higher rates of infection are found in inner city areas or in individuals originating from high prevalence countries in the Far East and sub-Saharan Africa. China has the largest burden of HBV infection, with more than 5% of the pregnant population infected in 2020.

SCREENING

Serological screening for HBV should be performed in pregnancy (UK National Screening Committee recommendation). Infants are at high risk of becoming chronic carriers if their mothers are positive for the hepatitis B e antigen (HBeAg positive) or have a high HBV viral load or high quantitative HBsAg; the risk is markedly reduced if e-antibodies are present. It has been estimated that chronic carriers of HBsAg are 22 times more likely to die from hepatocellular carcinoma or cirrhosis than non-carriers.

MANAGEMENT

Pregnant women who are HBsAg positive should be further assessed by a specialist, alongside detailed serology to ascertain their transmission risk, and should be screened for coinfection with other blood-borne viruses. Ongoing monitoring will also be needed for the long-term consequences of chronic infection, for example hepatocellular carcinoma.

Pregnancy in individuals with the highest risk of vertical transmission, such as those with a high viral DNA load, may be offered antiviral therapy (such as tenofovir disoproxil). Caesarean section is not recommended solely to avoid vertical transmission of hepatitis B. However, use of fetal scalp electrodes and fetal blood sampling in labour should be avoided where possible. After birth for infants at high risk of transmission, passive immunization with hepatitis B Ig is advised. This provides immediate protection against any virus transmitted to the baby from contact with blood during delivery, and should be given immediately after delivery. All infants born to HBsAg-positive mothers should be given HBV vaccination as soon after birth as possible and further doses should be given during the first year of life. This provides protection for 95% of infants.

HEPATITIS C

INFECTIVE ORGANISM

The hepatitis C virus (HCV) is an RNA virus. Acquisition of the virus occurs predominantly through infected blood products and injection of drugs. It can also occur with tattooing and body piercing. Vertical transmission can occur due to contact with infected maternal blood around the time of delivery, and the risk is higher in those coinfected with HIV. Sexual transmission is extremely rare.

PREVALENCE

In the UK, the overall antenatal prevalence has been estimated to be around 1%, with regional variation. The risk of vertical transmission is estimated to lie between 3% and 5%, and it is estimated that 70 births each year are infected with HCV as a result of vertical transmission in the UK, the risk of which increases with increasing maternal viral load.

SCREENING

Current recommendations vary between countries about whether pregnant women should be offered routine screening for HCV or if it should be offered only to those with risk factors such as individuals known to be injecting drug users. In the UK, universal screening is not currently offered. The rationale for this is a lack of evidence-based effective interventions for the treatment of HCV during pregnancy, and a lack of evidence about which interventions reduce vertical transmission of HCV. Other countries offer screening so that pregnant women can be made aware of their status, can receive counselling and risk stratification, and can consider treatment before a future pregnancy.

CLINICAL FEATURES

HCV is a major public health concern due to its long-term consequences for health. It is one of the major causes of liver cirrhosis, hepatocellular carcinoma and liver failure. Following initial infection, only 20% of individuals will have hepatic symptoms, 80% being asymptomatic. The majority of pregnant women with hepatitis C will not have reached the phase of having the chronic disease and may well be unaware that they are infected.

MANAGEMENT

Testing for HCV in the UK involves detection of anti-HCV antibodies in serum with subsequent confirmatory testing by PCR for the virus, if a positive result is obtained. Upon confirmation of a positive test, post-test counselling and referral to a hepatologist for management should be offered.

Antiviral curative treatment for hepatitis C is now readily available, but the existing treatment regimens are not recommended for use in pregnancy. Ribavirin is teratogenic, so pregnant women and their partners receiving ribavirin are recommended to avoid pregnancy during treatment and for 6 months after the completion of treatment.

There is no strong evidence regarding the impact of the mode of delivery on hepatitis C transmission. Therefore, elective caesarean section is not recommended for all women with hepatitis C, although it is recommended if the individual is also HIV

> **KEY LEARNING POINTS**
>
> - Screening for infections in pregnancy is associated with a reduction in the burden of some long-term viral conditions, particularly HIV and hepatitis B.
> - Active management of HIV infection in pregnancy dramatically reduces the risk of vertical transmission.
> - Most treatments for infections are suitable for use in pregnancy (with a small number of exceptions) and treatment should not be withheld because of the pregnancy.
> - A small number of infections can cause congenital anomalies in the fetus that can be identified on antenatal ultrasound.

positive. Breastfeeding is also not contraindicated in women with HCV infection, except if the mother has cracked or bleeding nipples or in the context of HIV coinfection.

FURTHER READING

British HIV Association guidelines for the management of HIV infection. https://www.bhiva.org/pregnancy-guidelines.

Public Health England (2013). *Fetal Anomaly Screening Programme.* Last updated: 27 July 2021. https://www.gov.uk/guidance/fetal-anomaly-screening-programme-overview.

NICE (2021). *Antenatal Care.* NICE guideline [NG201]. https://www.nice.org.uk/guidance/ng201

RCOG Clinical Guidelines. https://www.rcog.org.uk/guidelines.

SELF-ASSESSMENT

For interactive SBAs and EMQs relating to this chapter, visit www.routledge.com/cw/mccarthy.

CASE HISTORY 1

A 26-year-old teacher attends the antenatal clinic complaining of reduced fetal movements at 28 weeks' gestation having been in contact with slapped cheek syndrome 6 weeks previously. She has an ultrasound scan performed that shows fetal ascites.

A What is the likely diagnosis and how might this be confirmed?

B What assessment using Doppler ultrasound should be performed on the baby?

C What therapy could be considered for the fetus that may improve the outcome?

ANSWERS

A The diagnosis is likely to be acute parvovirus B19 infection. This can be confirmed with a maternal blood test confirming IgM and/or new IgG antibodies. In addition, amniotic fluid can be tested for parvovirus by PCR.

B A middle cerebral artery Doppler velocity can be performed, which may be consistent with fetal anaemia caused by aplastic anaemia.

C If the fetus is confirmed to be anaemic, intrauterine blood transfusion can be considered. This can potentially prolong the pregnancy until the fetus has recovered or has reached a gestation at which it is safe to consider delivery. Normally, only one transfusion is required, as the fetus can recover from the infection and haematopoiesis will restart.

CASE HISTORY 2

Mrs L, a 36-year-old woman, presents to labour ward. She is 36 weeks' pregnant and gives a history consistent with premature prelabour rupture of membranes for 28 hours. She labours spontaneously after developing a temperature of 38.2°C and delivers a 2.5-kg baby boy. Shortly after delivery, the baby has several 'dusky' episodes. Ten minutes later, the mother rings the alarm bell as her baby has become unresponsive and requires resuscitation.

A What is the likely diagnosis?

B What risk factors does Mrs L have for this complication? What are the other risk factors for this complication?

C What is the treatment?

ANSWERS

A The likely diagnosis is sepsis secondary to GBS. This will be confirmed by neonatal septic screening, which will show GBS in the blood with or without cerebrospinal fluid. The acute deterioration of the baby is consistent with the aggressive nature of GBS infection.

B Mrs L had prolonged rupture of membranes and was preterm. She also developed a pyrexia intrapartum. Other risk factors include a previous infant with GBS, incidental detection of GBS in current pregnancy and GBS bacteriuria.

C Neonatal management following resuscitation is focused mainly around the supportive treatment and administration of intravenous antibiotics.

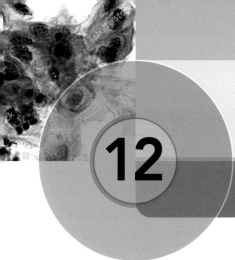

Labour: Normal and abnormal

12

DEIRDRE J MURPHY

> **Learning Objectives**
> - Understand the maternal and fetal anatomy relevant to labour and birth.
> - Understand the physiological principles of labour and birth.
> - Understand the contributors to normal labour and its management.
> - Understand the contributors to abnormal labour and its management.
> - Introduce the social, psychological and governance elements of labour and birth.

INTRODUCTION

Labour or human parturition is the physiological process that results in the birth of a baby, the delivery of the placenta and the signal for lactation to begin. At a human level, it is a major life event for the pregnant woman and her partner that heralds the start of parenting. In terms of providing care to a woman in labour, attention must be paid to safety and clinical outcomes, but also to the patient's emotional wellbeing and desire for a fulfilling birth experience. Normal labour requires observation, monitoring and support, and falls within the scope of midwifery care. Abnormal labour must be recognized and acted upon, and requires a multidisciplinary approach including midwifery, obstetrics, anaesthetics and neonatology. While most labours result in a positive outcome, some labours result in tragedy, and each healthcare team needs to have the skillset to care for women and their families through all types of events.

Health professionals who manage labour must understand the anatomy and physiology of the pregnant woman and fetus, what distinguishes normal from abnormal labour, when it is appropriate to intervene, how to intervene safely and how to support the woman and her partner through unexpected labour events. The first important step is to make an accurate diagnosis of labour. Labour is then divided into three stages:

1. The first stage begins when labour is diagnosed and ends when full cervical dilatation is reached.

10.1201/9781003196112-12

2. The second stage begins with full cervical dilatation and ends with the birth of the baby.

3. The third stage begins with the birth of the baby and ends with complete delivery of the placenta and membranes.

Complications can occur during any of the three stages and can be divided into maternal and perinatal (fetal-neonatal) complications.

An understanding of the physiological and anatomical principles involved in normal and abnormal labour is best summarized using the '3 Ps', which are the powers, the passages and the passenger. The 'powers' refers to forces: firstly, the contractions of the uterine muscle that result in the passage of the fetus through the birth canal and, secondly, the maternal effort of pushing in the second stage of labour. The 'passages' refers to the birth canal itself, which is made up of the bony pelvis and ligaments, the muscles of the pelvic floor and the soft tissues of the perineum. The 'passenger' refers to the fetus in terms of its size (small, average or large), presentation (the part of the fetus entering the pelvis first; e.g. vertex of head, face, brow or breech) and position (the orientation of the presenting part in relation to the maternal pubic symphysis; e.g. occipito-anterior (OA) or occipito-posterior [OP]). When the 3Ps are favourable (average size baby, vertex presentation and OA position), normal labour is likely to ensue, resulting in a spontaneous vaginal birth. When any of the 3Ps are unfavourable, labour is likely to be abnormal and require intervention, which can result in morbidity or mortality.

It is important that labour and birth outcomes are audited locally, nationally and internationally to ensure that optimal outcomes are achieved and that lessons are learned when adverse events occur. Priorities, choice and outcomes differ greatly depending on whether a birth occurs in a high-income or low-income setting. Even within settings, there can be marked differences in the perspectives of pregnant women and their care providers, reflected in the planned place of birth, choice of care provider, analgesia use, mode of delivery and outcomes for women and their babies. Childbirth has physical, psychological, social, cultural and political dimensions, which makes it a very interesting area to work in.

MATERNAL AND FETAL ANATOMY

BONY PELVIS

PELVIC INLET

The pelvic inlet or brim is bounded anteriorly by the upper border of the symphysis pubis (the joint separating the two pubic bones); laterally by the upper margin of the pubic bone, the iliopectineal line and the ala of the sacrum; and posteriorly by the promontory of the sacrum (**Figure 12.1**). The normal transverse diameter in this plane is 13.5 cm and is wider than the anterior–posterior (AP) diameter, which is normally 11.0 cm (**Figure 12.2**). For this reason, the fetal head typically enters the pelvis orientated in a transverse position in keeping with the wider transverse diameter. The angle of the inlet is normally 60° to the horizontal in the erect position, but in Afro-Caribbean women this angle may be as much as 90°. This increased angle may delay the head entering and descending through the pelvis compared with labour in Caucasian women.

MID-PELVIS

The mid-pelvis, also known as the mid-cavity, can be described as an area bounded anteriorly by the middle of the symphysis pubis; laterally by the pubic bones, the obturator fascia and the inner aspect of the ischial

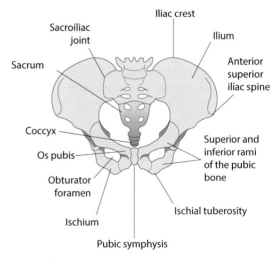

Figure 12.1 The bony pelvis.

Sacroiliac joint

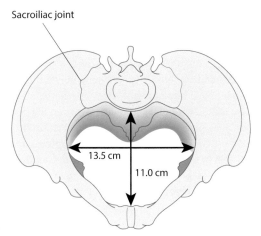

Figure 12.2 The pelvic brim.

bone and spines; and posteriorly by the junction of the second and third sections of the sacrum. The mid-pelvis is almost round, as the transverse and anterior diameters are similar at 12 cm. The ischial spines are palpable vaginally and are used as important land-marks for two purposes: (1) to assess the descent of the presenting part on vaginal examination (e.g. sta-tion zero is at the level of the ischial spines, –1 is 1 cm above the spines and +1 is 1 cm below the spines) and (2) when administering a local anaesthetic pudendal nerve block. The pudendal nerve passes behind and below the ischial spine on each side. A pudendal nerve block may be used for a vacuum or forceps-assisted birth. Station zero is an important landmark clini-cally because assisted vaginal birth can be performed only if the fetal head has descended to the level of the ischial spines or below.

PELVIC OUTLET

The pelvic outlet is bounded anteriorly by the lower margin of the symphysis pubis; laterally by the descending ramus of the pubic bone, the ischial tuber-osity and the sacrotuberous ligament; and posteriorly by the last piece of the sacrum. The AP diameter of the pelvic outlet is 13.5 cm and the transverse diam-eter is 11 cm (**Figures 12.3** and **12.4**). Therefore, the transverse is the widest diameter at the inlet, but at the outlet it is the AP diameter, and the fetal head must rotate from a transverse to an AP position as it passes through the pelvis. Typically, this happens in the

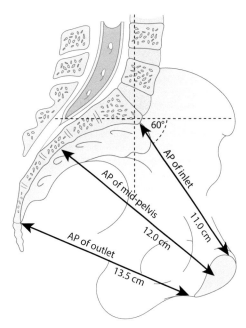

Figure 12.3 Sagittal section of the pelvis demonstrating the anterior–posterior (AP) diameters of the inlet and outlet.

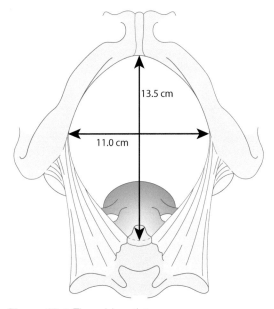

Figure 12.4 The pelvic outlet.

mid-pelvis where the transverse and AP diameters are similar. In addition, the pelvic axis describes an imagi-nary J-shaped curved line, a path that the centre of the fetal head must take during its passage through the

195

pelvis, from entry at the inlet and descent and rotation in the mid-pelvis to exit at the outlet. Recognizing the important features of the maternal pelvis is central to understanding the mechanism of labour.

PELVIC SIZE AND SHAPE

The pelvic measurements described previously are average values and relate to bony points. The pelvic ligaments at the pubic ramus and the sacroiliac joints loosen towards the end of the third trimester and these diameters may increase as the pelvis becomes more flexible. It is also possible to enhance the pelvic dimensions with more favourable positions for the woman in labour (e.g. squatting or kneeling).

A variety of pelvic shapes are described, and these may contribute to difficulties encountered in labour. The gynaecoid pelvis is the most favourable and the most common (**Figure 12.5**). Other pelvic shapes are shown in **Figures 12.6** to **12.8**. An android-type pelvis is said to predispose to failure of rotation and deep transverse arrest, and

the anthropoid shape encourages an OP position. A platypelloid pelvis is also associated with an increased risk of obstructed labour due to failure of the head to engage, rotate or descend.

Short stature, ethnicity, previous pelvic fractures and metabolic bone disease, such as rickets, may all be associated with measurements less than the population average. It is now uncommon to perform X-rays or computed tomography/magnetic resonance imaging scans of the pelvis to measure the pelvic dimensions because pelvic imaging has proven to be of little clinical use in predicting the outcome of labour.

PELVIC FLOOR

This is formed by the two levator ani muscles, which, with their fascia, form a musculofascial gutter during the second stage of labour (**Figure 12.9**). The configuration of the bony pelvis together with the gutter-shaped pelvic floor muscles encourage the fetal head to flex and rotate as it descends through the mid-pelvis towards the pelvic outlet.

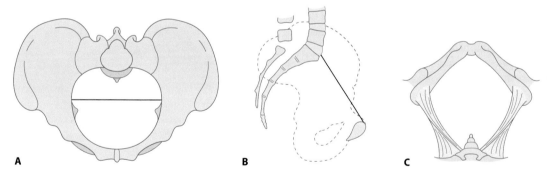

A   B   C

Figure 12.5 The gynaecoid pelvis: (**A**) brim, (**B**) lateral view and (**C**) outlet.

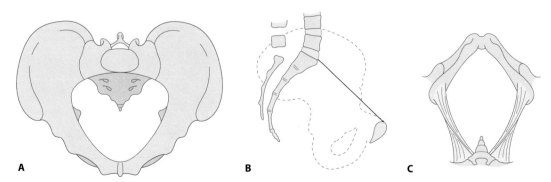

A   B   C

Figure 12.6 The android pelvis: (**A**) brim, (**B**) lateral view and (**C**) outlet.

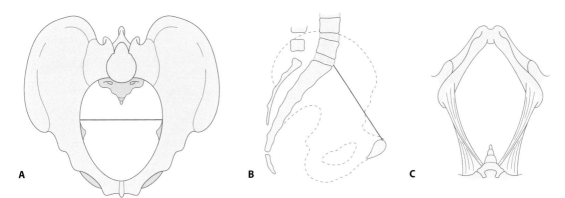

Figure 12.7 The anthropoid pelvis: (**A**) brim, (**B**) lateral view and (**C**) outlet.

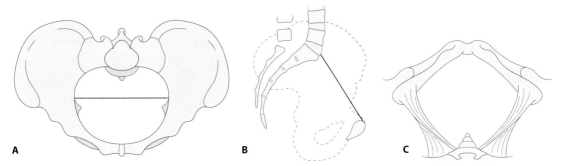

Figure 12.8 The platypelloid pelvis: (**A**) brim, (**B**) lateral view and (**C**) outlet.

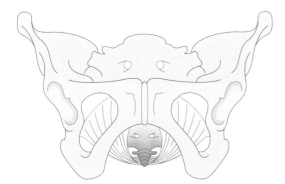

Figure 12.9 The musculofascial gutter of the levator sling.

PERINEUM

The final obstacle to be overcome by the fetus during labour is the perineum. The perineal body is a condensation of fibrous and muscular tissue lying between the vagina and the anus (**Figure 12.10**). It receives attachments of the posterior ends of the bulbo-cavernous muscles, the medial ends of the superficial and deep transverse perineal muscles and the anterior fibres of the external anal sphincter. The perineum is taut and relatively resistant in the nulliparous individual and pushing can be prolonged. Vaginal birth may result in tearing of the perineum and pelvic floor muscles, or an episiotomy (surgical cut) may be required. The perineum is stretchy and less resistant in multiparous individuals, resulting in faster labour and a higher probability of delivering with an intact perineum.

FETAL SKULL

SKULL BONES, SUTURES AND FONTANELLES

The fetal skull is made up of the vault, the face and the base. The sutures are the lines formed where the individual bony plates of the skull meet one another. At term, the sutures joining the bones of the vault

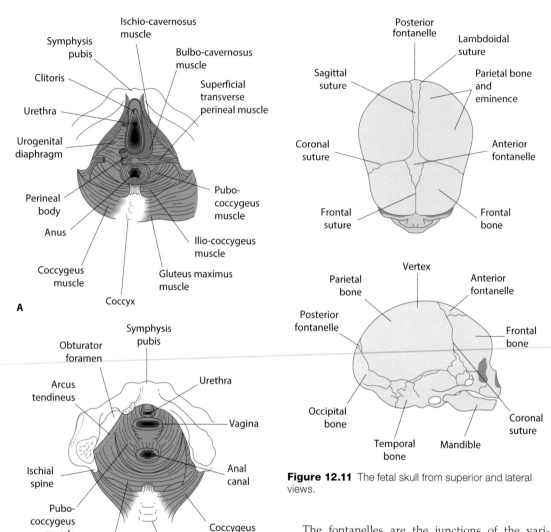

Figure 12.10 The perineum, perineal body and pelvic floor from below, showing superficial (**A**) and deeper (**B**) views. The pelvic floor muscles are made up of the levator ani (pubo-coccygeus and ilio-coccygeus).

Figure 12.11 The fetal skull from superior and lateral views.

are soft, unossified membranes, whereas the sutures of the fetal face and the skull base are firmly united (**Figure 12.11**). The vault of the skull is composed of the parietal bones and parts of the occipital, frontal and temporal bones. Between these bones there are four membranous sutures: the sagittal, frontal, coronal and lambdoidal sutures.

The fontanelles are the junctions of the various sutures. The anterior fontanelle, also known as bregma, is at the junction of the sagittal, frontal and coronal sutures and is diamond shaped. On vaginal examination, four suture lines can be felt. The posterior fontanelle lies at the junction of the sagittal suture and the lambdoidal sutures between the two parietal bones and the occipital bone and is smaller and triangular shaped. On vaginal examination, three suture lines can be felt. The fact that the sutures are not fixed is important for labour. It allows the bones to move together and even to overlap. The parietal bones usually slide over the frontal and occipital bones. Furthermore, the bones themselves are compressible. Together, these characteristics of the fetal skull allow a process called 'moulding' to occur, which reduces

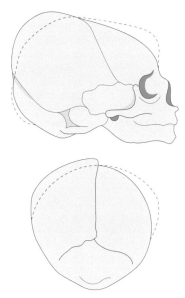

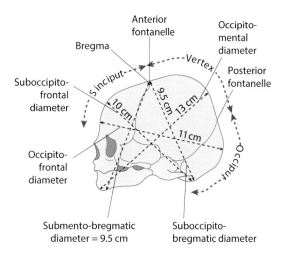

Figure 12.13 The diameters of the fetal skull.

Figure 12.12 A schematic representation of moulding of the fetal skull.

the diameters of the fetal head and encourages progress through the bony pelvis, while still protecting the underlying brain (**Figure 12.12**). However, severe moulding or moulding early in labour can be a sign of obstructed labour due to a fetal malposition (failure of the head to rotate to OA) or cephalopelvic disproportion (CPD), namely a fetal head that is disproportionately large compared with the maternal pelvis.

The area of the fetal skull bounded by the two parietal eminences and the anterior and posterior fontanelles is termed the 'vertex'. In normal labour, the vertex of the fetal head is the presenting part and the posterior fontanelle (indicating the occiput) is used to define the position of the fetal head in relation to the pubic symphysis. The anatomical differences between the anterior and posterior fontanelles on vaginal examination facilitate correct diagnosis of the fetal head position in labour. The OA position is the most favourable for a spontaneous vaginal birth. An occipito-transverse (OT) or OP position is considered a malposition and may result in prolonged labour, assisted vaginal birth or caesarean section.

DIAMETERS OF THE SKULL

The fetal head is ovoid in shape. The attitude of the fetal head refers to the degree of flexion and

extension at the upper cervical spine. Different longitudinal diameters are presented to the pelvis in labour depending on the attitude of the fetal head (**Figures 12.13** and **12.14**).

The longitudinal diameter that presents with a flexed attitude of the fetal head (chin on the chest) is the suboccipito-bregmatic diameter. This is usually 9.5 cm and is measured from beneath the occiput (suboccipital) to the centre of the anterior fontanelle (bregma). The longitudinal diameter that presents in a less well-flexed head, such as is found in an OP position, is the suboccipito-frontal diameter. It is measured from the suboccipital region to the prominence of the forehead and measures 10 cm.

With further extension of the head, the occipito-frontal diameter presents (deflexed OP). This is measured from the root of the nose to the posterior fontanelle and is 11.5 cm. The greatest longitudinal diameter that may present is the mento-vertical, which is taken from the chin to the furthest point of the vertex and measures 13 cm. This is known as a brow presentation that is usually too large to pass through the normal pelvis. Extension of the fetal head beyond this point results in a smaller diameter. The submento-bregmatic diameter is measured from below the chin to the anterior fontanelle and is 9.5 cm. This is termed a face presentation. A face presentation can deliver vaginally when the chin is anterior (mento-anterior position).

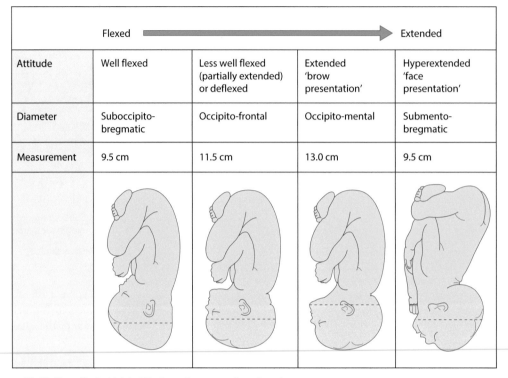

	Flexed			Extended
Attitude	Well flexed	Less well flexed (partially extended) or deflexed	Extended 'brow presentation'	Hyperextended 'face presentation'
Diameter	Suboccipito-bregmatic	Occipito-frontal	Occipito-mental	Submento-bregmatic
Measurement	9.5 cm	11.5 cm	13.0 cm	9.5 cm

Figure 12.14 The effect of fetal attitude on the presenting diameter.

KEY LEARNING POINTS

Maternal and fetal anatomy
- The pelvic inlet is wider in the transverse than in the AP diameter.
- The pelvic outlet is wider in the AP than in the transverse diameter.
- The ischial spines are in the mid-pelvis and denote station zero.
- The fetal head enters the pelvis in a transverse position, rotates in the mid-pelvis and delivers in an AP position.
- Pelvic dimensions may increase during labour due to pelvic ligament laxity.
- The shape of the pelvis and pelvic floor muscles aid flexion and rotation of the fetal head.
- The sutures and fontanelles are used to assess the position and attitude of the fetal head.
- Moulding of the skull bones during labour reduces the dimensions of the fetal head.
- A fetus in a flexed OA position with a gynaecoid pelvis is most favourable for vaginal birth.
- Perineal tissues present resistance to delivery especially in the nulliparous population.

PHYSIOLOGY OF LABOUR

The mechanisms underlying human labour are not fully understood and differ from other animal models that have been studied. In particular, the process that initiates labour is poorly understood. The cervix, which is initially long, firm and closed with a protective mucus plug, must soften, shorten, thin out (efface) and dilate for labour to progress. Passage of the mucus plug reflects this process and is termed a 'show'. The uterus must change from a state of relaxation to an active state of regular, strong, frequent contractions to facilitate transit of the fetus through the birth canal. Each contraction must be followed by a resting phase in order to maintain placental blood flow and adequate perfusion of the fetus. The pressure of the presenting part on the pelvic floor muscles as the fetus descends from the mid-pelvis to the pelvic outlet produces a maternal urge to push enhanced further by stretching of the perineum. The onset of labour occurs when the factors that inhibit contractions and maintain a closed cervix diminish and are overtaken by factors that do the opposite. Both the pregnant woman and the fetus appear to contribute to this process.

UTERUS

Myometrial cells of the uterus contain filaments of actin and myosin that bring about contractions in response to an increase in intracellular calcium. Prostaglandins and oxytocin increase intracellular free calcium ions, whereas beta-adrenergic compounds and calcium-channel blockers do the opposite. Separation of the actin and myosin filaments brings about relaxation of the myocyte; however, unlike any other muscle cell of the body, this actin–myosin interaction occurs along the full length of the filaments so that a degree of shortening occurs with each successive interaction. This progressive shortening of the uterine smooth muscle cells is called retraction and occurs in the cells of the upper part of the uterus. The result of this retraction process is the development of the thicker, actively contracting 'upper segment'. At the same time, the lower segment of the uterus becomes thinner and more stretched. Eventually, this results in the cervix being 'taken up' (effacement) into the lower segment of the uterus, thus forming a continuum with the lower uterine segment (**Figure 12.15**). The cervix then dilates and the fetus descends in response to this directional force.

It is essential that the myocytes of the uterus contract in a coordinated way. Individual myocytes are laid down in a mesh of collagen. There is cell-to-cell communication by means of gap junctions, which facilitate the passage of various products of metabolism and electrical current between cells. These gap junctions are absent for most of the pregnancy but appear in significant numbers at term. Gap junctions increase in size and number with the progress of labour and allow greater coordination of myocyte activity. Prostaglandins stimulate their formation, while beta-adrenergic compounds are thought to do the opposite. A uterine pacemaker from which contractions originate probably exists but has not been demonstrated histologically.

Uterine contractions are involuntary in nature and there is relatively little extrauterine neuronal control. The frequency of contractions may vary

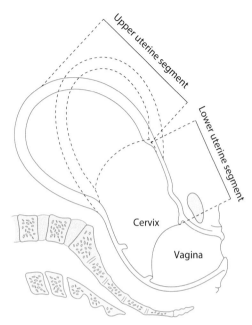

Figure 12.15 The thick upper segment and the thin lower segment of the uterus at the end of the first stage of labour. The dotted lines indicate the position assumed by the uterus during contraction.

during labour and with parity. Throughout the majority of labour, they occur at intervals of 2–4 minutes and are described in terms of the frequency within a 10-minute period (2 in 10 increasing to 4–5 in 10 in advanced labour). Their duration also varies during labour, from 30 to 60 seconds or occasionally longer.

CERVIX

The cervix contains myocytes and fibroblasts separated by a 'ground substance' made up of extracellular matrix molecules. Interactions between collagen, fibronectin and dermatan sulphate (a proteoglycan) during the earlier stages of pregnancy keep the cervix firm and closed. Contractions at this point do not bring about effacement or dilatation. Under the influence of prostaglandins and other humoral mediators, there is an increase in proteolytic activity and a reduction in collagen and elastin. Interleukins bring about a pro-inflammatory change with a significant invasion by neutrophils. Dermatan sulphate is replaced by the more hydrophilic hyaluronic acid, which results in an increase in water content of the cervix. This causes cervical softening or 'ripening', so that contractions, when they begin, can bring about the processes of effacement and dilatation.

HORMONAL FACTORS

Progesterone maintains uterine relaxation by suppressing prostaglandin production, inhibiting communication between myometrial cells and preventing oxytocin release. Oestrogen opposes the action of progesterone. Prior to labour, there is a reduction in progesterone receptors and an increase in the concentration of oestrogen relative to progesterone. Prostaglandin synthesis by the chorion and the decidua is enhanced, leading to an increase in calcium influx into the myometrial cells. This change in the hormonal milieu also increases gap junction formation between individual myometrial cells, creating a functional syncytium, which is necessary for coordinated uterine activity. The production of corticotrophin-releasing hormone by the placenta increases towards term and potentiates the action of prostaglandins and oxytocin on myometrial contractility. The fetal pituitary secretes oxytocin and the fetal adrenal gland produces cortisol, which stimulates the conversion of progesterone to oestrogen. As labour becomes established, the output of oxytocin increases through the Ferguson reflex. Pressure from the fetal presenting part against the cervix is relayed via a reflex arc involving the spinal cord and results in increased oxytocin release from the maternal posterior pituitary.

NORMAL LABOUR

DIAGNOSIS OF LABOUR

The onset of labour can be defined as the presence of strong, regular, painful contractions resulting in progressive cervical change. In practice, the diagnosis is suspected when a pregnant woman presents with contraction-like pains and is confirmed when the midwife performs a vaginal examination that reveals effacement and dilatation of the cervix. Loss of the 'show' (blood-stained plug of mucus passed from the cervix) or spontaneous rupture of the membranes (SROM) does not define the onset of labour, although these events may occur around the same time. Labour can be well established before either of these events occurs, and both may precede labour by many days.

STAGES OF LABOUR

Labour can be divided into three stages. The definitions of these stages rely predominantly on anatomical criteria and, in real terms, the exact time of transition from first to second stage may not be apparent. The important events in normal labour are the diagnosis of labour and the maternal urge to push, which usually corresponds with full dilatation of the cervix and the baby's head distending the pelvic floor. Defining the three stages of labour becomes more relevant if labour is not progressing normally. The average duration of first labours is 8–12 hours and that of subsequent labours is 4–6 hours. First labours rarely last more than 18 hours and second and subsequent labours do not usually last more than 12 hours.

FIRST STAGE

This describes the time from the diagnosis of labour to full dilatation of the cervix (10 cm). The first stage of labour can be divided into two phases. The 'latent phase' is the time between the onset of regular painful contractions and 3–4 cm cervical dilatation. During this time, the cervix becomes 'fully effaced'. Effacement is a process by which the cervix shortens in length as it becomes incorporated into the lower segment of the uterus. The process of effacement may begin during the weeks preceding the onset of labour but will be complete by the end of the latent phase. Effacement and dilatation should be thought of as consecutive events in the nulliparous population but may occur simultaneously in the multiparous. Dilatation is expressed in centimetres from 0 to 10 cm. The duration of the latent phase is variable and time limits are arbitrary. However, it usually lasts between 3 and 8 hours, being shorter in multiparous women.

The second phase of the first stage of labour is called the 'active phase' and describes the time between the end of the latent phase (3–4 cm dilatation) and full cervical dilatation (10 cm). It is also variable in length, usually lasting between 2 and 6 hours, and is shorter in multiparous women. Cervical dilatation during the active phase occurs typically at 1 cm/hour or more in a normal labour and is considered abnormal only if it occurs at less than 1 cm in 2 hours.

SECOND STAGE

This describes the time from full dilatation of the cervix to delivery of the fetus or fetuses. The second stage of labour may also be subdivided into two phases. The 'passive phase' describes the time between full dilatation and the onset of involuntary expulsive contractions. There is no maternal urge to push and the fetal head is still relatively high in the pelvis. The second phase is called the 'active second stage'. There is a maternal urge to push because the fetal head is low (often visible), causing a reflex need to 'bear down'. In normal labour, the second stage is often diagnosed at this late point because the maternal urge to push prompts the midwife to perform a vaginal examination. If a pregnant woman never reaches a point of involuntary pushing, the active second stage is said to begin when she starts making voluntary pushing efforts directed by the midwife. Conventionally, a normal active second stage should last no longer than 2 hours in a nulliparous woman and 1 hour in a parous individual. Although these definitions are arbitrary, there is evidence that a second stage of labour lasting more than 3 hours is associated with increased maternal and fetal morbidity. Use of epidural anaesthesia will influence the length and management of the second stage of labour. A passive second stage of 1 or 2 hours is usually recommended to allow the head to rotate and descend prior to active pushing.

THIRD STAGE

This is the time from birth of the fetus or fetuses until complete delivery of the placenta(e) and membranes. The placenta is typically delivered within a few minutes of the birth of the baby. A third stage lasting more than 30 minutes is defined as abnormal, unless the woman has opted for 'physiological management' (see the section 'Management of third stage' later in this chapter), in which case it is reasonable to extend this definition to 60 minutes.

DURATION OF LABOUR

There is no ideal length of labour, but morbidity increases when labour is too fast (precipitous) or too slow (prolonged). Precipitous labour is defined as birth of the fetus within less than 3 hours of the onset of regular contractions. From a psychological perspective, the morale of most pregnant women starts to deteriorate after 6 hours in active labour and, after 12 hours, the rate of deterioration accelerates. There is a greater incidence of fetal hypoxia and need for operative delivery associated with long labours. It is difficult to define prolonged labour, but it would be reasonable to suggest that labour lasting longer than 12 hours in the nulliparous population and 8 hours in the multiparous population should be regarded as prolonged.

MECHANISMS OF LABOUR

This refers to the series of changes in position and attitude that the fetus undergoes during its passage through the birth canal. It is described here for the vertex presentation and the gynaecoid pelvis. The relation of the fetal head and body to the maternal pelvis changes as the fetus descends through the pelvis. This is essential so that the smallest diameters of the fetal skull are present at each stage of the descent.

Engagement

The fetal head normally enters the pelvis in the transverse position or some minor variant of this, taking advantage of the widest pelvic diameter. Engagement is said to have occurred when the widest part of the presenting part has passed successfully through the inlet. The number of fifths of the fetal head palpable abdominally is used to describe whether engagement has taken place. If more than two-fifths of the fetal head is palpable abdominally, the head is not yet engaged. Engagement occurs in the majority of nulliparous women prior to labour, usually by 37 weeks' gestation, but it occurs in labour for the majority of multiparous women.

Descent

Descent of the fetal head is needed before flexion, internal rotation and extension can occur (**Figure 12.16**). During the first stage and passive phase of the second stage of labour, descent of the fetus occurs with

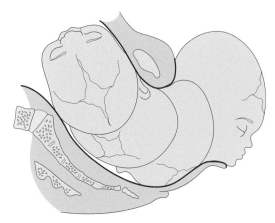

Figure 12.16 Descent and flexion of the head followed by internal rotation and ending in birth of the head by extension.

uterine contractions. In the active phase of the second stage of labour, descent of the fetus is assisted by voluntary efforts of the woman using her abdominal muscles and the Valsalva manoeuvre ('pushing').

Flexion

The fetal head is not always completely flexed when it enters the pelvis. As the head descends into the narrower mid-pelvis, flexion occurs (chin onto chest). This passive movement occurs due, in part, to the surrounding structures and is important in reducing the presenting diameter of the fetal head.

Internal rotation

If the head is well flexed, the occiput will be the leading point and, on reaching the sloping gutter of the levator ani muscles, it will be encouraged to rotate anteriorly so that the sagittal suture now lies in the AP diameter of the pelvic outlet (the widest diameter). If the fetus has engaged in the OP position, internal rotation can occur from an OP position to an OA position. This long internal rotation may explain the increased duration of labour associated with OP position. Alternatively, an OP position may persist, resulting in a 'face to pubes' delivery. Furthermore, the persistent OP position may be associated with extension of the fetal head and a resulting increase in the diameter presented to the pelvic outlet. This may lead to obstructed labour and the need for assisted vaginal birth by vacuum or forceps or caesarean section.

Extension

Following completion of internal rotation, the occiput is beneath the symphysis pubis and the bregma is near the lower border of the sacrum. The well-flexed head now extends and the occiput escapes from underneath the symphysis pubis and distends the vulva. This is known as 'crowning' of the head. The head extends further and the occiput underneath the symphysis pubis acts as a fulcrum point as the bregma, face and chin appear in succession over the posterior vaginal opening and perineal body. This extension process if controlled reduces the risk of perineal trauma. However, the soft tissues of the perineum offer resistance and some degree of tearing occurs in the majority of first births.

Restitution

When the head is delivering, the occiput is directly anterior. As soon as it crosses the perineum, the head aligns itself with the shoulders, which have entered the pelvis in the oblique position. This slight rotation of the occiput through one-eighth of the circle is partial restitution.

In order to be delivered, the shoulders have to rotate into the direct AP plane (the widest diameter at the outlet). When this occurs, the occiput rotates through a further one-eighth of a circle to the transverse position. This completes restitution (**Figure 12.17**).

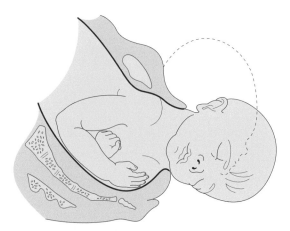

Figure 12.17 Restitution of the head after delivery as the anterior shoulder rotates forwards to pass under the subpubic arch.

Delivery of the shoulders and fetal body

When restitution has occurred, the shoulders will be in the AP position. The anterior shoulder is under the symphysis pubis and delivers first, and the posterior shoulder delivers subsequently.

Normally, the rest of the fetal body is delivered easily, with the posterior shoulder guided over the perineum by gentle upwards traction in the opposite direction, so delivering the baby on to the maternal abdomen.

MANAGEMENT OF NORMAL LABOUR

Women are advised to contact their local labour suite or their community midwife if they think their waters may have broken (SROM) or when their contractions are occurring every 5 minutes or more. It is important to recognize that women have very different thresholds for seeking advice and reassurance. The need for pain relief may result in admission to hospital before either of these two criteria is reached. Whether at home or in hospital, the attending midwife will then make an assessment based on the history and clinical examination, as well as the preferences of the woman.

HISTORY

A detailed history should be taken, including past obstetric history, history of the current pregnancy, relevant medical history and events leading up to hospital attendance. The admission history and examination provide an initial screen for labour and potential maternal and/or fetal risk. If all features are normal and reassuring, the woman will remain under midwifery care. If there are risk factors identified, medical involvement in the form of the on-call obstetric team may be appropriate.

ADMISSION EXAMINATION

It is important to identify women who have a raised body mass index, as this may complicate the management of labour. The temperature, pulse and blood pressure must be recorded on admission and a sample of urine tested for protein, blood, ketones, glucose and nitrates.

BOX 12.1: Admission history

- Previous births and size of previous babies
- Previous caesarean section(s)
- Onset, frequency, duration and perception of strength of the contractions
- Whether membranes have ruptured and, if so, colour and amount of amniotic fluid seen
- Presence of abnormal vaginal discharge or bleeding
- Recent activity of the fetus (fetal movement)
- Medical or obstetric issues of note (e.g. diabetes, hypertension, fetal growth restriction)
- Any special requirements (e.g. an interpreter or particular emotional/psychological needs)
- Maternal expectations of labour and birth/birth preferences or a birth plan

---

ABDOMINAL EXAMINATION

After the initial inspection for scars indicating previous surgery, it is important to determine the lie of the fetus (longitudinal, transverse or oblique) and the nature of the presenting part (cephalic or breech). If it is a cephalic presentation, the degree of engagement must be determined in terms of fifths palpable abdominally. A head that remains high (four- to five-fifths palpable) is a poor prognostic sign for successful vaginal birth. If there is any doubt as to the presentation or if the head is high, an ultrasound scan should be performed to confirm the presenting part or the reason for the high head (e.g. OP position, deflexed head, placenta praevia, fibroid, etc.).

Abdominal examination also includes an assessment of the contractions; this takes time (at least 10 minutes) and is done by palpating the uterus directly. The tocograph provides reliable information on the frequency, regularity and duration of contractions, but not the strength.

VAGINAL EXAMINATION

The purpose and technique of vaginal examination is explained to the woman and her consent must be obtained. The examination should be conducted in a manner that maintains the woman's dignity and privacy. The index and middle fingers are passed to the top of the vagina and the cervix. The cervix is examined for position, length and effacement, consistency, dilatation and application to the presenting part. The length of the cervix at 36 weeks is about 3 cm. It gradually shortens by the process of effacement and may still be uneffaced in early labour. The dilatation is estimated digitally in centimetres. At about 4 cm of dilatation, the cervix should be fully effaced. Providing the cervix is at least 4 cm dilated, it should be possible to determine both the position and the station of the presenting part. When no cervix can be felt, this means the cervix is fully dilated (10 cm).

A vaginal examination also allows assessment of the fetal head position, station and attitude and the presence of caput or moulding. In normal labour, the vertex will be presenting and the position can be determined by locating the occiput. The occiput is identified by feeling for the triangular posterior fontanelle and the three suture lines. Normally, the occiput will be transverse (OT) or anterior (OA). Failure to feel the posterior fontanelle may be because the head is deflexed (abnormal attitude), the occiput is posterior (malposition) or there is so much caput and moulding that the sutures cannot be felt. All of these indicate the possibility of a prolonged labour or a degree of mechanical obstruction. Relating the leading part of the head to the ischial spines will give an estimation of the station. This vaginal assessment of station should always be taken together with assessment of the degree of engagement by abdominal palpation. If the head is fully engaged (no fifths palpable) at or below the ischial spines (0 to +1 cm or more) and the occiput is anterior (OA), the outlook is favourable for vaginal birth.

The condition of the membranes should also be noted. If they have ruptured, the colour and amount of amniotic fluid draining should be noted. A generous amount of clear fluid is a good prognostic feature; scanty, heavily blood-stained or meconium-stained fluid is a warning sign of possible fetal compromise.

FETAL ASSESSMENT IN LABOUR

A healthy term fetus is usually able to withstand the demands of normal labour. However, with each contraction, placental blood flow and oxygen transfer are temporarily interrupted and a fetus that is compromised prior to labour will deteriorate. Insufficient oxygen delivery to the fetus causes a switch from aerobic to anaerobic metabolism and results in the generation of lactic acid and hydrogen ions. In excess, these saturate the buffering systems of the fetus and cause a metabolic acidosis, which, if prolonged and severe, can cause permanent neurological injury or perinatal death. Hypoxia and acidosis cause changes in the fetal heart rate (FHR) pattern, which can be detected by auscultation and cardiotocography (CTG). Meconium (fetal stool) is often passed by a healthy fetus at or after term as a result of maturation of the gastrointestinal tract; in this scenario, it is usually thin and a very dark green or brown colour. However, it may also be expelled from a fetus exposed to intrauterine hypoxia or acidosis; in this scenario, it is often thicker and much brighter green in colour.

In labour, the FHR should be auscultated with a Pinard stethoscope or by using a hand-held Doppler device. It should be listened to for at least 1 minute, immediately after a contraction. This should be repeated every 15 minutes during the first stage of labour and at least every 5 minutes in the second stage. The practice of performing an 'admission CTG' on all women is no longer recommended; however, a CTG should be performed if there are issues that might complicate labour and birth. Most of these women will be advised to have continuous EFM throughout labour using CTG. Women who begin labour with intermittent auscultation will be advised to change to continuous CTG if complications occur during labour.

> **BOX 12.2: Fetal assessment options in labour**
>
> - Amniotic fluid – fresh meconium, absence of fluid and blood-stained fluid or bleeding are markers of potential fetal compromise
> - Intermittent auscultation of the fetal heart using a Pinard stethoscope or a hand-held Doppler ultrasound
> - Continuous external electronic fetal monitoring (EFM) using CTG
> - Continuous internal EFM using a fetal scalp electrode (FSE) and CTG
> - Fetal scalp stimulation
> - Fetal scalp blood sampling

- Meconium staining of the amniotic fluid
- Abnormal FHR detected by intermittent auscultation
- Maternal pyrexia (temperature ≥38.0°C or ≥37.5°C on two occasions)
- Fresh vaginal bleeding
- Augmentation of contractions with an oxytocin infusion
- Maternal request
- Epidural analgesia

The interpretation of the FHR pattern on a CTG is discussed in **Chapter 4**. In brief, features of a normal FHR pattern include a baseline heart rate of between 110 and 160 beats per minute (bpm, averaged over a 20-minute interval or more), variability of between 5 and 25 bpm (variation in the FHR above and below the baseline), accelerations (a transient increase in FHR of at least 15 bpm lasting at least 15 seconds) and the absence of decelerations (transient decrease in the FHR of 15 bpm or more).

Each feature of the CTG (baseline rate, variability, accelerations and decelerations) should be assessed each time a CTG is reviewed. Each feature can be described as 'reassuring', 'non-reassuring' or 'abnormal' according to certain nationally agreed definitions outlined in the National Institute for Health and Care Excellence (NICE) guideline on intra-partum management. If all four features are reassuring, then the CTG is classified as 'normal' (**Figure 12.18**). If only one feature is non-reassuring, then the CTG is classified as 'suspicious'. If there are two or more non-reassuring features or any one abnormal feature, then the CTG is 'pathological'. The CTG can be difficult to interpret and it carries a significant false-positive rate (i.e. it often raises the possibility of fetal compromise when in fact the fetus is still in good condition or compensating well). Any reversible causes must be considered and addressed (e.g. dehydration, woman lying flat) and, if it persists, further assessment of the fetus may be necessary with fetal scalp stimulation or fetal scalp blood sampling (see the section 'Management of possible fetal compromise' later in this chapter). If this is not possible or safe, then the baby should be delivered without delay. Education and training are crucial in the interpretation and response to CTG monitoring in labour.

The quality of a CTG recording is sometimes poor because of the fetal position or maternal obesity. A fetal scalp electrode (FSE) may overcome this problem. It is fixed onto the skin of the fetal scalp and picks

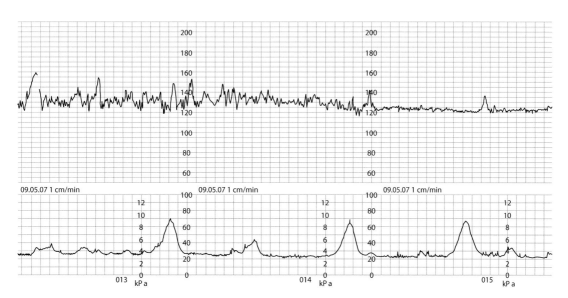

Figure 12.18 A normal cardiotocograph showing a baseline fetal heart rate of approximately 120 beats per minute (bpm), baseline variability of 10–15 bpm, frequent accelerations, and no decelerations. The uterus is contracting approximately once every 5 minutes (or 2 in 10).

up the FHR directly. It is contraindicated in the presence of significant maternal infection (e.g. human immunodeficiency virus (HIV) or hepatitis C).

PARTOGRAM

The introduction of a graphic record of labour in the form of a partogram has been an important development. This record allows an instant visual assessment of the progress of labour based on the rate of cervical dilatation compared with an expected norm, according to the parity of the woman, so that slow progress can be recognized and appropriate actions taken to correct it where possible. Other key observations are entered onto the chart, including the frequency and strength of contractions, the descent of the head in fifths palpable and station, the amount and colour of the amniotic fluid draining, and basic observations of maternal well-being, such as blood pressure, heart rate and temperature (**Figure 12.19**).

A line can be drawn on the partogram at the end of the latent phase demonstrating progress of 1 cm dilatation per hour. Another line ('the action line') can be drawn parallel and 4 hours to the right of it. If the plot of actual cervical dilatation reaches the action line, indicating slow progress, then consideration should be given to measures that aim to improve progress such as hydration, mobility, maternal position, artificial rupture of membranes (ARM) or oxytocin (see the section 'Management during the first stage'). Progress can also be considered slow if the cervix dilates at less than 1 cm every 2 hours.

MANAGEMENT DURING THE FIRST STAGE

Women who are in the latent phase of labour should be encouraged to mobilize and should be managed away from the labour suite where possible. Indeed, they may well go home to return later when the contractions are stronger or more frequent. Encouragement and reassurance are extremely important. Intervention during this phase is best avoided unless there are risk factors identified. Simple analgesics are preferred over nitrous oxide gas and epidurals. Vaginal examinations are usually performed every 4 hours to determine when the active phase has been reached (approximately 4 cm

> ### KEY LEARNING POINTS
>
> **Management of the first stage of labour**
> - The first stage of labour is the time from the diagnosis of labour to full dilatation of the cervix.
> - One-to-one midwifery care should be provided.
> - Additional emotional support from a birth partner should be encouraged.
> - Obstetric and anaesthetic care should be available as required.
> - Maternal and fetal well-being should be monitored.
> - Vaginal examinations are performed 4 hourly or as clinically indicated.
> - Progress of labour is monitored using a partogram with timely intervention if abnormal.
> - Appropriate pain relief should be provided consistent with the woman's wishes.
> - Ensure adequate hydration and light diet to prevent ketosis.

dilatation and full effacement). Thereafter, the timing of examinations should be decided by the midwife in consultation with the woman: 4 hourly is standard practice, but this frequency may be increased if the midwife thinks that progress is unusually slow or fast or if there are fetal concerns. The lower limit of normal progress is 1 cm dilatation every 2 hours once the active phase has been reached. Descent of the presenting part through the pelvis is another crucial component of progress and should be recorded at each vaginal examination.

During the first stage, the membranes may be intact, may have ruptured spontaneously or may be ruptured artificially. If the membranes are intact, it is not necessary to rupture them if the progress of labour is satisfactory. Artificial rupture of membranes (ARM) may be appropriate if progress in labour is slow.

Maternal and fetal observations are carried out and recorded on the partogram. Women should receive one-to-one care (i.e. from a dedicated midwife) and should not be left alone for any significant period of time once labour has established. Women should be able to choose their preferred birth partner and should be able to adopt whatever positions they find most comfortable. Mobility during labour is encouraged and it is likely that standing upright encourages progress. This can be more challenging

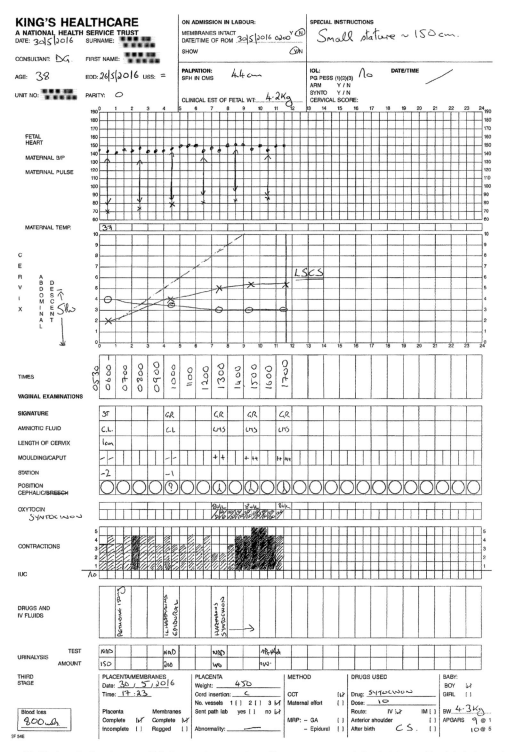

Figure 12.19 A typical partogram. This is a partogram of a nulliparous woman of short stature with a big baby and an augmented labour. The labour culminates in an emergency caesarean section for cephalopelvic disproportion.

with continuous CTG monitoring. Women may drink during established labour and those who are becoming dehydrated may benefit from intravenous fluids to prevent ketosis, which can impair uterine contractility. Light diet is acceptable if there is no obvious risk factor for needing a general anaesthetic and if the woman has not had pethidine or diamorphine for pain relief, which can cause vomiting. Shaving and enemas are unnecessary and antacids need only be given to women with risk factors for complications or to those who have had opioid analgesia. A variety of methods of pain relief are available, depending on the location of the birth (these are discussed in the section 'Pain relief in labour' later in this chapter).

'Active management of labour' is a collection of interventions that was routinely recommended to nulliparous women to maximize the chances of a normal birth. It included one-to-one midwifery care, 2-hourly vaginal examinations, early ARM and use of oxytocin augmentation if progress fell more than 2 hours behind the schedule of 1 cm dilatation per hour. A variety of studies failed to show any obvious benefit of active management, except that derived from one-to-one care, which is now the only component recommended for all women in normal labour.

MANAGEMENT DURING THE SECOND STAGE

If the labour has been normal, the first sign of the second stage is likely to be an urge to push experienced by the woman. Full dilatation of the cervix should be confirmed by a vaginal examination if the head is not visible. The woman will get an expulsive reflex with each contraction and will generally take a deep breath, hold it and strain down (the Valsalva manoeuvre). Women will be guided by their own urge to push; however, the midwife has an important role to play, with advice, support and reassurance if progress is slow. Women should be discouraged from lying supine or semi-supine and should adopt any other position that they find comfortable. Lying in the left lateral position, squatting and 'all fours' are particularly effective options. Maternal and fetal surveillance intensifies in the second stage, as described previously. The development of fetal acidaemia may accelerate, and maternal exhaustion and ketosis increase in line with the duration of active pushing.

Use of regional analgesia (epidural or spinal) may interfere with the normal urge to push, and the second stage is more often diagnosed on a routine scheduled vaginal examination. Pushing is usually delayed for at least an hour and up to 2 hours if an epidural is in situ (the 'passive second stage'); however, in all cases, guidelines recommend that the baby should be delivered within 4 hours of reaching full dilatation.

DESCENT AND DELIVERY OF THE FETAL HEAD

The progress of descent of the fetal head can be judged by watching the perineum. At first, there is a slight general bulge as the woman bears down. When the head stretches the perineum, the anus will begin to open, and soon after this the baby's head will be seen at the vulva at the height of each contraction. Between contractions, the elastic tone of the perineal muscles will push the head back into the pelvic cavity. The perineal body and vulva will become more and more stretched, until eventually the head is low enough to pass forwards under the subpubic arch. When the head no longer recedes between contractions it is described as crowning. This indicates that it has passed through the pelvic floor and delivery is imminent. Vaginal and perineal tears are common consequences of vaginal birth, particularly during first births. The 'hands-on' approach has been very popular. As crowning occurs, the hands of the accoucheur (midwife or obstetrician) are used to flex the fetal head and guard the perineum. The belief is that controlling the speed of delivery of the fetal head will limit maternal soft tissue damage. Once the head has crowned, the woman should be discouraged from bearing down by telling them to take rapid, shallow breaths ('panting').

DELIVERY OF THE SHOULDERS AND REST OF THE BODY

Once the fetal head is born, a check is made to see whether the cord is wound tightly around the neck, thereby making delivery of the body difficult. If this is the case, the cord may need to be clamped and divided before delivery of the rest of the body. With the next contraction, there is restitution of the head, and the shoulders can be delivered. To aid the delivery of the shoulders, there should be gentle traction on the head downwards and forwards until the anterior shoulder appears beneath the pubis. The head is then lifted gradually until the posterior shoulder appears over the perineum and the baby is then swept upwards to deliver the body and legs. Shoulder dystocia (difficulty in delivering the shoulders) is discussed in **Chapter 14**.

IMMEDIATE CARE OF THE NEONATE

After the baby is born, it lies between the mother's legs or is delivered directly on to her abdomen. The baby will usually take its first breath within seconds. There is no need for immediate clamping of the cord, and indeed about 80 mL of blood will be transferred from the placenta to the baby before cord pulsations cease, reducing the chances of later neonatal anaemia and iron deficiency. The baby's head should be kept dependent to allow mucus in the respiratory tract to drain, and oropharyngeal suction should be applied only if necessary. Delayed cord clamping is recommended for at least 3 minutes unless the baby needs immediate resuscitation. The baby should have an Apgar score calculated at 1 minute of age (see **Chapter 16**), which is then repeated at 5 minutes. Immediate skin-to-skin contact between the mother and the baby will help bonding and promote the further release of oxytocin, which will encourage uterine contractions. The baby should be dried and covered with a warm blanket or towel, maintaining maternal contact. Initiation of breastfeeding should be encouraged within the first hour of life, and routine newborn measurements of head circumference, birthweight and temperature are usually performed soon after this hour has elapsed. Before being transferred from the delivery room, a prophylactic dose of vitamin K should be given (if parental consent has been given) and the infant should have a general examination for abnormalities and a wrist label attached for identification.

MANAGEMENT OF THE THIRD STAGE

The third stage is the interval between the birth of the baby and the complete expulsion of the placenta and membranes. This normally takes between 5 and 10 minutes and is considered prolonged after 30 minutes unless a physiological approach is preferred.

BOX 12.4: Signs of placental separation

- Apparent lengthening of the cord
- A small gush of blood from the placental bed
- Rising of the uterine fundus to above the umbilicus (**Figure 12.20**)
- Uterine contraction resulting in firm globular feel on palpation

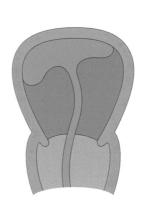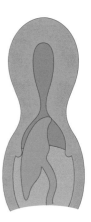

Figure 12.20 Signs of separation and descent of the placenta. After separation, the uterine upper segment rises and feels more rounded.

BOX 12.5: Active management of the third stage

- Intramuscular or intravenous injection of 10 IU oxytocin, immediately after delivery of the baby
- Clamping and cutting of the umbilical cord (delayed cord clamping is now recommended)
- Controlled cord traction (**Figure 12.21**)

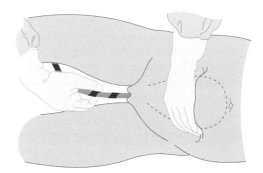

Figure 12.21 Delivering the placenta by controlled cord traction.

Separation of the placenta occurs because of the reduction of volume of the uterus due to uterine contraction and the retraction (shortening) of the lattice-like arrangement of the myometrial muscle fibres. A cleavage plane develops within the decidua basalis and the separated placenta lies free in the lower segment of the uterine cavity. Management of the third stage can be described as 'active' or 'physiological'.

ACTIVE MANAGEMENT

Active management of the third stage should be recommended to all women because high-quality evidence shows that it reduces the incidence of post-partum haemorrhage from 15% to 5%. When the signs of placental separation are recognized, controlled cord traction is used to expedite delivery of the placenta. When a contraction is felt, the left hand should be moved suprapubically and the fundus elevated with the palm facing towards the woman. At the same time, the right hand should grasp the cord and exert steady traction so that the placenta separates and is delivered gently, care being taken to peel off all the membranes, usually with a twisting motion. Uterine inversion is a rare complication, which may occur if the uterus is not adequately controlled with the left hand and excessive traction is exerted on the cord in the absence of complete separation and a uterine contraction (see **Chapter 14**).

In approximately 2% of cases, the placenta will not be expelled by this method. If no bleeding occurs, a further attempt at controlled cord traction should be made after 10 minutes. If this fails, the placenta is 'retained' and will require manual removal under general or regional anaesthesia in the operating theatre.

It is now recognized that a modified approach to active management of the third stage may be preferable with delayed cord clamping for between 1 and 3 minutes. This approach allows autotransfusion of placental blood to the neonate while maintaining the benefit of a reduced risk of post-partum haemorrhage. It is of particular importance in preterm birth.

PHYSIOLOGICAL MANAGEMENT

In physiological management of the third stage, the placenta is delivered by maternal effort and no uterotonic drugs are given to assist this process. It is associated with heavier bleeding, but women who are not at increased risk of post-partum haemorrhage should be supported if they choose this option. In the event of haemorrhage (estimated blood loss >500 mL) or if the placenta remains undelivered after 60 minutes of physiological management, active management should be recommended.

After completion of the third stage, the placenta should be inspected for missing cotyledons or a succenturiate lobe. If these are suspected, examination under anaesthesia and manual removal of placental tissue should be arranged, because the risk of post-partum haemorrhage is high.

Finally, the genital tract of the mother should be inspected for any tears or lacerations. Minor tears do not require suturing, but tears extending into the perineal muscles (or, indeed, an episiotomy) will require careful repair (see **Chapter 13**).

⊙━ KEY LEARNING POINTS

Features of normal labour:

- spontaneous onset at 37–42 weeks' gestation
- singleton pregnancy
- cephalic vertex presentation
- no artificial interventions
- cervical dilatation of at least 1 cm every 2 hours in the active phase of the first stage
- an active second stage of no more than 2 hours in nulliparous women and 1 hour in multiparous women
- spontaneous vaginal birth
- a third stage lasting no more than 30 minutes with active management or 60 minutes with physiological management

ABNORMAL LABOUR

Labour becomes abnormal when there is poor progress (as evidenced by a delay in cervical dilatation or descent of the presenting part) and/or when the fetus shows signs of compromise. In addition, if there is a fetal malpresentation, a multiple pregnancy or a uterine scar, or if labour has been induced, labour cannot be considered normal. Progress in labour is dependent on the 3Ps as described previously (powers, passages, passenger). Abnormalities in one or more of these factors can slow the normal progress of

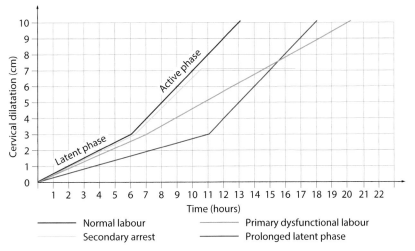

Figure 12.22 Abnormalities of the partogram.

labour. Plotting the findings of serial vaginal examinations on the partogram will help to highlight slow progress during the first and second stages of labour.

PATTERNS OF ABNORMAL PROGRESS IN LABOUR

The use of a partogram to plot the progress of labour improves the detection of slow progress. Three patterns of abnormal labour are commonly described (**Figure 12.22**).

'Primary arrest' is the term used to describe poor progress in the active first stage of labour (<2 cm cervical dilatation/4 hours) and is also more common in nulliparous women. It is typically caused by inefficient uterine contractions, but can also result from CPD, malposition and malpresentation of the fetus. 'Secondary arrest' occurs when progress in the active first stage is initially good but then slows, or stops altogether, typically after 7 cm dilatation. Although inefficient uterine contractions may be the cause, fetal malposition, malpresentation and CPD feature more commonly than in primary arrest. 'Arrest in the second stage of labour', not to be confused with 'secondary arrest', occurs when birth is not imminent after the usual interval of pushing in the second stage of labour. This may be due to inefficient uterine activity, malposition, malpresentation, CPD or a resistant perineum. It may also be due to maternal exhaustion, fear or pain.

MANAGEMENT OF ABNORMAL LABOUR

POOR PROGRESS IN THE FIRST STAGE OF LABOUR

DYSFUNCTIONAL UTERINE ACTIVITY ('POWERS')

This is the most common cause of poor progress in labour. It is more common in nulliparous and older women and is characterized by weak, irregular and infrequent contractions. The assessment of uterine contractions is carried out by clinical examination and by using external uterine tocography. Intrauterine pressure catheters are available and these do give a more accurate measurement of the pressure being generated by the contractions, but they are invasive and rarely necessary. A frequency of four contractions per 10 minutes is usually considered ideal. Fewer contractions than this does not necessarily mean progress will be slow, but more frequent examinations may be indicated to detect poor progress earlier. When poor progress in labour is suspected, it is usual to recommend repeat vaginal examination at 2 hours, rather than 4 hours after the last. If delay is confirmed, the woman should be offered ARM and, if there is still poor progress in a further 2 hours, advice should be sought from an obstetrician regarding the use of an oxytocin

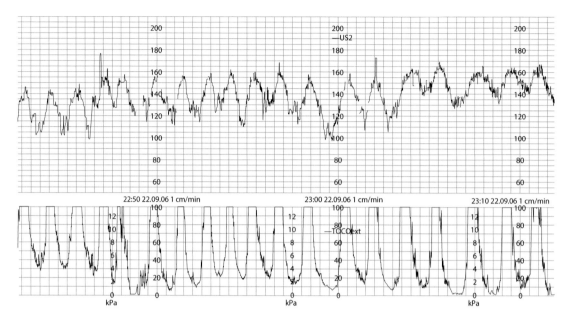

Figure 12.23 A pathological cardiotocograph secondary to uterine hyperstimulation.

infusion to augment the contractions. The infusion is commenced at a low rate initially and increased every 30 minutes, according to a well-defined protocol. Continuous EFM is necessary, as excessively frequent strong contractions may cause fetal compromise (**Figure 12.23**). Women should be offered an epidural before oxytocin is started, along with ongoing hydration and emotional support.

Multiparous women are less likely to experience poor progress in labour secondary to dysfunctional uterine activity. Extreme caution must be exercised when making this diagnosis in a multiparous woman when an alternative explanation, such as malposition, malpresentation or obstructed labour due to CPD, is more likely. An obstetrician must be closely involved in the assessment of such a situation and the decision to augment with oxytocin must be considered very carefully. Excessive uterine contractions in a truly obstructed labour may result in uterine rupture in a multiparous woman, a complication that is extremely rare in a nulliparous woman. Augmentation with oxytocin is contraindicated if there are concerns regarding the condition of the fetus. If progress fails to occur despite 4–6 hours of augmentation with oxytocin, a caesarean section will usually be recommended.

CEPHALOPELVIC DISPROPORTION ('PASSAGES' AND 'PASSENGER')

CPD implies anatomical disproportion between the fetal head and the maternal pelvis. It can be due to a large head, a small pelvis or a combination of the two relative to each other. Women of short stature (<1.60 m) with a large baby in their first pregnancy are potential candidates to develop this problem. The pelvis may be unusually small because of previous fracture or metabolic bone disease. Rarely, a fetal anomaly will contribute to CPD. Obstructive hydrocephalus may cause macrocephaly (abnormally large fetal head), and fetal thyroid and neck tumours may cause extension at the fetal neck. Relative CPD is more common and occurs with malposition of the fetal head. The OP position is associated with deflexion of the fetal head and presents a larger skull diameter to the maternal pelvis (**Figure 12.24**; see also **Figure 12.14**).

Oxytocin can be given carefully to a primigravida with mild to moderate CPD if the CTG is normal. Relative disproportion may be overcome if the malposition is corrected (i.e. rotation to a flexed OA position). Oxytocin must never be used in a multiparous woman when CPD is suspected, and it should be used with caution in women with a uterine scar.

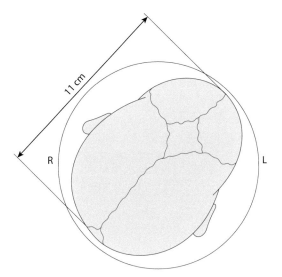

Figure 12.24 Vaginal palpation of the head in the right occipito-posterior position. The circle represents the pelvic cavity, with a diameter of 12 cm. The head is poorly flexed so that the anterior fontanelle is easily felt.

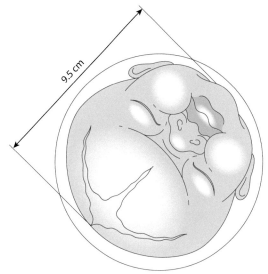

Figure 12.25 Vaginal examination in the left mento-anterior position. The circle represents the pelvic cavity, with a diameter of 12 cm.

BOX 12.6: Findings suggestive of CPD

- Fetal head is not engaged in labour
- Progress is slow or arrests despite efficient uterine contractions
- Vaginal examination shows severe moulding and caput formation
- Head is poorly applied to the cervix
- Haematuria

MALPRESENTATION ('PASSENGER')

A firm application of the fetal presenting part on to the cervix is necessary for good progress in labour. A face presentation (**Figures 12.25** and **12.26**) may apply poorly to the cervix and the resulting progress in labour may be slow, although vaginal birth is still possible. Brow presentation is associated with the mento-vertical diameter presenting, which is simply too large to fit through the bony pelvis unless flexion occurs or hyperextension to a face presentation (**Figures 12.27** and **12.28**). Brow presentation therefore often manifests as slow progress in the first stage, often in a multiparous woman. Shoulder presentations cannot deliver vaginally and, once again, slow progress will occur. Malpresentations are more common in women

Figure 12.26 The mechanism of labour with a face presentation. The head descends with increasing extension. The chin reaches the pelvic floor and undergoes forwards rotation. The head is born by flexion.

of high parity and carry a risk of uterine rupture if labour is allowed to continue without progress.

ABNORMALITIES OF THE BIRTH CANAL ('PASSAGES')

The bony pelvis may cause delay in the progress of labour as discussed earlier (CPD). Abnormalities of the uterus and cervix can also delay labour. Unsuspected

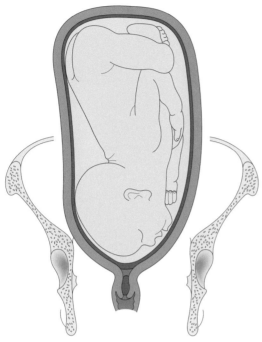

Figure 12.27 Brow presentation. The head is above the brim and not engaged. The mento-vertical diameter of the head is trying to engage in the transverse diameter at the brim.

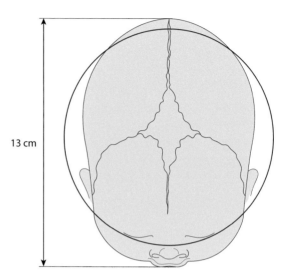

13 cm

Figure 12.28 Vaginal examination with brow presentation. The circle represents the pelvic cavity, with a diameter of 12 cm. The mento-vertical diameter of 13 cm is too large to permit engagement of the head.

fibroids in the lower uterine segment can prevent descent of the fetal head. Delay can also be caused by 'cervical dystocia', a term used to describe a non-compliant cervix that effaces but fails to dilate because of severe scarring or rigidity, usually because of previous cervical surgery such as a cone biopsy. Caesarean section may be necessary.

POOR PROGRESS IN THE SECOND STAGE OF LABOUR

Birth of the baby is expected to take place within 3 hours of the start of the active second stage (pushing) in nulliparous women and 2 hours in parous women. Delay is diagnosed if delivery is not imminent after 2 hours of pushing in a nulliparous labour and 1 hour for a parous woman. The causes of second-stage delay can again be classified as abnormalities of the powers, the passages and the passenger. Secondary dysfunctional uterine activity ('powers') is a common cause of second-stage delay and may be exacerbated by epidural analgesia. Having achieved full dilatation, the uterine

contractions may become weak and ineffectual and this is sometimes associated with maternal dehydration and ketosis. If no mechanical problem is anticipated and the woman is nulliparous, the treatment is with rehydration and intravenous oxytocin. If the woman is multiparous, a full clinical assessment should be performed by a skilled obstetrician prior to considering oxytocin due to the risks described previously.

Delay in the second stage can occur because of a narrow mid-pelvis (android pelvis), which prevents internal rotation of the fetal head ('passages'). This may result in arrest of descent of the fetal head at the level of the ischial spines in the transverse position, a condition called deep transverse arrest (**Figure 12.29**). Delay can also occur because of a persistent OP position of the fetal head ('passenger'). In this situation, the head will have to either undergo a long rotation to OA or be delivered in the OP position (i.e. face to pubes). It may also occur due to a resistant perineum, particularly in a nulliparous woman.

Assisted vaginal birth should be considered for prolonged second stage if the safety criteria have been fulfilled. If the safety criteria for assisted vaginal birth are not met, then delivery will be by caesarean section. A resistant perineum resulting in significant delay may be an indication for an episiotomy (see **Chapter 13**).

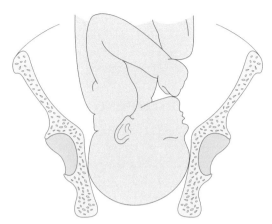

Figure 12.29 Deep transverse arrest of the head.

⊙━ KEY LEARNING POINTS

Management options for delay in the second stage of labour:

- continued pushing with encouragement
- regular reviews of progress and fetal well-being
- oxytocin to augment contractions
- episiotomy for a resistant perineum
- assisted vaginal birth (vacuum or forceps)
- caesarean section

FETAL COMPROMISE IN LABOUR

Concern for the well-being of the fetus is one of the most common reasons for medical intervention during labour. The fetus may have been compromised before labour, and the reduction in placental blood flow associated with contractions may reveal this and over time lead to fetal hypoxia and acidosis. Fetal compromise may present as fresh meconium staining to the amniotic fluid or an abnormal CTG. However, neither of these findings confirms fetal hypoxia or acidosis. Meconium can be passed for physiological reasons, such as fetal maturity, and it is well recognized that the abnormal CTG carries a high false-positive rate for the diagnosis of fetal compromise. 'Suspected fetal compromise' is therefore a more accurate term than 'fetal distress'. In many cases, babies delivered by vacuum, forceps or caesarean section for suspected fetal compromise are found to be in good condition.

BOX 12.7: Risk factors for fetal compromise in labour

- Placental insufficiency – intrauterine growth restriction and pre-eclampsia
- Prematurity (<37 weeks)
- Prolonged pregnancy (>42 weeks)
- Multiple pregnancy
- Prolonged labour
- Use of oxytocin/hyperstimulation
- Precipitate labour
- Intra-partum abruption
- Cord prolapse
- Uterine rupture/dehiscence
- Diabetes in pregnancy
- Cholestasis of pregnancy
- Maternal pyrexia/chorioamnionitis
- Oligohydramnios

RECOGNITION OF FETAL COMPROMISE

Meconium staining of the amniotic fluid is considered significant when it is either thick or tenacious and dark green, bright green or black. Any particulate meconium should also be of concern. Thin and light meconium is more likely to represent fetal gut maturity than fetal compromise. However, when any meconium is seen in the liquor, consideration should be given to starting continuous EFM with the CTG and this is mandatory if the meconium is thick and dark. Another reason for commencing the CTG is if a change in the heart rate is noted with intermittent auscultation, particularly fetal tachycardia, bradycardia or FHR decelerations. The CTG may have already been recorded throughout the labour because of underlying risk factors that predate the labour. Interpretation of the CTG is discussed in more detail in **Chapter 4**.

MANAGEMENT OF POSSIBLE FETAL COMPROMISE

A number of resuscitative manoeuvres should be considered when a CTG is classified as 'suspicious'. These include repositioning of the pregnant woman, intravenous fluids, reducing or stopping the oxytocin

> ### BOX 12.8: Resuscitating the fetus in labour
>
> - Maternal dehydration and ketosis can be corrected with intravenous fluids.
> - Maternal hypotension secondary to an epidural can be reversed by a fluid bolus, although a vasoconstrictor such as ephedrine is occasionally necessary.
> - Uterine hyperstimulation from excess oxytocin can be treated by turning off the infusion temporarily and using tocolytic drugs, such as terbutaline.
> - Venocaval compression and reduced uterine blood flow can be eased by turning the woman to a left lateral position.

infusion and correction of epidural-associated hypotension. It is reasonable to continue observation of the CTG and more complex intervention is not required. If a CTG becomes 'pathological', these reversible factors should also be considered, but it is also important to carry out an immediate vaginal examination to exclude malpresentation and cord prolapse and to assess the progress of the labour. If the cervix is fully dilated, it may be possible to assist the delivery of the baby vaginally using the forceps or vacuum. Alternatively, if the cervix is not fully dilated, fetal blood sampling can be considered. This is usually only possible when the cervix is dilated 3 cm or more. A normal result will support continuing labour, although it may need to be repeated every 30–60 minutes if the CTG abnormalities persist or worsen. An abnormal result mandates immediate delivery, by caesarean section if the cervix is not fully dilated.

FETAL SCALP STIMULATION

Digital fetal scalp stimulation is a second-line test of fetal well-being that may be indicated when there are concerns about the FHR pattern on a CTG. The test is performed during a vaginal examination by digital rubbing of the fetal scalp to elicit an FHR acceleration or an increase in variability. A gentle rubbing pressure should be applied to the fetal scalp with the examining fingers (index and middle fingers) for a duration of approximately 30 to 60 seconds. The FHR pattern on the CTG is monitored closely for 1 to 10 minutes following stimulation looking for evidence of an elicited FHR acceleration (defined as an increase in the FHR of ≥15 bpm for at least 15 seconds) and/or normal FHR variability (5 to 25 bpm).

FETAL BLOOD SAMPLING

Fetal blood sampling is a second-line test of fetal well-being that may be indicated when there are concerns about the FHR pattern on a CTG. The test involves collection of a capillary sample of blood from the fetal scalp to assess fetal pH and/or lactate. An amnioscope with a light source is inserted into the vagina, positioned through the cervix and applied directly onto the fetal scalp. The fetal scalp is visualized and dried using gauze and then ethyl chloride is sprayed by an assistant to induce a reactive hyperaemia. Once dry, a thin layer of paraffin is applied to the fetal scalp to facilitate droplet formation of the capillary sample. A shallow fetal scalp incision/puncture is performed and, once a blood droplet has formed, it is collected in a heparin-coated capillary tube. One or more samples may be required to get a reliable result. Following collection, the incision site is pressed with gauze to prevent further bleeding.

A normal pH value is above 7.25. A pH below 7.20 is confirmation of fetal compromise. Values between 7.20 and 7.25 are 'borderline'. The base deficit can also be useful in interpretation of the fetal scalp pH. A base excess of more than −12.0 demonstrates a significant metabolic acidosis, with increasing risk of fetal neurological injury beyond this level. More than one fetal scalp sample may be necessary over the course of the labour. A downwards trend in the fetal scalp pH values is to be expected and should be assessed together with how the labour is progressing. If an abnormal CTG persists in labour, then, despite normal values, fetal scalp sampling should be repeated every 60 minutes, or sooner if the CTG deteriorates. If the result is borderline, it should be repeated no more than 30 minutes later.

PLACE OF BIRTH

Most births in high-income countries take place in hospital. However, depending on the circumstances, women may have the opportunity to choose between hospital birth, home birth or birth in a midwifery unit or birth centre. Currently, less than 5% of women deliver at home in most areas of the UK. Some midwifery units are based within a hospital environment and some are stand-alone. The published evidence guiding women on the outcomes of birth in the different settings is limited to observational studies, the largest of which is the Birthplace in England study. The chance of a normal birth at home or in a midwifery unit is higher than in an obstetric unit, and the best outcomes are for women who are multiparous and without complicating factors. All women should be informed, however, that unexpected emergencies can occur in labour and that the outcome from these may be better in a hospital setting. It should also be made clear that the need for transfer into hospital, during labour, is possible from home or a midwifery unit. Women with issues that increase the chance of problems occurring during labour should be recommended to deliver in an obstetric unit, and local guidelines provide a list of obstetric, fetal and medical factors to assist midwives and obstetricians when counselling women. In addition, a variety of indications are listed for intra-partum transfer into an obstetric unit, including maternal pyrexia in labour, delayed progress in labour, concerns regarding fetal well-being, hypertension, retained placenta and complicated perineal trauma requiring suturing. Use of epidural pain relief is restricted to hospital settings. Some women will chose to labour or give birth in water. At present, there is insufficient good-quality evidence to either support or discourage water birth.

PAIN RELIEF IN LABOUR

There is a social and cultural dimension to the provision and uptake of analgesia in labour. Some women and their carers believe that there is an advantage in avoiding analgesia, whereas others will use all methods on offer to limit their pain. Professionals who are knowledgeable about labour and the available options for pain relief should give tailored advice according to the needs and priorities of the individual woman. The method of pain relief is to some extent dependent on the previous obstetric record of the woman, the course of labour and the anticipated

duration of labour. Although the final decision rests with the woman, there are certain circumstances in which particular forms of analgesia are contraindicated and should not be offered.

NON-PHARMACOLOGICAL METHODS

One-to-one care in labour from a midwife alongside a supportive birth partner has been shown to reduce the need for analgesia. Relaxation and breathing exercises may help the woman to manage her pain. Prolonged hyperventilation can make her dizzy and can cause alkalosis. Homeopathy, acupuncture and hypnosis are sometimes employed, but their use has not been associated with a significant reduction in pain scores or with a reduced need for conventional methods of analgesia.

Relaxation in warm water during the first stage of labour often leads to a sense of well-being and allows women to cope much better with pain. The temperature of the water should not exceed 37.5°C. Transcutaneous electrical nerve stimulation (TENS) works on the principle of blocking pain fibres in the posterior ganglia of the spinal cord by stimulation of small afferent fibres (the 'gate' theory). It may be of use in the latent phase of labour and is often used by women at home. It has been shown to be ineffective in reducing pain scores or the need for other forms of analgesia in established labour. It does not have any adverse effects.

PHARMACOLOGICAL METHODS

Opiates, such as pethidine and diamorphine, are still used in many obstetric units and indeed can be administered by midwives without the involvement

BOX 12.9: Side effects of opioid analgesia

- Nausea and vomiting (they should always be given with an anti-emetic)
- Maternal drowsiness and sedation
- Delayed gastric emptying (increasing the risks of general anaesthesia)
- Short-term respiratory depression of the baby
- Possible interference with breastfeeding

of medical staff. This may be one of the reasons for their popularity. They provide only limited pain relief during labour and may have significant side effects.

Opiates tend to be given as intramuscular injections; however, an alternative is a subcutaneous or intravenous infusion by a patient-controlled analgesic device. This allows the woman, by pressing a dispenser button, to determine the level of analgesia that they require. If a very short-acting opiate is used, the opiate doses can be timed with the contractions. This method of pain relief is particularly popular among women who cannot have an epidural and find non-pharmacological options insufficient.

INHALATIONAL ANALGESIA

Nitrous oxide in the form of entonox (an equal mixture of nitrous oxide and oxygen) is available on most labour wards. It has a quick onset, a short duration of effect and is more effective than pethidine. It may cause light-headedness and nausea. It is not suitable for prolonged use from early labour because hyperventilation may result in hypocapnoea, dizziness and, rarely, tetany and fetal hypoxia. It is most suitable in the active first stage of labour or while awaiting epidural analgesia.

EPIDURAL ANALGESIA

Epidural (extradural) analgesia is the most reliable means of providing effective analgesia in labour. Failure to provide an epidural is one of the most frequent causes of upset and disappointment among labouring women. The epidural service must be well organized to be effective, and fortunately resources are now available in most hospital settings so that a significant delay in the placement of an epidural is unusual.

The woman must be informed about the benefits and risks, and the final decision should rest with her unless there is a definite contraindication. It is important to warn her that she may lose sensation and movement in her legs temporarily, and that intravenous access and a more intensive level of maternal and fetal monitoring will be necessary, for example with CTG. The effect of epidural analgesia on labour duration and the operative delivery

> **BOX 12.10: Indications and contraindications for epidural analgesia**
>
> **Indications**
> - Prolonged labour/oxytocin augmentation
> - Gestational hypertensive disorders
> - Multiple pregnancy
> - Selected medical conditions affecting the pregnant woman
> - A high risk of operative intervention
>
> **Contraindications**
> - Coagulation disorders (e.g. low platelet count)
> - Local or systemic sepsis
> - Hypovolaemia
> - Logistical: insufficient numbers of trained staff (anaesthetic and midwifery)

rate has been a controversial issue. The evidence is now clear that epidural analgesia does not increase caesarean section rates; however, the second stage is longer with a delayed urge to push. In some clinical situations, an epidural in the second stage of labour may assist a vaginal birth by relaxing the woman and allowing time for the head to descend and rotate.

Complications of regional analgesia

Hypotension can occur with epidural analgesia although it is more common with spinal anaesthesia. It can usually be rectified with intravenous fluid boluses but may need vasopressors. Occasionally, hypotension in the pregnant woman will lead to fetal compromise.

Bladder dysfunction can occur if the bladder is allowed to overfill because the woman is unaware of the need to micturate, particularly after the birth while the spinal or epidural anaesthesia is wearing off. Over-distension of the detrusor muscle of the bladder can permanently damage it and leave long-term voiding problems. To avoid this, catheterization of the bladder should be carried out during labour.

Accidental dural puncture occurs in approximately 1% of cases. If the subarachnoid space is accidentally reached with an epidural needle, this may allow leakage of cerebrospinal fluid and results in a 'spinal headache'. This is characteristically experienced on the top of the head and is relieved by lying flat and exacerbated by sitting upright. If the headache is severe or persistent, a blood patch may be necessary. This involves injecting a small volume of the woman's blood into the epidural space at the level of the accidental dural puncture. The resulting blood clot is thought to block off the leak of cerebrospinal fluid.

Accidental total spinal anaesthesia (injection of epidural doses of local anaesthetic into the subarachnoid space) causes severe hypotension, respiratory failure, unconsciousness and death if not recognized and treated immediately. The woman requires intubation, ventilation and circulatory support. Hypotension must be treated with intravenous fluids, vasopressors and positioning of the woman on her left side. In some cases, urgent delivery of the baby may be required to overcome aorto-caval compression and so permit resuscitation of the woman.

Spinal haematomata and neurological complications are rare and are usually associated with other factors such as bleeding disorders. Drug toxicity can occur with accidental placement of a catheter within a blood vessel. This is normally noticed by aspiration prior to injection.

Short-term respiratory depression of the baby is possible because all modern epidural solutions contain opioids, which reach the circulation of the pregnant woman and may cross the placenta.

Technique

After detailed discussion, the woman's back is cleansed and local anaesthetic is used to infiltrate the skin. The woman may be in an extreme left lateral position or sitting upright but leaning over. Flexion at the upper spine and at the hips helps to open up the spaces between the vertebral bodies of the lumbar spine. Aseptic technique is used. The epidural catheter is normally inserted at the L2–L3, L3–L4 or L4–L5 interspace and should come to lie in the epidural space, which contains blood vessels, nerve roots and fat (**Figure 12.30**). The catheter is aspirated to check for position and, if no blood or cerebrospinal fluid is obtained, a 'test dose' is given to confirm the catheter position (**Figure 12.31**). This test dose is a small volume of dilute local anaesthetic that would not be expected to have any clinical effect. If indeed it has no obvious effect on sensation in the lower limbs, the

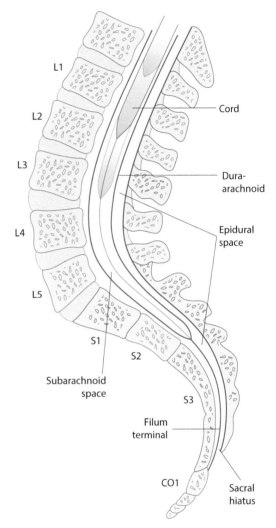

Figure 12.30 Sagittal section of the lumbo-sacral spinal cord.

catheter is correctly sited. If, however, there is a sensory block, leg weakness and peripheral vasodilatation, the catheter has been inserted too far and into the subarachnoid (spinal) space. Inserting the normal dose of local anaesthetic into the spinal space by accident would risk complete motor and respiratory paralysis. If none of these signs is observed 5 minutes after injection of the test dose, a loading dose can be administered. The epidural solution is usually a mixture of low-concentration local anaesthetic (e.g. 0.0625–0.1% bupivacaine) with an opioid such as fentanyl. Combining the opioid with the local

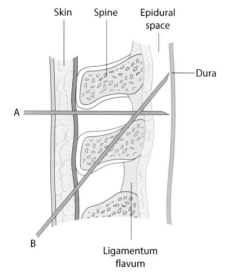

Skin   Spine   Epidural space

Dura

A

B

Ligamentum flavum

Figure 12.31 Needle positioning for an epidural anaesthetic: midline (**A**) and paramedian (**B**) approaches.

anaesthetic reduces the amount of local anaesthetic required and this reduces the motor blockade and peripheral autonomic effects of the epidural (e.g. hypotension).

After the loading dose is given, the woman should be kept in the right or left lateral position and her blood pressure should be measured every 5 minutes for 15 minutes.

A fall in blood pressure may result from the vasodilatation caused by blocking of the sympathetic tone to peripheral blood vessels. This hypotension is usually short lived but may cause a fetal bradycardia due to redirection of blood away from the uterus. It should be treated with intravenous fluids and, if necessary, vasoconstrictors such as ephedrine. The woman should never lie supine, as aorto-caval compression can reduce their cardiac output and so compromise placental perfusion. Hourly assessment of the level of the sensory block using a cold spray is critical in the detection of a block that is creeping too high and risking respiratory compromise. Regional analgesia can be maintained throughout labour with either intermittent boluses or continuous infusions. Patient-controlled epidural analgesia is an option. Women should be encouraged to move around and adopt whichever upright position suits them best. Full mobility is more difficult. Regional

anaesthesia should be continued until after completion of the third stage of labour, including repair of any perineal injury.

SPINAL ANAESTHESIA

A spinal block is considered more effective than that obtained by an epidural and is of faster onset. A fine-gauge atraumatic spinal needle is passed through the epidural space, through the dura and into the subarachnoid space, which contains the cerebrospinal fluid. A small volume of local anaesthetic is injected, after which the spinal needle is withdrawn. This may be used as anaesthesia for caesarean sections, for the trial of assisted vaginal births (in theatre), for manual removal of a retained placenta and for the repair of difficult perineal and vaginal tears. Spinal anaesthesia is not used for routine analgesia in labour.

Combined spinal–epidural analgesia has gained in popularity. This technique has the advantage of producing a rapid onset of pain relief and the provision of prolonged analgesia. Because the initiating spinal dose is relatively low, this is an option for immediate pain relief in labour.

LABOUR IN SPECIAL CIRCUMSTANCES

WOMEN WITH A UTERINE SCAR

Some women will have a pre-existing uterine scar, usually because of a previous caesarean section. Approximately 25–35% of all deliveries in high-income countries are by caesarean section and 99% of these are performed through the lower segment of the uterus because blood loss is less, healing is better and the risk of subsequent uterine rupture is lower than following an upper segment or 'classical' caesarean section. There are still a few indications for upper segment caesarean section (e.g. extreme prematurity) and it is important that these women are counselled appropriately. It is estimated that uterine rupture or dehiscence (scar separation) occurs in approximately 1 in 200 women who labour spontaneously with a pre-existing lower segment uterine

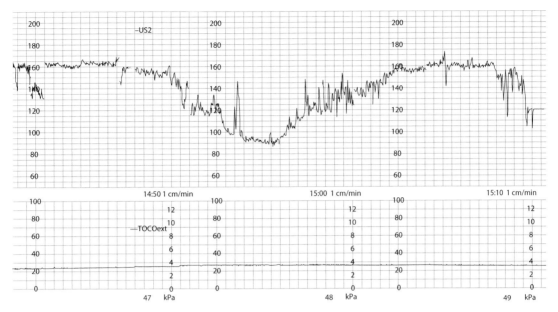

Figure 12.32 Fetal bradycardia to a heart rate of 90 beats per minute, lasting approximately 11 minutes.

scar. The risk is two to three times higher in women with a previous upper segment incision.

Signs of uterine rupture include severe lower abdominal pain, vaginal bleeding, haematuria, cessation of contractions, tachycardia in the pregnant woman and fetal compromise (often a bradycardia; **Figure 12.32**). Uterine rupture carries serious risks (shock, need for blood transfusion and operative repair, possibly a hysterectomy) to the pregnant woman and serious fetal risks (hypoxia, permanent neurological injury and perinatal death). Rupture of the uterus is more likely to occur late in the first stage of labour, with induced or accelerated labour, and in association with a large baby.

Labour after a previous caesarean section is known as vaginal birth after caesarean (VBAC). Approximately 60–70% of women who attempt a VBAC will give birth vaginally and the remainder will need repeat caesarean delivery. The chance of a successful vaginal birth depends on a number of factors, including a previous vaginal birth, size of the baby and the original indication for a caesarean birth.

If a woman with a previous history of a caesarean section is admitted in labour, close surveillance is required to identify early signs of uterine rupture. Continuous CTG monitoring is strongly

> **BOX 12.11: Relative contraindications to VBAC**
>
> - Two or more previous caesarean section scars
> - Need for induction of labour (IOL)
> - Previous labour outcome suggestive of CPD
> - Previous classical caesarean section (absolute contraindication)

recommended and there should be a low threshold for urgent delivery by repeat caesarean section.

Some women will have scars on the uterus as a result of a previous myomectomy. In general, there is low risk of rupture of a myomectomy scar unless the uterine cavity was opened during the procedure.

MALPRESENTATION

BREECH PRESENTATION

The antenatal management of breech presentation and the mechanics of the delivery are discussed in **Chapter 6**. Most breech presentations recognized at term (≥37 weeks) are delivered by caesarean section. Although this is evidence based, and it is probably safer for breech babies to be delivered this way, there is still a place for a vaginal breech birth in certain circumstances. Individual choice and the failure to detect breech presentation until very late in labour mean that obstetricians need to be competent in the skills of vaginal breech delivery and aware of the potential complications. Poor progress in a breech labour is taken by most to be an indication for caesarean section. However, some obstetricians support the use of augmentation with oxytocin if contractions are infrequent.

FACE PRESENTATION

Face presentation occurs in about 1 in 500 labours and is due to complete extension of the fetal head. In the majority of cases, the cause for the extension is unknown, although it is frequently attributed to excessive tone of the extensor muscles of the fetal neck. Rarely, extension may be due to a fetal anomaly such as a thyroid tumour. The presenting diameter is the submento-bregmatic, which measures 9.5 cm, and is approximately the same in dimension as the sub-occipito-bregmatic (vertex) presentation. Despite this, engagement of the fetal head is late and progress in labour is frequently slow, possibly because the facial

bones do not mould. It is diagnosed in labour by palpating the nose, mouth and eyes on vaginal examination (see **Figure 12.25**). If progress in labour is good and the chin remains mento-anterior, vaginal birth is possible, with the head being delivered by flexion (see **Figure 12.26**). If the chin is posterior (mento-posterior position), delivery is impossible, as extension over the perineum cannot occur. In this circumstance, caesarean section is performed. Oxytocin should not be used and, if there is any concern about the fetal condition, caesarean section should be carried out. Forceps delivery is acceptable for low mento-anterior face presentation but vacuum extraction is contraindicated.

BROW PRESENTATION

Brow presentation arises when there is less extreme extension of the fetal neck than that with a face presentation. It can be considered a midway position between vertex and face. It is the least common malpresentation, occurring in 1 in 1,500–2,000 labours. The causes are similar to those of face presentation, although some brow presentations arise as a result of exaggerated extension associated with an OP position. The presenting diameter is the mento-vertical (measuring 13.5 cm) (see **Figures 12.14** and **12.27**). This is incompatible with a vaginal birth. It is diagnosed in labour by palpating the anterior fontanelle, supra-orbital ridges and nose on vaginal examination (see **Figure 12.28**). If this presentation persists, delivery can be achieved only by caesarean section.

SHOULDER PRESENTATION

This is reported as occurring in 1 in 300 pregnancies at term, but few of these women will go into labour. Shoulder presentation occurs as the result of a transverse or oblique lie of the fetus and the causes of this abnormal presentation include placenta praevia, high parity, pelvic tumour and uterine anomaly (see **Chapter 6**). Delivery should be by caesarean section. Delay in making the diagnosis risks cord prolapse and uterine rupture.

MULTIPLE PREGNANCY

The mechanics of the delivery of twins is discussed in greater detail in **Chapter 7**.

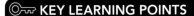

KEY LEARNING POINTS

Normal and abnormal labour management

- Most labours are uncomplicated and the outcomes are good.
- Labour can be a hazardous journey for the baby and the woman.
- Labour is divided into three stages.
- Progress in the first and second stage of labour is monitored with a partogram.
- Fetal well-being is monitored using the FHR, amniotic fluid and, where necessary, fetal blood sampling.
- The term 'suspected fetal compromise' should be used if there are concerns about fetal well-being.
- Abnormalities of the uterine contractions (the 'powers'), the pelvis and lower genital tract (the 'passages') and the fetus (the 'passenger') can cause abnormal labour.
- Augmentation of labour with an oxytocin infusion will often correct inefficient uterine contractions and may help correct a fetal malposition.
- Augmentation of labour with oxytocin can be dangerous in multiparous women, in those with a uterine scar, in cases of a malpresentation and when there are concerns about fetal well-being.
- Abnormal progress in the first stage of labour can be managed with ARM, oxytocin augmentation or emergency caesarean section.
- Abnormal progress in the second stage of labour can be managed with oxytocin augmentation, episiotomy, assisted vaginal birth (vacuum or forceps) or caesarean section.
- An abnormal third stage of labour may result in manual removal of placental tissue and/or post-partum haemorrhage.

INDUCTION OF LABOUR

Induction of labour (IOL) is the planned initiation of labour prior to its spontaneous onset. Approximately 20–30% of births in the UK occur following IOL. The common reasons for IOL are listed in this section. Broadly speaking, an IOL is performed when the risks of continuing to the fetus and/or the woman outweigh those of bringing the pregnancy to an end.

It should be performed only if there is a reasonable chance of success and if the risks of the process to the woman and/or fetus are acceptable. If either of these is not the case, the woman should be advised to await spontaneous labour or a caesarean section should be performed.

The most common reason for IOL is prolonged pregnancy (previously described as 'post-term' or 'post-dates'). There is evidence that pregnancies extending beyond 42 weeks' gestation are associated with a higher risk of stillbirth, fetal compromise in labour, meconium aspiration and mechanical problems at delivery. Because of this, women are usually recommended IOL at around 41 weeks' gestation. Induction for prolonged pregnancy does not increase the rate of caesarean section. The evidence is high quality and the recommendation is a strong one; however, 300–400 pregnancies need to be induced to prevent one perinatal death that would have occurred if the pregnancies had been managed expectantly beyond 42 weeks' gestation. Women who choose not to be induced for this reason are offered more intensive serial fetal monitoring (see **Chapter 6**).

Pre-labour rupture of membranes (PROM) is another common indication for IOL. It is not uncommon for the membranes to rupture and the subsequent onset of labour to be significantly delayed. The longer the delay between membrane rupture and delivery of the baby, the greater the risk of ascending infection (chorioamnionitis) and infectious morbidity in both the mother and the neonate. At term (beyond 37 weeks), good-quality evidence supports IOL approximately 24 hours following membrane rupture. This policy, endorsed in the NICE guideline on IOL, reduces rates of chorioamnionitis, endometritis and admissions to the neonatal unit. The evidence is less clear at present when PROM occurs preterm (PPROM). Before 34 weeks, some other additional indication is needed to justify IOL if the membranes rupture (e.g. suspected infection in the mother, fetal compromise, growth restriction). Between 34 and 37 weeks, in an otherwise straightforward pregnancy, the risks and benefits of IOL need to be assessed on an individual basis.

Pre-eclampsia and other hypertensive disorders often indicate earlier delivery. Pre-eclampsia at term is normally managed with IOL; however, at very preterm gestations (<34 weeks) or when there is rapid deterioration of the woman or significant fetal compromise, caesarean delivery may be a better option. Diabetes (both pre-existing and gestational diabetes), twin gestation and intrahepatic cholestasis of pregnancy are all common reasons for IOL at 38 weeks' gestation, and sometimes earlier. The published evidence is limited, and several randomized controlled trials are in progress to address these issues.

Suspected fetal macrosomia (>90th percentile), in the absence of diabetes, is now considered an indication for IOL following publication of a large randomized controlled trial. The difficulty with this approach is that the estimation of fetal weight by ultrasound has an error margin of 10–20%, and some inductions may subsequently prove to have been unnecessary.

'Social' IOL is controversial and is performed to satisfy the domestic and organizational needs of the woman and her family. It is mostly discouraged, and there must be careful counselling as to the potential risks involved. These are determined essentially by the parity and the cervical condition. If the situation is favourable for vaginal birth, with higher parity and a favourable cervix (see the next section, 'Bishop score'), social indications are more acceptable.

There are a number of absolute contraindications to IOL, including placenta praevia and severe fetal compromise. A deteriorating condition of the mother with major antepartum haemorrhage, pre-eclampsia or cardiac disease may favour caesarean delivery. Breech presentation is a relative contraindication to IOL, and women with a previous history of caesarean birth need to be informed of the greater risk of uterine rupture. Preterm gestation is not an absolute contraindication, but induction at <34 weeks is associated with a much higher risk of failure and the need for subsequent caesarean section.

> ## BOX 12.13: Indications for IOL
>
> - Prolonged pregnancy (usually offered after 41 completed weeks)
> - PROM >24 hours
> - Pre-eclampsia and other gestational hypertensive disorders
> - Fetal growth restriction
> - Diabetes mellitus
> - Fetal macrosomia
> - Deteriorating illness in the mother
> - Unexplained antepartum haemorrhage
> - Twin pregnancy continuing beyond 38 weeks
> - Intrahepatic cholestasis of pregnancy
> - Iso-immunization against red cell antigens in the mother
> - 'Social' reasons

BISHOP SCORE

As the time of spontaneous labour approaches, the cervix becomes softer, shortens, moves forwards, effaces and starts to dilate. This reflects the natural preparation for labour. If labour is induced before this process has occurred, the induction process will tend to take longer. Bishop produced a scoring system to quantify this process prior to IOL (**Table 12.1**). A high Bishop score (a 'favourable' cervix) is associated with an easier, shorter induction process that is less likely to fail. A low score (an 'unfavourable' cervix) is associated with a longer IOL that is more likely to fail and result in caesarean section.

METHODS

IOL was traditionally performed by ARM. In the mid-1950s, synthetic oxytocin (Syntocinon®) became available and was then used as an intravenous infusion

Table 12.1 Modified Bishop score

Score	0	1	2	3
Dilatation of cervix (cm)	0	1–2	3–4	5 or more
Consistency of cervix	Firm	Medium	Soft	–
Length of cervical canal (cm)	>2	1–2	0.5–1	<0.5
Position of cervix	Posterior	Mid	Anterior	–
Station of presenting part	–3	–2	–1 or 0	Below spines

after rupture of the membranes. In unfavourable cases, it was often unsuccessful and sometimes it was impossible to rupture the membranes. In the late 1960s, synthetic prostaglandin became available. Various routes and preparations have been used, but the most common formulation in current use is prostaglandin E_2, inserted vaginally into the posterior fornix as a tablet, gel or controlled-release pessary. Two doses of tablets or gel are often required, given at least 6 hours apart. The controlled-release pessary is left in place for up to 24 hours. Prostaglandins can be used even when the cervix is favourable. Labour may ensue following the administration of prostaglandin, but ARM and oxytocin are often also necessary, particularly in nulliparous women. Oxytocin has a short half-life and is given intravenously, as a dilute solution. The response to oxytocin is highly variable and a strict protocol exists for its use. The starting infusion rate is low and defined increments follow every 30 minutes until three to five contractions are achieved in every 10 minutes.

Mifepristone (an anti-progesterone) and misoprostol (prostaglandin E_1) can be used to induce labour, but complication rates seem higher and this drug combination is currently used in the UK only to induce labour following intrauterine fetal death.

'Membrane sweeping' describes the insertion of a gloved finger through the cervix and its rotation around the inner rim of the cervix. This strips the chorionic membrane from the underlying decidua and releases natural prostaglandins. It can be uncomfortable for the woman and is possible only if the cervix is beginning to dilate and efface. It can be performed more than once and evidence shows that it reduces the need for formal induction. It is usually performed only at term, and placenta praevia must be excluded before it is offered. It should be considered an adjunct to the normal processes of induction.

BOX 12.14: Methods of induction

- Membrane sweep (offer weekly from 40 weeks)
- Prostaglandin gel, tablet or pessary to ripen cervix and initiate contractions
- ARM (cervix must be favourable)
- Oxytocin infusion (membranes ruptured first, spontaneous or artificial)
- Mifepristone and misopostol (for intrauterine fetal death)

COMPLICATIONS OF INDUCTION OF LABOUR

It is generally agreed that a woman is likely to experience more pain with an induced labour, and the use of epidural analgesia is more common in induced labour. Long labours augmented with oxytocin predispose to post-partum haemorrhage secondary to uterine atony. Fetal compromise may occur during induced labours and this, in part at least, is due to uterine hyperstimulation as a side effect of the use of prostaglandins and oxytocin (see **Figure 12.23**). A contraction frequency of more than five contractions per 10 minutes should be treated by stopping the oxytocin and, if necessary, administration of a tocolytic drug, most commonly a subcutaneous injection of the beta-2 agonist terbutaline. Uterine hyperstimulation may precipitate a fetal bradycardia and the need for emergency caesarean section if the FHR fails to resolve promptly. If ARM is performed while the fetal head is high, then cord prolapse may occur, again precipitating the need for emergency caesarean section. Women with a previous caesarean section scar are at greater risk of uterine rupture if they are induced. The risk of scar rupture increases from 1 in 200 in a spontaneous labour to as high as 1 in 50 if IOL is performed using prostaglandins.

IOL may fail and this is said to have occurred if an ARM is still impossible after the maximum number of doses of prostaglandin have been given or if the cervix remains uneffaced and less than 3 cm dilated after an ARM has been performed and oxytocin has been administered for 6–8 hours with regular contractions. When an induction fails, the options include a rest period followed by attempting induction again or performing a caesarean section. Delaying delivery further is acceptable only if there is no major threat to the fetal or maternal condition. This may be the case with a failed social induction, for example. Failed induction in the setting of pre-eclampsia or fetal growth restriction will usually necessitate a caesarean delivery.

CLINICAL RISK MANAGEMENT

Risk management is an approach to healthcare provision that aims to limit harm occurring to patients and to improve the quality of care. Clinical risk management (CRM) can be applied to all areas of medicine, but the labour ward provides one of the best illustrations of its importance to modern healthcare.

Labour and birth carry a serious risk of harm. Trauma to the mother (both physical and psychological) and infant neurological injuries are examples of poor outcomes following birth that can potentially be avoided in many cases. Legal action is frequently taken after outcomes such as these, and this is expensive for the NHS in litigation payments and is distressing for all involved. The aim of CRM is to improve standards of care and subsequently reduce the harm occurring to women and their babies. This in turn should reduce the number of complaints made against hospitals and the financial costs of litigation.

Shoulder dystocia, for example, can result in brachial plexus injury, intra-partum asphyxia and serious perineal trauma in the mother. In many cases, these poor outcomes following shoulder dystocia can be avoided by appropriate management. Regular staff education and the performance of shoulder dystocia 'drills' can limit adverse outcomes. In these drills, the manoeuvres used to safely overcome shoulder dystocia are rehearsed to facilitate timely skilled intervention in the event of a real emergency. The use of guidelines and protocols drawn from evidence-based medicine is another tool of CRM. These help to reduce errors and to prevent erratic or incorrect decision-making.

Medical and midwifery staff are encouraged to report when things 'go wrong'. Once a 'near-miss' or an adverse outcome has occurred, careful documentation is vital if claims of negligence are to be defended. Good communication between the staff and the patient involved may help to clear up misunderstandings and minimize the chances of a formal complaint or legal action. Root-cause analysis is a technique that serves to examine in detail a poor outcome, or near-miss, so that every step of the patient journey is scrutinized to see if the outcome could have been prevented. This approach allows

assessment of both systemic (organizational) and individual (doctor/midwife) contributors to errors. In this way, lessons are learned for the future and unit policies and guidelines can be adjusted accordingly. It is usually the case that a whole series of failings or errors need to occur together for an avoidable poor outcome to result (a cascade effect). Organizational systems as a whole often contribute, and one individual is rarely solely responsible for a poor outcome.

Audit of labour ward outcomes is an important tool in CRM. If guidelines are not being followed and certain standards are not being met, this will be detected by audit and steps will be taken to address the problem. A repeat audit should show that improvements have occurred as a result of the actions taken.

KEY LEARNING POINTS

Important elements of CRM

- Focus on safety and quality of care
- Clinical audit
- Education and training
- Clinical incident reporting
- Root-cause analysis of adverse events
- Systems for complaints and claims handling
- Guidelines and research
- Service development

FURTHER READING

Birthplace in England Collaborative Group (2011). Perinatal and maternal outcomes by planned place of birth for healthy women with low risk pregnancies in England national prospective cohort study. *BMJ*, 343: d7400.

NICE (2021). *Inducing Labour*. NICE clinical guideline [NG207].

NICE (2023). *Intrapartum Care*. NICE guideline [NG235].

SELF-ASSESSMENT

For interactive SBAs and EMQs relating to this chapter, visit www.routledge.com/cw/mccarthy.

CASE HISTORY

Ms A is a 28-year-old woman who booked for antenatal care in her first pregnancy. She attended for shared care between her midwife and obstetrician and her pregnancy was uncomplicated. She was aiming for a physiological approach to labour and birth. Her membranes ruptured spontaneously at 40 weeks and 4 days. The liquor was clear, the baby was active and her vital signs were normal. She was advised that she could wait for 24 hours to allow spontaneous labour to establish if all was well. Regular contractions started after 4 hours and she presented to the labour ward later that night. On abdominal examination, she was assessed to have an average size fetus with one-fifth of the head palpable, confirming engagement. She had regular painful contractions at a rate of 3–4 in 10 and was coping well. The cervix was soft, central, effaced and 4 cm dilated with the vertex 2 cm above the ischial spines. The liquor continued to be clear. She was transferred to a labour room in spontaneous labour. She was monitored with intermittent auscultation of the FHR at 15-minute intervals and her vital signs were checked every 4 hours. The contractions spaced out to 2 in every 10 minutes and, 8 hours after admission, she was found to be 6 cm dilated.

What is the diagnosis and what are the management options?

ANSWER

This is arrest of labour in the first stage (primary arrest), most likely due to inefficient uterine contractions. The membranes have ruptured spontaneously and therefore the next option is to commence an oxytocin infusion to augment labour. In this case, Ms A progressed to full dilatation 4 hours after commencing oxytocin and progressed to a spontaneous vaginal birth.

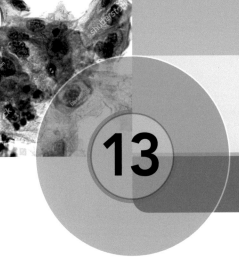

Operative delivery

13

DEIRDRE J MURPHY

Learning Objectives
- Understand the assessment and management of perineal tears.
- Understand the assessment and management of episiotomy.
- Understand the indications, contraindications, procedures and complications of assisted vaginal birth with vacuum or forceps.
- Understand the indications, procedure, complications and consequences of caesarean section.
- Introduce the concept of risk management in relation to operative delivery.

INTRODUCTION

Operative delivery encompasses caesarean section, assisted vaginal birth by vacuum or forceps, episiotomy and repair of perineal tears. While most women aim for a spontaneous vaginal birth with an intact perineum, referred to as a "normal birth", this outcome is achieved in barely half of all women who labour in high-income settings. The most common form of operative intervention is suturing of a perineal tear or episiotomy. Uncomplicated perineal tears and episiotomies are usually repaired by a midwife but, if the tear is complex, it will require repair in an operating theatre by an obstetrician. Women who encounter complications that require urgent delivery in the first stage of labour (for either maternal or fetal indications) will need an emergency caesarean section. Complications that require expedited birth in the second stage of labour present a choice between assisted

vaginal birth with a vacuum or forceps and delivery by caesarean section. A further group of women will have a scheduled caesarean section performed before the onset of labour. In all cases, operative intervention should be performed only when the benefits outweigh the potential risks. The needs of the mother and the baby should be balanced with careful consideration of the potential consequences in the short term and long term. Operative deliveries should be performed only by clinicians who have competency in the procedure or under direct supervision of an experienced trainer.

PERINEAL REPAIR

The first important step following the birth of a baby and the delivery of the placenta is to assess the woman carefully to identify and classify any perineal tearing. A complete assessment includes both vaginal and

10.1201/9781003196112-13

- First-degree tears are lacerations of the skin or vaginal epithelium only.
- Second-degree tears involve perineal muscles and includes episiotomy.
- Third-degree tears involve any part of the anal sphincter complex (external or internal):
    - 3a: less than 50% of the external anal sphincter is torn
    - 3b: more than 50% of the external anal sphincter is torn
    - 3c: the tear involves the internal anal sphincter and/or complete disruption of the external sphincter
- Fourth-degree tears involve the anal sphincter complex extending into the rectal mucosa.

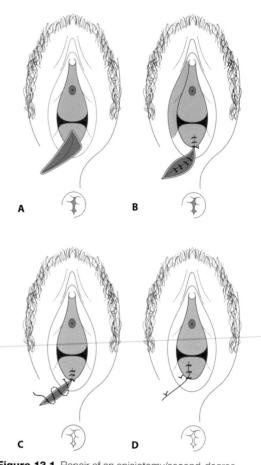

Figure 13.1 Repair of an episiotomy/second-degree perineal tear. (**A**) The perineum prior to the repair. (**B**) Continuous repair of the vaginal mucosa. (**C**) Subcutaneous suture of the skin. (**D**) Completed repair.

rectal examination. Eighty-five per cent of women who have a vaginal birth will have some degree of perineal trauma and 60–70% will require suturing. Perineal tears should be classified as first-, second-, third- or fourth-degree tears and, when in doubt, the operator should classify according to a higher rather than a lower grade (see **Box 13.1**, 'Classification of perineal tears'). This will ensure that the woman receives optimal care.

Perineal massage can be performed in the antenatal period and this may reduce the risk or extent of tearing. Similarly, the use of warm compresses, gentle perineal support and controlled crowning of the fetal head may reduce trauma at the time of birth. Perineal tears occur more commonly with prolonged labour, especially prolonged pushing, with big babies, malposition such as occipito-posterior and in association with forceps or vacuum-assisted delivery. Third- and fourth-degree tears are grouped together and termed obstetric anal sphincter injuries (OASIs). OASIs are reported in approximately 3% of nulliparous and 0.5% of multiparous individuals. In general terms, external anal sphincter incompetence causes faecal urgency, whereas internal anal sphincter incompetence causes faecal incontinence.

SURGICAL TECHNIQUE

First-degree tears or minor lacerations with minimal or no bleeding may not require surgical repair and will heal spontaneously. Second-degree tears and episiotomies require surgical repair. A systematic approach should be followed for perineal repair (**Figure 13.1**). An explanation should be provided to the mother and verbal consent should be documented or, if a complex tear requires repair in an operating theatre, written consent should be gained. Adequate analgesia should be provided by infiltration with local anaesthetic or topping up an epidural. The operator should recheck the extent of grazes and lacerations with a vaginal and rectal examination. Sometimes, the anatomy is distorted and assessment is improved following positioning in lithotomy with effective anaesthesia. If a tear is more complex than initially appreciated, a more experienced operator may be required.

It may be helpful to place a pad or tampon high in the vagina to prevent blood loss from the uterus obscuring the view. Care needs to be taken that this is removed at the end of the procedure. The vaginal mucosa is repaired first using rapidly absorbable suture material on a large, round body needle. A knot should be tied above the apex of the cut or tear (as severed vessels retract slightly) and a continuous stitch should be used to close the vaginal mucosa. Interrupted sutures are then placed to close the muscle layer. Closure of the perineal skin follows with either interrupted sutures or a continuous subcuticular stitch, which produces more comfortable results. A gentle vaginal examination should be performed to check for any missed tears and to ensure that good apposition has been achieved. A rectal examination should be performed to confirm that the sphincter feels intact and to ensure that no sutures have been inadvertently placed through the rectal mucosa. If sutures are felt in the rectum they must be removed and replaced. The pad or tampon should be removed and a careful count of swabs, instruments and needles should be completed and documented in the records alongside the operation note and post-operative instructions. Analgesia should be prescribed.

OBSTETRIC ANAL SPHINCTER INJURY REPAIR

Repair of third- and fourth-degree tears should be performed or directly supervised by a trained practitioner. There must be adequate analgesia. In practice, this means either a regional or a general anaesthetic, as local infiltration does not allow relaxation of the sphincter enough to allow a satisfactory repair. The lighting must be adequate and an assistant is usually needed. Repair of the rectal mucosa and/or internal anal sphincter should be performed first. The torn external sphincter is then repaired. It is important to ensure that the muscle is correctly approximated with long-acting sutures so that the muscle is given adequate time to heal. Some surgeons opt for an end-to-end repair, while others use an overlap technique; current evidence suggests that the outcome is similar with both methods. The remainder of the perineal repair is the same as for second-degree trauma. The surgical repair should be documented and a clinical incident form should be completed for risk assessment purposes.

OBSTETRIC ANAL SPHINCTER INJURY AFTERCARE

Lactulose (laxative) and a bulk agent, such as ispaghula husk, are recommended for 5–10 days and the woman should remain in hospital until she has had a first bowel motion. An oral broad-spectrum antibiotic should be prescribed for 5 to 7 days to reduce the risk of infection. Regular oral analgesia should also be prescribed. All women who have sustained a third- or fourth-degree tear should be offered follow-up in the postnatal period. A team approach via a specialist perineal clinic is ideal; physiotherapy should include augmented biofeedback, as this has been shown to improve continence. At 6–12 weeks, a full evaluation of the degree of symptoms should take place. This must include careful questioning regarding urinary and faecal symptoms and advice in relation to future pregnancy and delivery. Asymptomatic women should be advised that the risk of recurrence in a future pregnancy is 6–8% and that vaginal birth is safely achievable. Symptomatic women should be offered investigation including endoanal ultrasound and manometry (see **Chapter 15**). Women with ongoing troublesome symptoms should be offered an elective caesarean section for future deliveries.

EPISIOTOMY

An episiotomy is a surgical incision of the perineum performed during the second stage of labour to enlarge the vulval outlet and assist vaginal birth. Although episiotomies were described in textbooks dating back to the mid-18th century, widespread use of the procedure increased during the early 20th century. By the 1970s, rates were as high as 90% and it was widely believed that episiotomy was preferable to tearing. A number of randomized controlled trials were conducted comparing restrictive versus routine use of episiotomy. The evidence was collated in a Cochrane systematic review, which demonstrated that a restrictive approach resulted in less posterior perineal trauma and less need for suturing with no difference in pain, urinary incontinence or dyspareunia. A routine episiotomy was not protective of more severe perineal tears (OASIs). In the UK, rates now approximate the World Health Organization recommendation of 10% of spontaneous vaginal births; however, there remains considerable international variation (rates are 50% in the USA and 99% in Eastern Europe). Episiotomy is more commonly indicated as part of assisted vaginal birth, particularly for forceps and nulliparous women.

SURGICAL TECHNIQUE

An episiotomy is performed in the second stage of labour, usually when the perineum is being stretched and it is deemed necessary, for example when the birth needs to be expedited for a fetal bradycardia or pushing is prolonged due to a tight perineum. The issue of consent to episiotomy should be addressed as part of antenatal education; when the fetal head is crowning, it is difficult to obtain true informed consent. If epidural anaesthesia is in place and time allows, it should be topped up prior to cutting with the patient upright to get best coverage of the perineal area. In the absence of an effective epidural, the perineum should be infiltrated with local anaesthetic.

A mediolateral episiotomy at a 60° angle to the midline is recommended. A midline episiotomy is an incision in a comparatively avascular area and results in less bleeding, quicker healing and less pain; however, there is an increased risk of extension to involve the anal sphincter (OASI). A mediolateral episiotomy should start at the posterior part of the fourchette and be angled at 60° away from the anal sphincter, so that any extension will avoid the sphincter (**Figure 13.2**). The episiotomy should be repaired in the same way as a second-degree tear unless there has been involvement of the anal sphincter complex requiring an OASI repair in theatre.

COMPLICATIONS

Short-term complications of perineal trauma or episiotomy include pain, infection and haemorrhage. Long-term effects include dyspareunia, incontinence of urine and incontinence of flatus or faeces. The risks are highest with OASI, especially if an anal sphincter injury has been missed. These morbidities can have a profound impact on women's health, relationships and self-esteem.

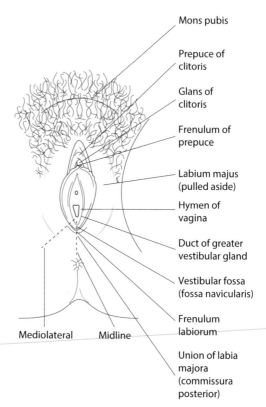

Figure 13.2 A right mediolateral episiotomy.

KEY LEARNING POINTS

- First- or second-degree tearing and uncomplicated episiotomy can be repaired under epidural or local anaesthesia in a labour room by a midwife or obstetrician.
- Assessment of the anal sphincter complex is essential in all cases to ensure that a third- or fourth-degree tear (OASI) has not been missed.
- Third- or fourth-degree tears require regional anaesthesia and are usually repaired in an operating theatre by an obstetrician with good lighting and an assistant.
- Either 'end-to-end' or overlap repair of the anal sphincter muscle with a long-acting suture material is acceptable.
- Aftercare is important for all women who tear, but women with OASI should receive antibiotics,

(Contd.)

(Contd.)
stool softeners and follow-up specialist review including physiotherapy.

- Women who experience significant pelvic floor symptoms following OASI should be offered an elective caesarean section in a future pregnancy.
- Mediolateral episiotomy should be performed in preference to midline, and it should be used restrictively.

ASSISTED VAGINAL BIRTH

Assisted vaginal birth (AVB) refers to a vaginal birth with the use of any type of forceps or vacuum extractor (ventouse). The terms instrumental delivery, operative vaginal delivery and AVB are used interchangeably. The latter is preferred, as the focus is on assisting the mother. The goal of AVB is to expedite the birth with a minimum of maternal or neonatal morbidity. As with other forms of intrapartum intervention, AVB should be performed only when the safety criteria have been met and when the benefits outweigh the risks. The guidelines of the Royal College of Obstetricians and Gynaecologists (RCOG) advise that obstetricians should achieve experience in spontaneous vaginal birth prior to commencing training in AVBs. AVBs should be conducted by obstetricians with competency in the chosen procedure or by trainees under direct supervision of an experienced trainer. When these conditions are adhered to, the outcomes of AVB are good.

In the UK, between 10% and 15% of deliveries are assisted with forceps or ventouse. The rate in nulliparous women is as high as 30%. The incidence of AVB varies widely both within and between countries and this has an impact on rates of second-stage caesarean section. Different strategies have been employed to help lower rates of AVB, including provision of one-to-one midwifery care in labour, the presence of a birth partner, delayed pushing in the second stage of labour especially with epidural analgesia, the use of oxytocin to enhance expulsive contractions in the second stage of labour and maternal repositioning to increase the effects of gravity and the maternal urge to push.

HISTORICAL PERSPECTIVE

The history of AVB is fascinating. Although the use of birth instruments was initially limited to the extraction of dead fetuses via destructive techniques, from as early as 1500 BC there have been reports of successful deliveries of live infants in obstructed labour. In the 16th and 17th centuries, the male midwife appeared as a new health practitioner and frequently dealt with obstructed labour. The development of the modern obstetric forceps by the Chamberlens, a Huguenot family practising in England, dramatically changed the role of assisted delivery in favour of a live infant. The Chamberlens kept their secret for more than a century; however, it is thought that Peter Chamberlen the elder was the pioneer in the development of forceps. Hugh Chamberlen, his son, unsuccessfully tried to persuade the great French obstetrician François Mauriceau to adopt obstetric forceps. Hugh Chamberlen's visit to Paris failed miserably when Mauriceau mischievously challenged him to deliver the baby of a mother in obstructed labour with a contracted pelvis due to rickets; Chamberlen's futile efforts had disastrous effects and both mother and baby succumbed. Nonetheless, forceps-assisted delivery became more widely accepted in part due to the work of William Smellie, a Scottish doctor working in the poorer parts of London. Smellie was a great teacher and described the use of forceps in his *Treatise on the Theory and Practice of Midwifery*, published in 1752. In 1849, the Edinburgh professor of obstetrics James Young Simpson, subsequently known for pioneering the use of chloroform in childbirth, designed the Air Tractor, which consisted of a metal syringe attached to a soft rubber cup. This was the earliest known vacuum extractor to assist childbirth. However, it did not gain widespread use until the 1950s, when it was popularized in a series of studies by Tage Malmstrom, a Swedish obstetrician. AVB remains controversial to this day.

INDICATIONS

The indications for AVB can be divided into fetal and maternal indications, although in many cases these factors coexist. The most common fetal indication is suspected fetal compromise usually based on cardiotocograph (CTG) abnormalities. The most common maternal indication is a prolonged active second stage of labour. The underlying aetiology for a prolonged second stage should be evaluated in terms of the 3Ps ('powers', 'passages' and 'passenger'; see **Chapter 12**). It may relate to inefficient uterine activity or poor maternal pushing ('powers'), short maternal stature, a less favourable pelvic shape or a tight perineum ('passages'), a macrosomic fetus, malposition or malpresentation ('passenger'). A mismatch between the passages and the passenger may result in cephalopelvic disproportion. Depending on the overall clinical findings, it may be appropriate to use an oxytocin infusion, change the maternal position and offer further encouragement, or proceed directly to AVB. In some cases, the findings will be a contraindication to AVB and favour delivery by caesarean section. The indications are summarised in **Table 13.1**. The complexity of the procedure is

Table 13.1 Indications for AVB

Type	Indication
Fetal	Suspected fetal compromise (pathological cardiotocograph, abnormal pH or lactate on fetal blood sampling, meconium)
Maternal	Nulliparous women: lack of continuing progress for 3 hours (total of active and passive second stage of labour) with regional anaesthesia or 2 hours without regional anaesthesia
	Multiparous women: lack of continuing progress for 2 hours (total of active and passive second stage of labour) with regional anaesthesia or 1 hour without regional anaesthesia
	Maternal exhaustion/distress
	Medical indications to avoid prolonged pushing or Valsalva (e.g. cardiac disease, hypertensive crisis, cerebral vascular disease, uncorrected cerebral vascular malformations, myasthenia gravis, spinal cord injury)
Combined	Fetal and maternal indications for assisted vaginal birth often coexist

Source: International guidelines (Royal College of Obstetricians and Gynaecologists, American Congress of Obstetricians and Gynecologists and UK National Institute for Health and Care Excellence) largely agree on second stage duration. Note, no indication is absolute and each case should be considered individually.

Table 13.2 Classification of AVB

Type	Classification
Outlet	Fetal scalp visible without separating the labia
	Fetal skull has reached the pelvic floor
	Rotation does not exceed 45°
Low	Leading point of the skull is at station +2 cm or more but not on the pelvic floor
	Two subdivisions: (a) rotation of 45° or less and (b) rotation more than 45°
Mid	Fetal head is no more than one-fifth palpable per abdomen, usually zero fifths
	Leading point of the skull is above station +2 cm but not above the ischial spines (station 0 to +1)
	Two subdivisions: (a) rotation of 45° or less and (b) rotation of more than 45°
High	Not appropriate; therefore, not included in classification (station −1 or above)

Source: Adapted from Royal College of Obstetricians and Gynaecologists (2020) and American Congress of Obstetricians and Gynecologists (2015).

reflected in how low the fetal head has descended within the pelvis (station) and whether rotation is required. The classification system is described in **Table 13.2**.

CONTRAINDICATIONS

A careful assessment should take place to ensure that the safety criteria for AVB have been fulfilled (**Table 13.3**). When the safety criteria are not met, AVB is contraindicated, for example a high fetal head two-fifths palpable abdominally with station above the ischial spines. The vacuum should not be used in gestations of less than 34 completed weeks because of the risk of cephalohaematoma and intracranial haemorrhage. It is relatively contraindicated at gestational ages of 35–36 weeks. It should not be used for a face or breech presentation. There is minimal additional risk of fetal haemorrhage if the vacuum extractor is employed following fetal blood sampling or application of a fetal scalp electrode. Forceps and vacuum extractor deliveries before full dilatation of the cervix are contraindicated.

Table 13.3 Safety criteria for assisted vaginal birth

Area	Criteria
Full abdominal and vaginal examination	Head is fully engaged (zero fifths palpable) or no more than one-fifth palpable per abdomen
	Cervix is fully dilated and the membranes ruptured
	Station at level of ischial spines or below (0/+1/+2/+3)
	Exact position of the head has been determined so correct placement of the instrument can be achieved
	Caput and moulding is no more than moderate (+ or ++)
	Pelvis is deemed adequate
Preparation of the mother	Clear explanation given and informed consent obtained
	Trust has been established and the woman offers full cooperation
	Appropriate anaesthesia is in place; for mid-pelvic rotational delivery this will usually be a regional block; a pudendal block may be appropriate, in the context of urgency; a perineal block may be sufficient for low-pelvic or outlet delivery
	Maternal bladder has been emptied recently
	In-dwelling catheter has been removed or balloon deflated
	Aseptic technique
Preparation of staff	Operator has the knowledge, experience and skill necessary
	Adequate facilities are available (appropriate equipment, bed, lighting) and access to an operating theatre
	Back-up plan in place in case of failure to deliver. For mid-pelvic deliveries, theatre staff should be available immediately to allow a caesarean section to be performed without delay (<30 minutes); senior obstetrician should be present if a junior obstetrician is conducting the delivery
	Anticipation of complications that may arise (e.g. shoulder dystocia, post-partum haemorrhage)
	Personnel present that are trained in neonatal resuscitation

Source: Adapted from RCOG Guidelines 2020.

CHOICE OF INSTRUMENT

The guidelines of the RCOG in the UK recommend that obstetricians should be competent and confident in the use of both forceps and vacuum and that practitioners should choose the most appropriate instrument for the individual circumstances. The choice of instrument should be based on a combination of indication, experience and training. The aim should be to complete the delivery successfully with the lowest possible morbidity, and the preferences of the mother should be taken into account. Vacuum and forceps have been compared in a number of randomized controlled trials within a Cochrane systematic review.

The incidence of maternal pelvic floor trauma in deliveries performed with the vacuum is significantly less than with forceps and OASI in particular is twice as common with forceps delivery (8% versus 3–4%). While long-term follow-up data are limited, one of the largest randomized controlled trials showed no difference in pelvic floor symptoms between women delivered by forceps or vacuum when assessed at approximately 5 years after the birth. Vacuum is preferred as a first-line instrument by many obstetricians in terms of reduced maternal trauma, but this needs to be balanced with a failure rate of 10–20% compared with a failure rate with forceps of 5% or less for similar deliveries. The morbidities for the baby differ, with a higher incidence of cephalohaematoma and cerebral haemorrhage with vacuum and a higher incidence of lacerations and facial palsy with forceps.

Vacuum (compared with forceps) is significantly more likely to be associated with:

- failure to achieve a vaginal birth
- cephalohaematoma (subperiosteal bleed)
- retinal haemorrhage
- maternal worries about the baby

Vacuum (compared with forceps) is significantly less likely to be associated with:

- the use of maternal regional/general anaesthesia
- significant maternal perineal and vaginal trauma
- severe perineal pain at 24 hours

Vacuum and forceps are similar in terms of:

- delivery by caesarean section (where failed vacuum is completed by forceps)
- low 5-minute Apgar scores

PLACE OF DELIVERY/RISK OF FAILURE

AVBs in the mid-pelvis (station 0/+1) are more difficult either because there is a malposition and rotation is required or because there is relative cephalopelvic disproportion (see **Table 13.2**). These deliveries require a higher degree of skill and there is a higher risk of failure. The alternative is to deliver by caesarean section, which can also be very challenging with the head deep in the pelvis, resulting in fetal impaction where the head is wedged and difficult to elevate into the abdominal wound. The safest approach for mid-pelvic or rotational AVB is to perform these deliveries in an operating theatre with timely recourse to caesarean section if required.

There have been no randomized controlled trials comparing AVB with second-stage caesarean section and the decision relies on clinical judgement. A prospective cohort study in the UK reported that women who were delivered by caesarean section in the second stage of labour were more likely to have a major haemorrhage and prolonged hospital stay than women delivered by AVB, whereas babies delivered by caesarean section were less likely to have trauma but were more likely to require admission to the neonatal unit than those delivered by AVB. What was striking was the outcome of subsequent births, with almost 70% of women who had a second-stage caesarean section going on to have a repeat caesarean section in the next birth, compared with only 10% of women whose first birth was successful AVB. It is therefore usual to aim for AVB in the second stage of labour rather than caesarean section, unless there are contraindications or the woman expresses a clear preference for caesarean section. It is essential that skilled obstetricians are present to supervise complex operative deliveries performed by trainees, whatever the time of day or night.

PROCEDURE

The anatomy of the birth canal and its relationship to the fetal head must be understood as a prerequisite to becoming skilled in the safe use of forceps or vacuum (see **Chapter 12**).

ASSESSMENT

A thorough abdominal and vaginal examination should take place to confirm the fetal lie, presentation, engagement, station, position, attitude and degree of caput or moulding. This will confirm whether the basic safety criteria for AVB have been met. A pelvic examination will determine whether there are any 'mechanical' contraindications to performing an AVB. If, for example, a contracted pelvis is the cause of failure to progress in the second stage, then consideration should be given to the choice of instrument or whether it may be more prudent to perform a caesarean section. The angle of the subpubic arch, the curve of the sacral hollow and the presence of flat or prominent ischial spines all contribute to the decision of whether an AVB may be safely performed. Anthropoid (narrow), android (male/funnel-shaped) or platypelloid (elliptical) pelvises all make instrumental deliveries more difficult and may preclude the use of rotational forceps. Assessment during a trial push is very helpful in determining whether descent occurs, and it may also be possible to attempt manual rotation of a fetal malposition at this point.

ANALGESIA

Analgesic requirements are greater for forceps than for vacuum-assisted births. When rotational forceps or mid-pelvic direct traction forceps are needed, regional analgesia is preferred. For a rigid cup vacuum-assisted delivery, a pudendal block with perineal infiltration may be all that is needed and, if a soft cup is used, analgesic requirements may be limited to perineal infiltration with local anaesthetic.

POSITIONING

AVBs are traditionally performed with the patient in the lithotomy position. The angle of traction needed requires that the bottom part of the bed be removed. In patients with limited abduction (such as those with symphysis pubis dysfunction), it may be necessary to limit abduction of the thighs to a minimum. The bladder should be emptied with a catheter to avoid injury.

CONTINGENCY PLANNING

With any AVB, there is the potential for failure with the chosen instrument and the operator must have a back-up plan for such an event. It may be possible to complete a failed vacuum-assisted birth with low-pelvic forceps, but failed or abandoned forceps delivery will almost always result in caesarean section. With any difficult AVB, the risk of shoulder dystocia after successful delivery of the fetal head should be considered, as should the potential for post-partum haemorrhage. The operator must develop the skills necessary to anticipate such events and to manage the consequences in a logical and calm manner. If the AVB is being performed for suspected fetal compromise, then the need for neonatal resuscitation should be anticipated and a neonatologist should have been called to attend.

INSTRUMENT TYPES

VENTOUSE/VACUUM EXTRACTORS

The basic premise of vacuum extraction is that a suction cup, of a silastic or rigid construction, is connected, via tubing, to a vacuum source (**Figure 13.3**). Either directly through the tubing or via a connecting 'chain', direct traction can then be applied to the

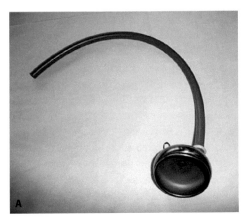

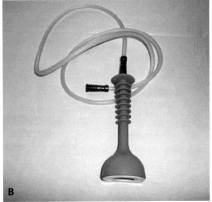

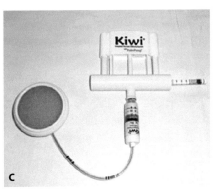

Figure 13.3 Ventouse/vacuum extractor cups. (**A**) Metal ventouse cup. (**B**) Silicone rubber cup. (**C**) OmniCup™.

239

presenting part coordinated with maternal pushing to expedite birth. Recent developments have removed the need for cumbersome external suction generators and have incorporated the vacuum mechanism into 'hand-held' pumps (e.g. OmniCup™). Initial clinical trials suggested that the failure rate is higher with hand-held disposable devices, but this may have related to the learning curve of adapting to new instruments. More recent large case series have reported success rates similar to that of standard vacuum devices.

Technique

Soft vacuum cups are significantly more likely to fail to achieve vaginal delivery than rigid cups; however, they are associated with less scalp injury. There appears to be no difference in terms of maternal trauma. The soft cups are appropriate for uncomplicated deliveries with an occipito-anterior position; metal or rigid cups appear to be more suitable for occipito-posterior, transverse and potentially difficult occipito-anterior position deliveries in which the infant is larger or there is more caput.

For successful use of the vacuum, determination of the flexion point is vital. This is located at the vertex, which, in an average term infant, is on the sagittal suture 3 cm anterior to the posterior fontanelle and thus 6 cm posterior to the anterior fontanelle. The centre of the cup should be positioned directly over this, as failure to do so will lead to progressive deflexion of the fetal head during traction and an inability to deliver the baby safely.

The operating vacuum pressure for nearly all types of device is between 0.6 and 0.8 kg/cm². It is prudent to increase the suction to 0.2 kg/cm² first and then to recheck that no maternal tissue is caught under the cup edge. When this is confirmed, the suction can then be increased.

Traction must occur in the plane of least resistance along the axis of the pelvis – the traction plane (**Figure 13.4**). This will usually be at exactly 90° to the cup and the operator should keep a thumb and forefinger on the cup and fetal scalp to ensure that the traction direction is correct and to feel for slippage. Safe and gentle traction is then applied coordinated with uterine contractions and voluntary maternal expulsive efforts. There is a descent phase, bringing the head onto the perineum, which is usually

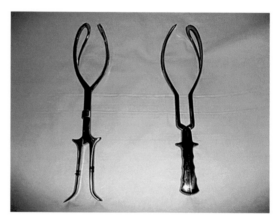

Figure 13.4 Kielland rotational forceps (left) and Simpson non-rotational forceps (right).

achieved in at most three pulls. The crowning phase should occur shortly afterwards and, depending on the resistance of the perineum, may occur with one further pull or some operators prefer to use up to three very small pulls to minimize perineal trauma. With any vacuum, the operator should allow no more than two episodes of breaking the suction 'pop-offs' in a vacuum-assisted birth, and the maximum time from application to delivery should ideally be less than 15 minutes. Rotation is achieved by the natural progression of the head through the pelvis.

It is not acceptable to use a vacuum when the position of the fetal head is unknown, there is a significant degree of caput that may either preclude correct placement of the cup or, more sinisterly, indicate a substantial degree of cephalopelvic disproportion, or the operator is inexperienced in the use of the instrument. For a demonstration video, please see https://www.youtube.com/watch?v=OMFa0gtpBQc.

FORCEPS

Types of forceps

The basic forceps design has not changed radically over many years and all types in use today consist of two blades with shanks, joined together at a lock, with handles to provide a point for traction. The specific details of construction vary between instruments. Non-rotational forceps are used when the head is occipito-anterior with no more than 45° deviation to the left or right. Examples such as Neville Barnes or Simpson forceps (see **Figure 13.4**) have a pelvic curve and a non-sliding lock. If the head is positioned more than 45° from the vertical, rotation must be accomplished before traction. Forceps designed for rotation, such as Kielland forceps, have minimal pelvic curve to allow rotation around a fixed axis; the sliding lock of the Kielland forceps (see **Figure 13.4**) facilitates correction of asynclitism (lateral tilt).

TECHNIQUE

For forceps, all of the usual prerequisites for safe AVB apply, but, in addition, it is essential that the operator checks the pair of forceps to ensure that a matching pair has been provided and that the blades lock with ease (both before and after application). By convention, the left blade is inserted before the right with the operator's hand protecting the vaginal wall from the blades. With proper placement of the forceps blades, they come to lie parallel to the axis of the fetal head and between the fetal head and the pelvic wall. The operator then articulates and locks the blades, checking their application before applying traction (**Figure 13.5**).

Traction should be applied intermittently, coordinated with uterine contractions and maternal expulsive efforts. The axis of traction changes during the delivery and is guided along the J-shaped curve of the pelvis. As the head begins to crown, the blades

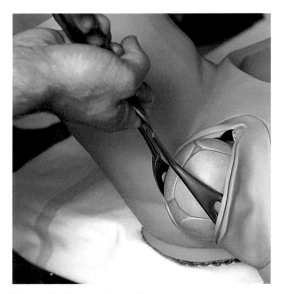

Figure 13.5 Application of forceps.

are directed to the vertical and the head is delivered. Forceps-assisted births should be completed in no more than three pulls. Specific techniques are required for rotational forceps deliveries and only those who have been properly trained in their use should employ them. Rotation occurs between contractions and the descent phase is similar to non-rotational forceps.

The role of episiotomy at vacuum and forceps delivery is controversial, with conflicting studies reported. A randomized controlled trial reported that a routine approach to episiotomy was neither protective nor associated with an increased risk of OASI, but the sample size was insufficient to draw definitive conclusions. In practice, most obstetricians cut an episiotomy routinely for forceps-assisted delivery especially in nulliparous births where anal sphincter damage is more likely. In parous women, particularly those requiring vacuum-assisted birth, an episiotomy may not be necessary. For a demonstration video, please see https://pie.med.utoronto.ca/TVASurg/project/routine-forceps-delivery/.

SPECIAL CONSIDERATIONS

FAILURE OF THE CHOSEN INSTRUMENT

Failure to complete delivery vaginally can occur when the choice of instrument is wrong (e.g. silastic vacuum where there is marked caput), when the application of the instrument is wrong (e.g. vacuum cup application over the anterior fontanelle) or when the position has been wrongly defined (most commonly occipito-posterior/occipito-anterior errors), leading to inappropriately large diameters presenting to the pelvis. Failure is also more common if the fetus is large or maternal effort is poor.

There have been no randomized studies assessing the best approach to take following failure to deliver with the first choice of instrument. Observational studies show that outcomes for babies are worse with multiple or sequential use of instruments than if the instrument of first choice is successful. In addition, the rates of third- and fourth-degree tears are higher when a second instrument is used. The operator must choose the approach most likely to result in timely delivery with the least morbidity.

When the first instrument fails, a number of scenarios may apply. If the reason for failure was cup detachment of a vacuum and the fetal head is occipito-anterior and on the perineum, low-pelvic or lift-out forceps to complete delivery is acceptable and likely to be less traumatic than a second-stage caesarean section. If the instrument failed because there was little or no descent with the first pull of a correctly applied instrument with traction in the correct axis of the pelvis, then delivery must be by caesarean section, as the likely diagnosis is cephalopelvic disproportion. If the instrument failed because the position was incorrectly defined, then the next option will be either a rotational instrumental delivery or a caesarean section. If there is any uncertainty, senior help should be sought immediately and a full re-evaluation should take place, ideally in an operating theatre. In many cases, delivery by caesarean section will be the safer option for the fetus.

COMPLICATIONS

The risk of fetal trauma in relation to forceps-assisted birth, particularly rotational procedures, has been long established. There is now a growing recognition that vacuum-assisted birth can also be associated with significant morbidity. In addition, there has been a growing recognition of the short- and long-term morbidity of maternal pelvic floor injury following AVB. This can result in incontinence (urinary or faecal) or pelvic floor prolapse. It is not surprising, therefore, that there has been an increase in litigation relating to vacuum and forceps-assisted births. If we are to offer women the option of safe AVBs, we need to improve our approach to clinical care. The goal should be to minimize the risk of morbidity and, where morbidity occurs, to optimize early recognition and aftercare. It is also important to remember that caesarean section, particularly in the second stage of labour, carries significant morbidity and implications for future births.

AVBs with both vacuum and forceps can be associated with significant maternal and fetal complications. Traumatic vaginal birth is considered to be the most important risk factor for faecal incontinence in women and may occur not only after recognized third-degree perineal tears, but also as a consequence of unrecognized anal sphincter injury. Postpartum haemorrhage is more common in women needing AVB than in women who deliver spontaneously, but is less common than in women delivered by caesarean section in the second stage. Measures to limit this include early recognition of abnormal bleeding and the use of an oxytocin infusion post-delivery, prompt suturing and careful identification of high vaginal wall tears.

Fetal complications are no less important; the incidence of cephalohaematoma is increased with the use of the vacuum and there are rare reports of life-threatening intracranial injuries such as subgaleal haemorrhage. Forceps-assisted injuries include facial palsy, intra- or extra-cranial haemorrhage and skull fracture. Risks of trauma to the baby correlate with the duration of the procedure, the station of the fetal head at the commencement of the procedure, the need for rotation and the condition of the fetus immediately prior to attempted AVB. It is important to remember that the risks of traumatic injury increase significantly among babies who are exposed to multiple attempts at both vacuum and forceps-assisted delivery and this should be avoided by careful case selection and contingency planning.

🔑 KEY LEARNING POINTS

- AVB should be classified according to the position and station of the presenting part.
- Clinical assessment and confirmation that the safety criteria have been met are essential prior to AVB.
- Vacuum or forceps may be suitable depending on the clinical circumstances and operator's preference.
- AVBs with a higher chance of failure should be conducted in an operating theatre.
- Contingency planning is an essential part of any AVB.
- Anticipation and early management of maternal and neonatal complications is essential.

CAESAREAN SECTION

A caesarean section is a surgical procedure in which incisions are made through the abdomen (laparotomy) and uterus (hysterotomy) to deliver one or more babies. In the UK and other high-income countries, between 25% and 35% of all babies are now delivered by caesarean section. The principal aims should be to ensure that women who need delivery by caesarean section receive it and that those who do not avoid unnecessary intervention. In 1985, concern regarding the increasing frequency of caesarean section led the World Health Organization to hold a consensus conference. This conference concluded that there were no health benefits above a caesarean section rate of 10–15%. More recently it has been suggested that there is maternal and neonatal benefit with caesarean section rates up to 19%. Despite this, rates of caesarean section continue to increase year on year with marked variation both nationally and internationally.

HISTORICAL PERSPECTIVE

There are three theories about the origin of the name caesarean. It is said to derive from a Roman legal code called *Lex Caesarea*, which allegedly contained a law prescribing that the baby be cut out of its mother's womb if she died before giving birth. The derivation of the name is also attributed to an ancient story, told in the first century AD by Pliny the Elder, who claimed that an ancestor of Caesar was delivered in this way. An alternative etymology suggests that the procedure's name derives from the Latin verb *caedere*, to cut. Caesar's mother, Aurelia, lived through childbirth and successfully gave birth to her son, ruling out the possibility that the Roman dictator and general was born by caesarean section. However, the Catalan saint, Raymond Nonnatus (1204–1240), received his surname (from the Latin *non natus*, not born) because he was born by caesarean section; his mother died while giving birth to him. The first recorded incidence of a woman surviving a caesarean section was in 1500 in Switzerland: Jakob Nufer, a pig gelder, is supposed to have performed the operation on his wife after a prolonged labour. From the 16th century onwards, the procedure had a high mortality and was performed only when the mother was already dead or considered to be beyond help. In Great Britain and Ireland, the mortality rate in 1865 was 85%. On 5 March 2000, Inés Ramírez performed a caesarean section on herself and survived, as did her son. She is believed to be the only woman to have performed a successful caesarean section on herself.

Key steps in reducing mortality at caesarean section were:

- adherence to principles of asepsis
- introduction of uterine suturing by Max Sänger in 1882
- extraperitoneal caesarean section and then moving to low transverse incision
- anaesthetic advances
- blood transfusion
- antibiotic prophylaxis and treatment

CLASSIFICATION

Traditionally, caesarean sections have been classified as elective or emergency. Elective caesarean sections are usually booked days or weeks ahead of time and are conducted during daytime hours. There is sometimes confusion between elective caesarean section and emergency caesarean section prior to labour. This can be overcome by using the term scheduled caesarean section for procedures that are planned ahead of time. All other caesarean sections can be classified as emergency, irrespective of whether the woman was in labour or not. The degree of urgency should be described clearly using a standard classification to ensure that there is effective communication between the members of the multidisciplinary team, particularly the theatre staff, anaesthetist and obstetrician.

INDICATIONS

There are many different reasons for performing a delivery by caesarean section. The four major

---

BOX 13.2: Classification system for emergency caesarean section

- *Category 1*: immediate threat to the life of the woman or the fetus
- *Category 2*: maternal or fetal compromise that is not immediately life threatening
- *Category 3*: requires early delivery
- *Category 4*: at a time to suit the woman and maternity services

indications accounting for greater than 70% of operations are:

1. previous caesarean section
2. malpresentation (mainly breech)
3. failure to progress in labour
4. suspected fetal compromise in labour

Other indications, such as multiple pregnancy, placental abruption, placenta praevia, fetal disease and maternal disease are less common. No list can be truly comprehensive and, whatever the indication, the overriding principle is that whenever the risk to the mother and/or the fetus from vaginal birth exceeds that from abdominal delivery, a caesarean section should be undertaken. Absolute indications for recommending delivery by caesarean section are few, almost all indications are relative and there will be circumstances in which caesarean section may be best for one woman but not for another. Maternal requests for caesarean section need to be differentiated, namely women who request caesarean section because of a previous traumatic birth experience (e.g. emergency caesarean section, difficult AVB or third-degree tear) and women who request caesarean section because they wish to avoid labour and vaginal birth. There is also increasing recognition of a condition termed tokophobia, which describes an irrational fear of childbirth that can be very incapacitating for the woman. Legally, a lack of consent in a woman with the capacity to give consent will prohibit caesarean section regardless of the perceived clinical need.

PROCEDURE

INFORMED CONSENT

Informed consent must always be obtained prior to surgery and, ideally, the possibility of caesarean section and the potential indications will have been discussed as part of antenatal education. The level of information provided in the acute setting must be commensurate with the urgency of the procedure, and a common-sense approach is needed. Although it is difficult to impart complete and thorough information when caesarean sections are performed as urgent procedures, women must understand what is being planned and why. It is important to remember that no other adult may give consent for another (although it is good practice to keep the birth partner fully informed). When there is incapacity to consent (as may occur with conditions such as eclampsia), the doctor is expected to act in the woman's best interests. The national consent forms require both the benefits and the risks to be discussed with patients and recorded on the consent form.

PREPARATION

Most scheduled caesarean sections are performed under spinal anaesthesia with the mother awake and the partner present. If an epidural has been sited during labour, there is usually sufficient time to top-up the anaesthesia in preparation for emergency caesarean section. General anaesthesia is occasionally required when regional anaesthesia is contraindicated or ineffective or when general anaesthesia is indicated due to the degree of urgency. The bladder should be emptied before the procedure commences and a urinary catheter is usually left in situ. A left lateral tilt minimizes aorto-caval compression and reduces the incidence of hypotension (and diminished placental perfusion). The anaesthetic block is confirmed and the abdomen is cleaned and draped. Prophylactic antibiotics should be administered intravenously prior to the surgical incision.

ABDOMINAL INCISION

The skin and subcutaneous tissues are incised using either (1) a transverse curvilinear incision two fingerbreadths above the symphysis pubis extending from and to points lateral to the lateral margins of the abdominal rectus muscles (pfannenstiel incision) or (2) a transverse suprapubic incision with no curve. Subcutaneous tissues are separated by blunt dissection, and the rectus sheath is incised transversely along the middle 2 cm. This incision is then extended with scissors before the fascial sheath is separated from the underlying muscle by further blunt dissection. Separation is performed cephalad to permit adequate exposure of the peritoneum in a longitudinal plane. The recti are separated, the peritoneum is incised and the abdominal cavity is entered. The transverse suprapubic incision has the advantages of improved cosmetic results, decreased analgesic requirements and superior wound strength.

A vertical skin incision is indicated in cases of extreme maternal obesity, when there is suspicion of other intra-abdominal pathology necessitating surgical intervention or when access to the uterine fundus may be required (classical caesarean section). The lower midline incision is made from the lower border of the umbilicus to the symphysis pubis and may be extended caudally towards the xiphisternum. Sharp dissection to the anterior rectus sheath is performed and is then freed of subcutaneous fat. The rectus sheath is then incised, taking care to avoid damage to any underlying bowel, and extended inferiorly to the vesical peritoneal reflection and superiorly to the upper limit of the abdominal incision. The vertical incision provides greater ease of access to the pelvic and intra-abdominal organs and may be enlarged more easily; however, the incidence of wound dehiscence is increased.

UTERINE INCISION

A lower uterine segment transverse incision is used in over 95% of caesarean deliveries due to ease of repair, reduced blood loss and low incidence of dehiscence or rupture in subsequent pregnancies (**Figure 13.6**). The loose reflection of vesico-uterine serosa overlying the uterus is incised and divided laterally, the underlying lower uterine segment is reflected with blunt dissection, the developed bladder flap is retracted and the lower uterine segment is opened in a transverse plane for a distance of 1–2 cm; the incision is extended laterally to allow delivery of the fetus without extension into the broad ligament or uterine vessels. There are relatively few absolute

indications for classical caesarean section (which incorporates the upper uterine segment in a vertical incision; see **Figure 13.6**). These include a lower uterine segment obscured by fibroids or a lower segment covered with dense adhesions, both of which may make entry difficult. Other indications include placenta praevia, transverse lie with the back down, fetal abnormality (e.g. conjoined twins) or caesarean section in the presence of a carcinoma of the cervix (so as to avoid damage to the cervix and its vascular and lymphatic supply).

Once the uterus is incised, the membranes are ruptured if still intact and the operator's hand is positioned below the presenting part. If cephalic, the head is flexed and delivered by elevation though the uterine incision either manually or with forceps. Fundal pressure is applied by the assistant to aid delivery; this should not commence until the presenting part is located within the incision for fear of converting the lie from longitudinal to transverse. Once the fetus is delivered, an oxytocic agent (5 IU Syntocinon™ intravenously) is administered to aid uterine contraction and placental separation. The placenta is delivered by controlled cord traction; manual removal significantly increases the intraoperative blood loss and post-operative infectious morbidity.

CLOSURE

Closure of the uterus should be performed in either single or double layers with continuous or interrupted sutures. The initial suture should be placed just lateral to the incision angle and the closure should be continued to a point just lateral to the angle on the opposite side. A running stitch is often used and this may be locked to improve haemostasis. A second layer is commonly used as a means to improve haemostasis and with the aim to improve the integrity of the scar. Once repaired, the incision is assessed for haemostasis and additional 'figure-of-eight' sutures can be used to control any bleeding points. Peritoneal closure is not routine and depends on the operator's preference. Abdominal closure is performed in the anatomical planes with high-strength low-reactivity materials, such as polyglycolic acid or polyglactin. The skin can be closed with either absorbable or non-absorbable suture material or with clips, again depending on operator preference.

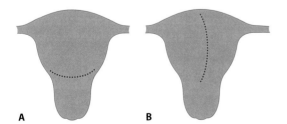

Figure 13.6 Uterine incisions for caesarean section. (**A**) Transverse lower segment incision. (**B**) Classical caesarean section incision.

COMPLICATIONS

Although caesarean section is relatively safe, the woman needs to be counselled about potential complications. Common complications include haemorrhage, infection of the wound, urinary tract or endometrium, and for the baby include transient tachypnea of the newborn. Confidential Enquiries into Maternal Deaths have enabled the risks associated with different methods of delivery to be analysed; the case fatality rate for all caesarean sections is five times that for vaginal birth, although for elective caesarean section the difference does not reach statistical significance. Some maternal deaths following caesarean section are not attributable to the procedure itself, but rather to medical or obstetric disorders that lead to the decision to deliver using this approach.

INTRAOPERATIVE COMPLICATIONS

Haemorrhage

Haemorrhage may be a consequence of damage to the uterine vessels or may be incidental as a consequence of uterine atony or placenta praevia. In patients with an anticipated high risk of haemorrhage (e.g. known cases of placenta praevia), blood should be routinely cross-matched. There are many manoeuvres to manage haemorrhage; these range from oxytocin infusion, administration of prostaglandins, bimanual compression and conservative surgical procedures (such as uterine compression sutures) to the more radical, but life-saving, hysterectomy.

Caesarean hysterectomy

The most common indication for caesarean hysterectomy is uncontrollable maternal haemorrhage; life-threatening haemorrhage requiring immediate treatment occurs in approximately 1 in 1,000 deliveries. The most important risk factor for emergency peri-partum hysterectomy is a previous caesarean section – especially when the placenta overlies the old scar, increasing the risks of placenta accreta (see **Chapter 14**). Other indications for hysterectomy are atony, uterine rupture, extension of a transverse uterine incision and fibroids preventing uterine closure and haemostasis. This operation, while a major

undertaking, should not be left too late, as the risk of operative complications, maternal morbidity and mortality increase with increasing haemorrhage.

Placenta praevia

The proportion of patients with a placenta praevia increases almost linearly after each previous caesarean section and, as the risks of such a complication increase with increasing parity, future reproductive intentions are very relevant to any individual decision for operative delivery.

Organ damage

Bowel damage may occur during a repeat procedure or if adhesions are present from previous surgery. The risk of bladder injury is increased after prolonged labours when the bladder is displaced caudally, after previous caesarean section when scarring obliterates the vesico-uterine space or when a vertical extension to the uterine incision has occurred. If damage is suspected, then transurethral instillation of methylene blue-coloured saline will help to delineate the defect. When such an injury is observed, repair with an absorbable suture as a single continuous or interrupted layer is appropriate. The urinary catheter should remain in situ for 7–10 days. Damage to the ureters is uncommon, as reflection of the bladder displaces them rostrally.

POST-OPERATIVE COMPLICATIONS

Infection

Women undergoing caesarean section have a 5–20-fold greater risk of an infectious complication than those undergoing a vaginal birth. Complications include fever, wound infection, endometritis, bacteraemia and urinary tract infection. Other common causes of post-operative fever include haematoma, atelectasis and deep vein thrombosis. Labour, its duration and the presence of ruptured membranes appear to be the most important risk factors, with obesity playing a particularly important role in the occurrence of wound infections. The most important source of microorganisms responsible for post-caesarean section infection is the genital tract, particularly if the membranes are ruptured preoperatively. Even in the presence of intact membranes, microbial invasion of the intrauterine cavity is common, especially with preterm labour. Infections are commonly polymicrobial and pathogens isolated from infected wounds and the endometrium include *Escherichia coli*, other aerobic Gram-negative rods and Group B *Streptococcus*. General principles for the prevention of any surgical infection include skin antisepsis, prophylactic antibiotics and good surgical technique.

Venous thromboembolism

Deaths from pulmonary embolism remain an important direct cause of maternal death, and caesarean section is a major risk factor. The signs and symptoms of pulmonary emboli and deep vein thrombosis are detailed in **Chapter 6**. The incidence of such complications can be reduced by adequate hydration, early mobilization and administration of prophylactic heparin. Early recognition and prompt initiation of treatment will reduce the consequences of venous thromboembolism.

Psychological

All difficult births carry increased maternal physical and psychological morbidity. The psychological well-being of women delivered by emergency caesarean section may be compromised by delayed contact with the baby – a factor that should be minimized wherever possible. The obstetrician who performed the surgery should review the woman prior to hospital discharge to discuss the indication for operative delivery, the potential for complications and the implications for the future, as well as to answer any questions the woman or her partner may have.

SUBSEQUENT BIRTH FOLLOWING CAESAREAN SECTION

In many units, caesarean section rates for primigravidae are 20–30%. Consequently, the problem of managing a woman with a previous caesarean section in a subsequent pregnancy is common. It is a vital part of antenatal care that women are given a clear understanding of the options for management from early on in their pregnancy, with the caveat that this may need to be adapted if pregnancy complications occur. The management in pregnancy following a caesarean section should be to review the previous delivery records, discuss the available options and select the appropriate choice through a shared decision-making process with the woman. The dictum popularized in the USA 'once a caesarean, always a caesarean' is misleading; up to 70% of women with a previous caesarean section who labour achieve a vaginal birth. It is important, however, to discuss the risks and benefits of elective repeat caesarean section (ERCS) compared with attempted vaginal birth after caesarean section (VBAC).

From a maternal perspective, ERCS avoids labour with its risk of pelvic floor trauma (urinary and faecal problems), the need to undergo emergency caesarean section, and scar dehiscence or rupture with subsequent morbidity and mortality. However, ERCS carries maternal risks: increased bleeding, febrile morbidity, prolonged recovery, thromboembolism, long-term bladder dysfunction and increased risks of placenta praevia/accreta in future pregnancies. From a fetal perspective, an ERCS reduces the risks associated with scar rupture, but increases the risk of transient tachypnoea or respiratory distress syndrome. There is limited robust evidence to inform decision-making, as most data relate to observational studies.

The risk of scar rupture is probably the most important clinical consideration when determining whether delivery should be by ERCS or by attempted VBAC. Most published studies do not differentiate between scar dehiscence and rupture; however, analysis of observational and comparative studies indicates that the excess risk of uterine rupture following attempted VBAC compared with women undergoing ERCS is between 0.5% and 1%.

Providing that the first operation was carried out for a non-recurrent indication and that the obstetric situation close to term in the subsequent pregnancy is favourable, then it is appropriate to offer a trial of labour after caesarean section to any woman with a single uncomplicated lower segment caesarean section and no other adverse obstetric feature. The predominant factors to consider when determining the preferred mode of delivery include the preferences of the mother, the risks of a repeat operation, the risks of labour to the baby and the risk of labour to the integrity of the uterine scar.

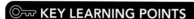

KEY LEARNING POINTS

- Caesarean section should be recommended when the benefits outweigh the risks.
- Informed written consent is required.
- Lower uterine segment caesarean section under regional anaesthesia is optimal.
- Common maternal complications include haemorrhage, infection and pain.
- Common neonatal complications include transient respiratory morbidity.
- The risks and benefits of ERCS versus VBAC require counselling on an ongoing basis.
- Up to 70% of women who labour following a single caesarean section achieve a VBAC.
- All adverse outcomes of attempted AVB and caesarean section require a clinical incident form and review.

CLINICAL RISK MANAGEMENT

Operative delivery, whether by vacuum, forceps or caesarean section, has never been free from controversy and is not without risks. Litigation is more likely to occur following perinatal death, cerebral palsy, brachial plexus injury and maternal pelvic floor damage. Common allegations against practitioners include inadequate indication for an operative delivery, inadequate supervision of less experienced operators, a lack of informed consent, excessive use of force with vacuum or forceps and delayed delivery by caesarean section. The fear of litigation should not dictate good medical practice. It is essential, however, that operators are appropriately trained in decision-making, operate within their competencies, have access to senior support (or a second opinion) and are effective communicators. Clinical incident forms should be completed as part of risk management procedures when adverse outcomes occur, and both individual and systems-based reviews are important elements of any organization with a learning culture.

FURTHER READING

Murphy DJ, Strachan BK, Bahl R; RCOG (2020). Assisted vaginal birth. *BJOG*, 127: e70–e112.

National Institute for Health and Care Excellence (NICE) (2011). *Caesarean Section*. Clinical guideline [CG 132].

RCOG (2015). Green-top Guideline No 45: Birth after previous Caesarean birth.

RCOG (2015). Green-top guideline No 29: Third- and fourth-degree perineal tears, management.

SELF-ASSESSMENT

For interactive SBAs and EMQs relating to this chapter, visit www.routledge.com/cw/mccarthy.

CASE HISTORY 1

Ms B, a 24-year-old nulliparous woman, went into spontaneous labour at 39 weeks' gestation. She had no relevant past medical history and findings on examination were unremarkable; vital signs were normal, the sympyhsis fundal height was appropriate for the gestational age, presentation was cephalic and the fetal head was engaged with one-fifth palpable abdominally. Delay in the first stage of labour led to artificial rupture of the membranes (clear liquor drained) and subsequent use of an oxytocin infusion. Ms B requested epidural analgesia, which was sited and effective. When the vaginal examination was repeated, the cervix was fully dilated, with the fetal head at the level of the ischial spines and in a right occipito-transverse position. There was minimal caput and moulding. Clear liquor continued to drain and there was a normal fetal heart rate pattern on the CTG. The midwife waited 1 hour for passive descent and then encouraged active pushing. After 50 minutes of pushing, the presenting part was just visible and there were late decelerations on the CTG. The registrar assessed Ms B and noted that the fetal head was zero fifths palpable abdominally and the fetal size was average; on vaginal examination, the fetal head position was occipito-anterior, station was +2cm with moderate caput and moulding, and pelvic dimensions were average. Ms B had been pushing well but was visibly tiring with slow progress over the previous 10 minutes. The late decelerations persisted on the CTG and the baseline had risen to 165 beats per minute. The registrar recommended AVB and verbal consent was given.

A Were the safety criteria for AVB met?
B What was the indication for AVB?
C What type of instrument should be used?

ANSWERS

A The findings on abdominal and vaginal examination are crucial to any consideration of this question. On examination, zero fifths of the fetal head were palpable, the position was occipito-anterior and at station spines +2cm with moderate caput and moulding. The pelvic dimensions were average. The patient had effective analgesia and gave verbal consent to AVB. The prerequisites for AVB were met and the procedure should be classified as low-pelvic not requiring rotation. This type of AVB should be within the skillset of an average registrar and can be conducted in a delivery room as the risk of failure is very low.

B The primary indication for AVB in this case relates to the finding of late decelerations and a rising baseline on the CTG, reflecting potential fetal hypoxia and the risk of fetal compromise. In addition, while the woman had been pushing for 50 minutes and this is not considered prolonged, she was visibly tiring and making little further progress, which is also an indication for assistance. As with many AVBs, the indication was based on both fetal and maternal factors.

C The choice here was between vacuum and forceps. If there was marked caput and moulding, a higher station of the presenting part or the mother was pushing poorly then forceps may be preferred. In this case, the baby had rotated and descended to spines +2cm and the caput and moulding was no more than moderate, with average pelvic dimensions. Vacuum-assisted birth is likely to be preferred in these circumstances, as the chance of success is high and the risk of significant perineal tearing (including OASI) is lower than with forceps.

CASE HISTORY 2

Following on from the first case history, Mrs B consents to an assisted vaginal birth.

A How should the delivery be conducted?
B What complications should be anticipated after the birth?

ANSWERS

A The procedure should be explained to Ms B and her partner. The neonatologist should be called in case resuscitation is required. The patient should be positioned in the lithotomy position with the end of the bed removed. The obstetrician should confirm that the epidural analgesia is effective and, if necessary, the perineum can be infiltrated with local anaesthesia. The bladder should be emptied with a catheter. The clinical findings should be confirmed once more. The choice is between a sialastic vacuum or a rigid disposable vacuum cup. The vacuum cup is applied over the flexion point of the fetal head and checked to ensure that no maternal tissues are trapped. The pressure is increased to 0.8 kg/cm^2 and the application of the cup is rechecked. The woman is encouraged to push with contractions while the obstetrician exerts traction along the axis of the pelvis. The head descends onto the perineum with two pulls and delivers with the assistance of a right mediolateral episiotomy with the next push. The head restitutes and the shoulders deliver easily on the next contraction. A healthy male infant of birthweight 3.4 kg is delivered onto his mother's abdomen and is vigorous at birth (Apgar score 9 at 1 minute and 10 at 5 minutes; paired cord bloods normal). There is delayed cord clamping after which the third stage is actively managed and the episiotomy is repaired. Antibiotics are administered and analgesia is prescribed. The AVB is documented on the standard proforma.

B There is a risk that the baby may be delivered in poor condition due to intra-partum hypoxia and may require resuscitation. There is a risk of trauma to the baby, which may include cephalohaematoma or scalp abrasions and much less commonly a serious complication such as subgaleal haemorrhage. There is a risk of an extended perineal or vaginal tear that may include the anal sphincter. There is an increased risk of post-partum haemorrhage, perineal infection, urinary retention or incontinence. Complications are mitigated by careful practice, active management of the third stage, administration of prophylactic antibiotics and education in relation to aftercare post-AVB.

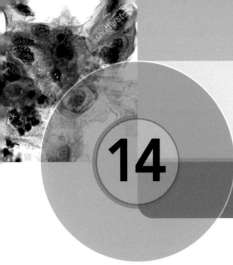

Obstetric emergencies

14

FERGUS McCARTHY

Learning Objectives
- Understand the incidence of common obstetric emergencies.
- Understand the risk factors for common obstetric emergencies.
- Understand the early warning signs in obstetric emergencies.
- Be able to provide a stepwise approach in the management of common obstetric emergencies.

INTRODUCTION

Obstetric emergencies are common and often result in significant maternal and fetal morbidity and mortality. Regardless of the emergency, it is essential that they are managed in a methodological, stepwise manner to limit morbidity and mortality and maintain safety for staff and patients. Accurate documentation is essential, as is the opportunity for a postnatal debrief to allow the woman (and partner if present) an opportunity to ask questions and understand what happened. This chapter covers common obstetric emergencies and also rare obstetric emergencies that may result in significant morbidity or mortality. A stepwise approach to managing these obstetric emergencies is suggested.

One maternal death occurs every minute worldwide. In the UK, it is estimated that 1 in every 100 births results in a high-dependency unit admission, while 1 in every 1,000 results in an intensive care unit admission. Maternal mortality is unacceptably high. Every day in 2017, approximately 810 women died worldwide from preventable causes related to pregnancy and childbirth, namely about 295,000 over the whole year. The vast majority of these deaths (94%) occurred in low-resource settings, and most could have been prevented. Leading causes of maternal mortality include thrombosis and thromboembolism, haemorrhage, sepsis, amniotic fluid embolism and cardiac disease.

An emergency is defined as a serious situation or occurrence that happens unexpectedly and demands

10.1201/9781003196112-14

Table 14.1 Incidence of obstetric emergencies

Obstetric emergency	Estimated rates
Maternal collapse	Collapse affects 0.14–6 in 1,000 (14–600 in 100,000) births in the UK
Sepsis	Worldwide, puerperal sepsis is estimated to complicate at least 75,000 maternal deaths every year (the majority in low-income countries) In the USA, sepsis is estimated to complicate approximately 1 in 3,000 deliveries
Major obstetric haemorrhage	The estimated incidence of haemorrhage in the UK is 3.7 in 1,000 pregnancies An estimated 125,000 women are thought to die annually worldwide as a consequence of haemorrhage
Amniotic fluid embolism	This affects 2.0 in 100,000 deliveries (95% CI 1.5–2.5), with maternal mortality rates of 0.33 per 100,000 pregnancies and perinatal mortality rates of 135 per 1,000 total births (95% CI 45–288) in the UK
Pre-eclampsia and eclampsia	In the UK, this occurs in 3–5% of first-time pregnancies and 2–3% of pregnancies overall, with mortality rates of 0.38 per 100,000 maternities Severe forms are estimated to affect up to 18% of pregnant women in parts of Africa, with a mortality rate of 10–25%
Thrombosis and thromboembolism	Approximately 50% of maternal venous thromboembolism events occur during pregnancy In the UK, overall prevalence is 1 in 1,600 pregnancies and the incidence of antenatal pulmonary embolism is 1.3 in 10,000, with a case fatality rate of 3.5% and overall mortality rates of 1.08 per 100,000 pregnancies
Cardiac disease	The prevalence of cardiac disease in pregnancy in the developed world is 0.2–3%, and the mortality rate in the UK is 2.25 per 100,000 pregnancies
Shoulder dystocia	The prevalence rate is 0.58–0.70%

CI, confidence interval.

immediate action. Prompt recognition and treatment of these emergencies/complications of pregnancy is essential to limit morbidity and mortality. The incidence and outcomes of obstetric emergencies varies hugely from country to country (e.g. deaths from complications such as pre-eclampsia are rare in the UK but are prevalent in Africa; Table 14.1). This chapter aims to cover all major obstetric emergencies including the incidence, risk factors and warning signs to recognize at-risk women, as well as suggested management strategies.

PREVENTION OF OBSTETRIC EMERGENCIES

It is not possible to prevent or predict all obstetric emergencies, but it is essential to recognize early warning signs, reduce risk factors and have

appropriate support present in anticipation of obstetric emergencies.

COLLAPSED/UNRESPONSIVE PATIENT

The general structured approach to the management of acute illness and trauma is the same for pregnant and non-pregnant patients and is summarized in **Figure 14.1**. Management consists of the following structured approach.

Identify life-threatening problems:

A *Airway* – with cervical spine control.
B *Breathing* – with ventilation. Look for chest movements, listen for breath sounds and feel for movement of air for a maximum of 10 seconds. If breathing is present, give high-flow oxygen. If breathing is absent, start ventilation.

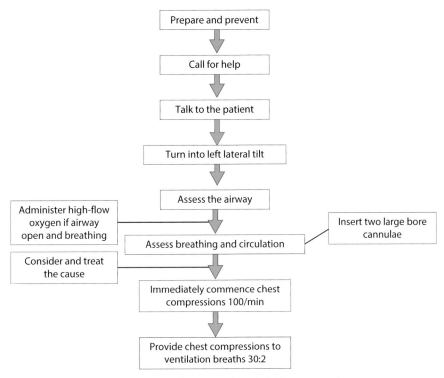

Prepare and prevent

Call for help

Talk to the patient

Turn into left lateral tilt

Assess the airway

Administer high-flow oxygen if airway open and breathing

Insert two large bore cannulae

Assess breathing and circulation

Consider and treat the cause

Immediately commence chest compressions 100/min

Provide chest compressions to ventilation breaths 30:2

Figure 14.1 The structured approach to managing obstetric emergencies.

C *Circulation* – with haemorrhage control. Minimize aorto-caval compression (**Figure 14.2**). Absence of breathing in the presence of a clear airway is now used as a marker of absence of circulation. If there is no circulation, start cardiopulmonary resuscitation (CPR): 30 chest compressions followed by two ventilations. Manage hypovolaemia/haemorrhage concurrently.

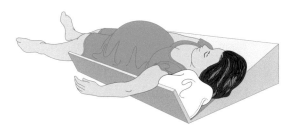

Figure 14.2 Left lateral tilt. The pregnant woman is tilted to the left to move the pregnant uterus off the abdominal vessels, thus improving cardiac output. There are various methods of achieving this; many hospitals have special wedge-shaped cushions, but pillows and blankets can be used.

D *Disability* – neurological status using the AVPU score: Alert, responds to Voice, responds to Pain, Unresponsive. Following initial resuscitation, perform a Glasgow coma score (GCS). GCS ≤8 indicates a compromised airway and will require intubation.

E *Exposure* – depending on environment. Perform full examination of patient, remembering risks of hypothermia (use warming blanket if needed) and patient's dignity. Monitoring may include non-invasive blood pressure, pulse oximetry, electrocardiogram (ECG), end tidal carbon dioxide and respiratory rate. Consider urinary catheter and nasogastric tube depending on circumstances (e.g. hourly urine output is essential in severe pre-eclampsia).

Resuscitation:

- Deal with any problems as you find them. Consider differential diagnosis (**Figure 14.3**).
- Assess fetal well-being and viability: deal with threat to life of fetus. Assess fetal well-being using cardiotocography (CTG).

253

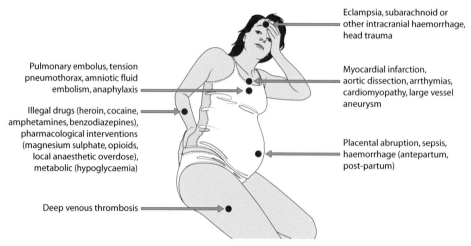

Figure 14.3 The differential diagnosis of acute maternal collapse.

Labels in figure:
- Eclampsia, subarachnoid or other intracranial haemorrhage, head trauma
- Myocardial infarction, aortic dissection, arrthymias, cardiomyopathy, large vessel aneurysm
- Pulmonary embolus, tension pneumothorax, amniotic fluid embolism, anaphylaxis
- Illegal drugs (heroin, cocaine, amphetamines, benzodiazepines), pharmacological interventions (magnesium sulphate, opioids, local anaesthetic overdose), metabolic (hypoglycaemia)
- Placental abruption, sepsis, haemorrhage (antepartum, post-partum)
- Deep venous thrombosis

- *Notes review*: review trends of vital signs/review notes.
- *Definitive care*: order investigations and plan treatment – specific management depending on underlying cause.

An anaesthetist experienced in obstetric care is critical in the successful management of obstetric emergencies. Difficulties that anaesthetists encounter in the resuscitation of the pregnant woman include increased risk of aspiration of gastric contents, increased metabolic oxygen consumption combined with a decreased functional residual capacity, pregnancy weight gain and increased breast size making optimal placement of head and intubation more difficult and, finally, aorto-caval compression and the effects of the gravid uterus on venous return.

☞ KEY LEARNING POINTS

Maternal collapse
- Obtain a left lateral tilt of at least 15–20° at the earliest opportunity to prevent/minimize aorto-caval compression in any patient.
- Resuscitation of a pregnant woman is more difficult due to reduced lung capacity, reduced venous return if supine, greater oxygen demand from the fetus and increased weight.
- The use of Modified Early Obstetric Warning System (MEOWS) scores are key in the early recognition of the clinical deterioration of a patient.

SEPSIS

Sepsis in the UK remains a significant cause of maternal death. The mortality rate for pregnancy-related sepsis has continued to increase steadily since its nadir in 2012–2014.

BOX 14.1: Sepsis: Prevention, risk factors and warning signs

- *Prevention*: all maternal observations should be documented on a MEOWS chart to allow early detection of sepsis and subsequent treatment.
- *Risk factors*: ruptured membranes, immunocompromised patients, immunosuppressants, obesity, diabetes, minority ethnic group origin, anaemia, urinary tract infections, vaginal discharge, previous pelvic infection, group B streptococcal infection, amniocentesis and other invasive procedures, cervical cerclage, group A streptococcal infection in close contacts.
- *Warning signs*: pyrexia, hypothermia, tachycardia, increased respiratory rate, hypotension, rise in MEOWS score and oliguria. Patients may rigor, have a rash, have reduced levels of consciousness and not respond to initial treatment.

MANAGEMENT

The Surviving Sepsis Campaign 'resuscitation bundles' set out key points in the timely management of sepsis:

- Obtain blood cultures prior to antibiotic administration.
- Administer broad-spectrum antibiotic within 1 hour of recognition of severe sepsis. Every 1 hour delay in administrating antibiotics increases mortality by approximately 8%.
- Measure serum lactate. A normal lactate level is generally less than 2.3 mmol/L.
- In the event of hypotension and/or a serum lactate level of ≥4 mmol/L, deliver an initial minimum 20 mL/kg of crystalloid or an equivalent.
- If there is no response, administer vasopressors for hypotension that is not responding to initial fluid resuscitation to maintain mean arterial pressure of ≥65 mmHg.
- In the event of persistent hypotension despite fluid resuscitation and/or a lactate level of ≥4 mmol/L, aim to achieve a central venous pressure of ≥8 mmHg, a central venous oxygen saturation of ≥70% or mixed venous oxygen saturation of ≥65%.

Involve a microbiologist or infectious disease physician early, particularly if the woman does not respond to first-choice antibiotics.

Severe sepsis may be defined by one or more of the following factors:

- temperature >38°C or <36°C
- heart rate >100 beats per minute
- respiratory rate >20 respirations per minute
- white cell count >17 × 10^9/L or <4 × 10^9/L with >10% immature band forms

Severe sepsis has a higher maternal mortality than sepsis/infection and requires aggressive prompt treatment and timely involvement of the multidisciplinary team.

ANTIBIOTIC USE

Each hospital should have its own antibiotic guidelines, as the incidence of resistant organisms varies both within and between countries. The selection of antibiotics should be guided by risk factors and potential sources of sepsis. A combination of either piperacillin/tazobactam or a carbapenem plus clindamycin provides very broad coverage for the treatment of severe sepsis. Other antibiotic options include:

- co-amoxiclav – provides Gram-positive and anaerobic cover; does not cover methicillin-resistant *Staphylococcus aureus* (MRSA), *Pseudomonas* or extended spectrum β-lactamase (ESBL)-producing organisms
- metronidazole – provides anaerobic cover
- clindamycin – covers streptococci and staphylococci including MRSA; also switches off exotoxin production
- gentamicin – provides Gram-negative cover against coliforms and *Pseudomonas*

🔑 KEY LEARNING POINTS

Management of sepsis

- Blood cultures should be performed before antibiotics are administered.
- Culture of other samples should be performed based on clinical suspicion (e.g. high vaginal swab, midstream urine, sputum culture).
- The key organisms involved in puerperal sepsis are Lancefield group A β-haemolytic streptococcus and *Escherichia coli*.
- Early diagnosis, rapid administration of broad-spectrum antibiotics and review by senior doctors and midwives is essential to reduce mortality and improve outcome.
- Lactate and haemoglobin should be measured and repeat measurements should be planned to help assess the response to initial treatment.
- Accurate hourly urine output should be measured.
- High-flow oxygen should be administered.

OBSTETRIC HAEMORRHAGE

Obstetric haemorrhage is a leading cause of maternal mortality worldwide and is responsible for up to 50% of maternal deaths in some countries. In the UK it is responsible for approximately 10% of all direct maternal deaths.

ANTEPARTUM HAEMORRHAGE

This is defined as vaginal bleeding after 20 weeks' gestation. It complicates 2–5% of pregnancies and most cases involve relatively small amounts of blood loss. However, significant blood loss poses a risk of mortality and morbidity to both the mother and baby. The causes can be classified into three groups:

1. *placental causes*: placental abruption, placenta praevia
2. *fetal cause*: vasa praevia
3. *maternal causes*: vaginal trauma, cervical ectropion, cervical carcinoma, vaginal infection and cervicitis

Placental causes are the most worrying, as potentially the mother's and/or fetus's life is in danger and often the bleeding may be more severe than with other causes such as cervical ectropion. However, any antepartum haemorrhage must always be taken seriously, and any woman presenting with a history of fresh vaginal bleeding must be investigated promptly and properly. The key question is whether the bleeding is placental and is compromising the mother and/or fetus or whether it has a less significant cause.

HISTORY

- How much bleeding is there?
- What were the triggering factors (e.g. post-coital bleed)?
- Is it associated with pain or contractions?
- Is the baby moving?
- When was the last cervical smear (date and normal/abnormal)?

EXAMINATION

- Take the pulse and blood pressure.
- Is the uterus soft or tender and firm?
- Undertake fetal heart auscultation/CTG.
- Undertake speculum vaginal examination, with particular importance placed on visualizing the cervix (having established that placenta is not a praevia, preferably using a portable ultrasound machine).

INVESTIGATIONS

- Depending on the degree of bleeding, full blood count, clotting and, if suspected praevia/abruption, cross-match 6 units of blood.
- Ultrasound (fetal size, presentation, amniotic fluid, placental position and morphology).

PLACENTAL ABRUPTION

Placental abruption is the premature separation of the placenta from the uterine wall. The bleeding is maternal and/or fetal and abruption is acutely dangerous for both the mother and the fetus (**Figure 14.4**).

> **BOX 14.2: Placental abruption: Prevention, risk factors and warning signs**
>
> - *Prevention*: avoidance of precipitating factors such as control of blood pressure and avoidance of precipitants such as cocaine and smoking
> - *Risk factors*: hypertension (including pre-eclampsia), smoking, trauma to the maternal abdomen, cocaine, polyhydramnios, multiple pregnancy, fetal growth restriction (FGR)
> - *Warning signs*: maternal collapse, feeling cold, light-headedness, restlessness, distress and panic, painful abdomen, vaginal bleeding

CLINICAL PRESENTATION

The characteristic presentation of placental abruption is that of painful bleeding associated with a tense rigid abdomen. The absence of a tense abdomen does not rule out a placental abruption. Placental abruption may be diagnosed on ultrasound but the absence of any ultrasound changes does not rule it out and patients should be managed on the basis of their clinical findings. Maternal signs and symptoms may include vaginal bleeding, abdominal pain, sweating, shock, hypotension, tachycardia, absence or reduced fetal movements and tense painful abdomen. CTG may reveal evidence of fetal distress.

The degree of vaginal bleeding does not necessarily correlate with the degree of abruption, as abruptions

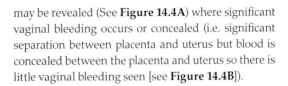

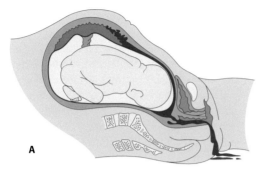

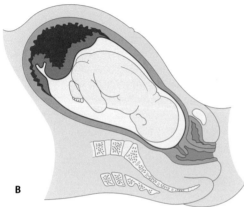

Figure 14.4 (**A**) Placental abruption with revealed haemorrhage. (**B**) Placental abruption with concealed haemorrhage.

may be revealed (See **Figure 14.4A**) where significant vaginal bleeding occurs or concealed (i.e. significant separation between placenta and uterus but blood is concealed between the placenta and uterus so there is little vaginal bleeding seen [see **Figure 14.4B**]).

PLACENTA PRAEVIA

A placenta covering or encroaching on the cervical os may be associated with bleeding, either provoked or spontaneous. The bleeding is from the mother and not the fetal circulation and is more likely to compromise the mother than the fetus (**Figure 14.5**).

> **BOX 14.3: Placenta praevia: Prevention, risk factors and warning signs**
>
> - *Prevention*: avoidance of non-clinically indicated caesarean section
> - *Risk factors*: multiple gestation, previous caesarean section, uterine structural anomaly, assisted conception
> - *Warning signs*: low-lying placenta at 20-week anomaly scan, maternal collapse, feeling cold, light-headedness, restlessness, distress and panic, painless vaginal bleeding

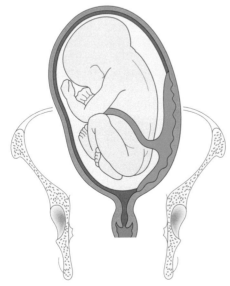

Minor placenta praevia

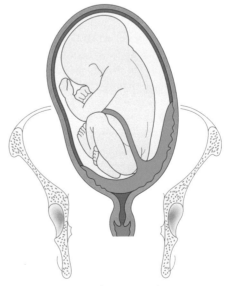

Major placenta praevia

Figure 14.5 Placenta praevia.

CLINICAL PRESENTATION AND DIAGNOSIS

The characteristic presenting complaint of bleeding associated with a placenta praevia is that of painless vaginal bleeding. The bleeding may trigger preterm labour so, often, patients with bleeding from placenta praevia will have irregular abdominal pain associated with uterine contractions. A placenta praevia is diagnosed using ultrasound, preferably transvaginal, to allow accurate measurement of the placental edge from the internal os. Often, patients will have been highlighted as having a low-lying placenta at their anomaly scan so there should be a high index of suspicion in any of these patients presenting with vaginal bleeding.

MANAGEMENT

If there is minimal bleeding and the cause is clearly local vaginal bleeding, symptomatic management may be given (for example antifungal preparations for candidiasis) as long as there is reasonable certainty that cervical carcinoma is excluded by smear history and direct visualization of the cervix. Placental causes of bleeding are a major concern. A large-gauge intravenous cannula is sited; blood is sent for full blood count, clotting and cross-match; and appropriate fetal and maternal monitoring is instituted. If there is major fetal or maternal compromise, decisions may have to be made about immediate delivery irrespective of gestation; an attempt at maternal steroid injection should still be made. If this is the situation, and bleeding is continuing, emergency management is required. If bleeding settles, the woman must be admitted for 48 hours, as the risk of re-bleeding is high within this time frame. Rhesus status is important: if the mother is rhesus negative, send a Kleihauer test (to determine whether any, or how much, fetal blood has leaked into the maternal circulation) and administer anti-D. When there is substantial vaginal bleeding (in excess of 500 mL), antenatal corticosteroids should be considered if gestation is under 35 weeks, as the risk of preterm delivery is significant.

VASA PRAEVIA

Vasa previa occurs when fetal vessels traverse the fetal membranes over the internal cervical os. These vessels may be either from a velamentous insertion of the umbilical cord or joining an accessory (succenturiate) placental lobe to the main disc of the placenta. The diagnosis is usually suspected when either spontaneous or artificial rupture of the membranes is accompanied by painless fresh vaginal bleeding from rupture of the fetal vessels. This condition is associated with a very high perinatal mortality from fetal exsanguination. If the baby is still alive, once the diagnosis is suspected the immediate course of action is delivery by emergency caesarean section.

🔑 KEY LEARNING POINTS

- Placenta praevia is most dangerous for the mother.
- Placental abruption is more dangerous for the fetus than for the mother.
- Vasa praevia is not dangerous for the mother but is nearly always fatal for the baby.
- Management involves resuscitation and stabilization of the mother and senior input regarding timing of delivery.

POST-PARTUM HAEMORRHAGE

Post-partum haemorrhage, defined as blood loss of ≥500 mL, affected 13% of all pregnancies in England in 2011 and 2012. In the UK and Ireland, there were 17 direct deaths due to obstetric haemorrhage between 2009 and 2012. This gives an overall mortality rate of 0.49 per 100,000 pregnancies (95% CI 0.29–0.78) and a case fatality rate for massive haemorrhage of approximately 1 per 1,200 women.

Major obstetric haemorrhage is defined as blood loss of ≥2,500 mL or requiring a blood transfusion of ≥5 units of red cells or treatment for coagulopathy. Major obstetric haemorrhage affected 0.6% of pregnancies in Scotland in 2011.

SIGNS AND SYMPTOMS OF HAEMORRHAGE

- *Symptoms*: anxiety, thirst, nausea, cold, pain, dizziness
- *Signs*: rising fundus, peritonism, reduced urine output, tachypnoea, tachycardia, hypotension, narrow pulse pressure

BOX 14.4: Post-partum haemorrhage: Prevention, risk factors and warning signs

- *Prevention*: haemoglobin levels below the normal range for pregnancy should be investigated and iron supplementation should be considered if indicated to optimize haemoglobin prior to delivery. Prophylactic use of oxytocin agents should be considered for high-risk patients.
- *Risk factors for uterine atony* (the most common cause of haemorrhage): macrosomia, multiple pregnancy, prolonged labour, oxytocin use, induction of labour, grand multiparity, polyhydramnios, antepartum haemorrhage, placental abruption.
- *Other risk factors for obstetric haemorrhage*: placenta praevia (see **Figure 14.5**) and accreata, previous multiple caesarean sections (risk of placenta accreata is greater than 60% for women who have had three or more previous caesarean sections), perineal trauma, full bladder, underlying haematological disorder (e.g. factor VIII deficiency), disseminated intravascular coagulation. There are three main areas from which haemorrhage occurs: uterus, placenta and cervix/vagina. Uterine causes of haemorrhage include atony (the most common cause of haemorrhage), uterine inversion and rupture. Remember, haemorrhage may be concealed.
- *Warning signs*: failure of uterus to contract following delivery of the placenta, maternal collapse.

© KEY LEARNING POINTS

Management of obstetric haemorrhage (Figure 14.6)

- Do not delay fluid resuscitation and blood transfusion because of false reassurance from a single haemoglobin result – treat the patient, not the result.
- Be proactive – young fit women compensate extremely well. Therefore, ongoing bleeding should be acted on without delay. Minimal signs of haemorrhage exist up to 1,000 mL of loss. The commonly used sign of hypotension is a very late sign in blood loss occurring after 2,000 mL of loss.
- Consider the administration of blood components before coagulation indices deteriorate if a woman is bleeding and is likely to develop a coagulopathy.
- Consider early recourse to hysterectomy if simpler medical and surgical interventions prove ineffective.
- In patients in whom complications are anticipated (e.g. placenta accreata), ideally obtain advanced consent (with partner present if possible) to cover possible interventions including blood transfusion, interventional radiology, leaving placenta in situ and hysterectomy.

ECLAMPSIA

Pre-eclampsia is a potentially life-threatening hypertensive disorder of pregnancy characterized by vascular dysfunction and systemic inflammation involving the brain, liver and kidneys of the mother. Eclampsia refers to the occurrence of one or more generalized convulsions and/or coma in the setting of pre-eclampsia and in the absence of other neurological conditions. The UK Obstetric Surveillance System report gives an estimated incidence of eclampsia of 27.5 cases per 100,000 pregnancies, with case fatality rate estimated to be 3.1%. Eclampsia is associated with significant maternal morbidity, in particular cerebrovascular events (2.3%). Cerebral haemorrhage has been reported to be the most common cause of death in patients with eclampsia (previously this was pulmonary oedema) and stroke is known to be the most common cause of death (45%) in women with haemolysis, elevated liver enzymes and low platelets (HELLP) syndrome.

- Initiate obstetric haemorrhage protocol
- Call for senior help
- Scribe to clearly document timing of events, people present and interventions administered

- Uterine compression/rub up contractions
- Empty uterus and vagina of clot
- Empty bladder
- Uterotonic agents
- Bimanual compression of uterus if atony is the cause
- Intravenous access ×2 large bore cannulae
- Full blood count/group and cross-match/coagulation profile
- Fluid replacement: cross-matched blood or O-negative blood if unavailable
- Rapid infuser with fluid warmer/cell saver set up

A stepwise approach to use of uteronic agents would be:

- 5–10 units IV/IM oxytocin
- 40 units oxytocin in 100 mL normal saline over 4 hours
- 800–1,000 µg rectal misoprostol
- Syntometrine (ergometrine 500 µg and Syntocinon™ 5 units)
- Repeat ergometrine (500 µg) IM or slow IV push
- Carbaprost 0.25 mg by IM repeated at intervals of not less than 15 minutes to a maximum of eight doses (contraindicated in women with asthma)

If ongoing bleeding consider:

- Disseminated intravascular coagulation and replacement of clotting agents
- Senior help – interventional radiology, gynaeoncology
- Transfer to operating theatre for surgical invention (uterine balloon insertion, iliac ligation, uterine artery embolization, hysterectomy)

- Clear documentation of sequence of events and cause of bleeding
- Debrief of staff, family members and patient
- Risk report

Figure 14.6 Algorithm for the management of obstetric haemorrhage. (IM, intramuscular; IV, intravenous.)

BOX 14.5: Eclampsia: Prevention, risk factors and warning signs

- *Prevention*: low threshold for administration of magnesium sulphate in women with pre-eclampsia who are thought to be unstable or suffering from severe pre-eclampsia. However, remember all patients with pre-eclampsia regardless of perceived severity are at risk of eclampsia.
- *Risk factors*: difficult to predict, uncontrolled hypertension, two or fewer prenatal care visits, primigravidity, obesity, Black ethnicity, history of diabetes, age <20 years.
- *Warning signs*: epigastric pain and right upper quadrant tenderness, headache, uncontrolled hypertension, agitation, hyper-reflexia and clonus, facial (especially periorbital) oedema, poor urine output, papilloedema.

MANAGEMENT

First, summon senior help and the emergency alert team. The initial approach is similar to that of the collapsed patient with a focus on airway, breathing and circulation. Magnesium sulphate is indicated as the first-line anticonvulsant and should be administered as soon as possible either in women at risk of eclampsia or when eclampsia occurs. A loading dose of 4 g is given followed by a maintenance infusion of 1 g/hour generally for 24 hours after delivery. Magnesium sulphate has a narrow therapeutic range and overdose can cause respiratory depression and ultimately cardiac arrest. The antidote is 10 mL 10% calcium gluconate given slowly intravenously.

AMNIOTIC FLUID EMBOLISM

Amniotic fluid embolism is a rare cause of maternal collapse and is believed to be caused by amniotic fluid entering the maternal circulation. This causes acute cardiorespiratory compromise and severe disseminated intravascular coagulation. In some cases, there may be an abnormal maternal reaction to amniotic fluid as the primary event. It is difficult to diagnose when it occurs and it is typically

- *Prevention*: unknown
- *Risk factors*: population proportional attributable risks are 35% for induction of labour, 13% for ethnic-minority women 35 years or older, and 7% for multiple pregnancy
- *Warning signs*: maternal collapse, shortness of breath, chest pain, feeling cold, light-headedness, restlessness, distress and panic, pins and needles in the fingers, nausea and vomiting

BOX 14.7: Umbilical cord prolapse: Prevention, risk factors and warning signs

- *Prevention*: with transverse, oblique or unstable lie, elective admission to hospital after 37+0 weeks' gestation allows for quick delivery should membranes rupture. Women with non-cephalic pre-labour preterm rupture of membranes should be managed as inpatients. Avoid artificial induction of labour when the presenting part is non-stable and/or mobile. When performing vaginal examination, avoid upwards pressure on the presenting part.
- *Risk factors*: polyhydramnios, multiparity, multiple pregnancy/second twin, unstable, transverse and oblique lie, fetal congenital abnormalities, low birthweight (<2.5 kg), internal podalic version, large balloon catheter induction of labour.
- *Warning signs*: signs of fetal distress on CTG following artificial or spontaneous rupture of membranes.

diagnosed at post-mortem, with the presence of fetal cells (squames or hair) in the maternal pulmonary capillaries.

MANAGEMENT

In the case of sudden collapse, management should be the structured ABC approach (airway, breathing and circulation). The prognosis is poor, with approximately 30% of patients dying in the first hour and only 10% surviving overall. Management is supportive, requiring intensive care, and there are no specific therapies available. Symptoms occurring just before the collapse may be helpful in diagnosis. Perimortem caesarean section should be carried out within 5 minutes or as soon as possible after cardiac arrest. This is for the benefit of the woman to improve the effect of resuscitation.

UMBILICAL CORD PROLAPSE

Umbilical cord prolapse may be defined as the descent of the umbilical cord through the cervix alongside or past the presenting part in the presence of ruptured membranes (**Figure 14.7**). It is estimated to occur in 0.1–0.6% of pregnancies with the perinatal mortality rate estimated to be 91 per 1,000.

MANAGEMENT

When suspected, perform speculum or digital examination immediately, as early detection is crucial for timely delivery and in the prevention of fetal morbidity and mortality (reported as high as 25–50% of cases). When diagnosed, summon senior help and prepare the operating theatre for emergency delivery. If diagnosed, attempt to prevent further cord compression by elevating the presenting part or filling the bladder. Avoid handling the cord, as this causes cord spasm. Place the mother in a knee-to-chest or left lateral position, ideally with the head slightly declined. Confirm fetal viability by auscultation of the fetal heart using CTG. Delivery is generally performed by emergency caesarean section (category 1 if pathological fetal heart pattern or category 2 if normal fetal heart pattern).

SHOULDER DYSTOCIA

Shoulder dystocia is defined as a vaginal cephalic delivery that requires additional obstetric manoeuvres to deliver the fetus after the head has delivered and gentle traction has been unsuccessful in delivering the shoulders (**Figure 14.8**). It is associated

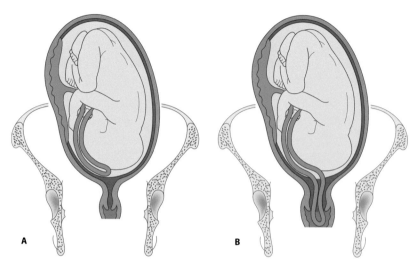

Figure 14.7 Cord prolapse. (**A**) Cord presentation: the cord is below the presenting party (head in this case but commonly a malpresentation) with the membranes intact. (**B**) Cord prolapse: the membranes have ruptured and the cord is below the presenting part and has prolapsed into the vagina.

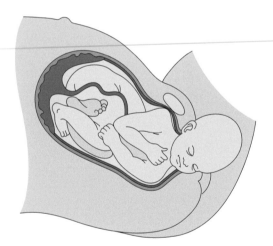

Figure 14.8 Shoulder dystocia. After delivery of the head, shoulder dystocia occurs due to the shoulders being unable to pass under the maternal symphysis pubis.

with significant morbidity for both the mother and the fetus.

Maternal complications include increased perineal trauma (third- and fourth-degree tear), post-partum haemorrhage and psychological trauma. Fetal complications include brachial plexus injury (2–7% at birth reducing to 1–3% at 12 months of age), fractured clavicle or humerus (1–2%) and hypoxic brain injury.

The suggested management algorithm for shoulder dystocia is shown in **Figure 14.9**.

- Call for senior help (neonatology, senior midwife, obstetric consultant)

- Drop the level of the delivery bed as low as it will go and flatten the back of the bed so the woman is completely flat. Remove the foot of the bed to allow access
- McRoberts position – using one assistant on each of the mother's legs, flex and abduct the legs at the hip (thighs to abdomen). This flattens the lumbosacral spine and will facilitate delivery in approximately 90% of cases
- Suprapubic pressure: apply over the posterior aspect of the anterior fetal shoulder. It can be used in a constant and then rocking motion
- Consider episiotomy
- Deliver posterior arm and shoulder or consider internal rotational manoeuvres, including Rubin II: insert a hand behind the anterior shoulder and push it towards the chest. This will adduct the shoulders then push them into the diagonal
- Woods' screw: pressure on the anterior aspect of the posterior shoulder to aid rotation. Reverse Woods' screw: rotate the baby in the opposite direction
- Change position to all fours
- Finally consider symphiotomy, cleidotomy or Zavanelli manoeuvre

- Debrief staff, patient and partner
- Write comprehensive notes
- Risk report and risk committe review

Figure 14.9 Algorithm for management of shoulder dystocia.

THROMBOSIS AND THROMBOEMBOLISM

Thrombosis and venous thromboembolism (VTE) continues to be the leading cause of direct deaths occurring within 42 days of the end of pregnancy. There has been a welcome decrease in the maternal mortality rate from VTE, which is now at a similar rate to what it was in 2012–2014 – an encouraging sign of improved detection of risk and better prevention. However, the Mothers and Babies: Reducing Risk through Audits and Confidential Enquiries across the UK (MBRRACE-UK) report published in 2021 into maternal deaths and morbidity in 2017–2019 demonstrates that more than two-thirds of maternal deaths could still be prevented with improvements to care. VTE is 10 times more common in pregnancy than in the non-pregnant population. Women with VTE may be asymptomatic or present with a range of symptoms (specific and non-specific) including calf or groin pain and/or swelling that is often unilateral, low-grade pyrexia to more extreme presentations including haemoptysis, shortness of breath, collapse and death.

When deep vein thrombosis is suspected clinically, compression duplex ultrasound should be undertaken. If this is negative and there is a low level of clinical suspicion, anticoagulant treatment can be discontinued. If clinical suspicion remains high or symptoms fail to resolve, ultrasound may be repeated or magnetic resonance venography may be performed. When pulmonary embolus is suspected, investigative options include chest X-ray (to rule out other respiratory causes of chest symptoms such as pneumonia), low limb Doppler to rule out lower limb VTE and finally a ventilation perfusion (V/Q scan) or computed tomography pulmonary angiography. The measurement of D-dimers is not helpful and should not be performed, as they are often elevated secondary to physiological changes in the coagulation system in pregnancy. Treatment of confirmed or suspected VTE is with therapeutic low-molecular-weight heparin given daily in two divided doses according to the patient's weight. In the case of a collapsed patient with pulmonary embolus, management options include intravenous unfractionated heparin, thrombolytic therapy or thoracotomy and surgical embolectomy. This complex management decision is taken by the multidisciplinary resuscitation team, including senior physicians, obstetricians and radiologists.

UTERINE INVERSION

Uterine inversion occurs when the uterus is partially or wholly inverted (**Figure 14.10**). Four degrees of

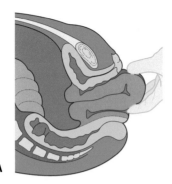

A

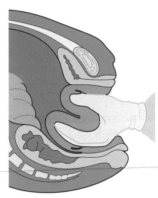

B

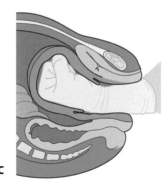

C

Figure 14.10 Uterine inversion.

inversion have been described: first degree, when the inverted fundus extends to but not through the cervix; second degree, when the inverted fundus extends through cervix but remains within the vagina; third degree, when the inverted fundus extends outside the vagina; and total inversion, when the vagina and uterus are inverted. Prompt recognition is essential, as the longer it is inverted the more difficult it becomes to replace, as a retraction ring forms, preventing eversion.

> **BOX 14.10: Uterine inversion: Prevention, risk factors and warning signs**
>
> - *Prevention*: senior in-house supervision and help to deal with this emergency
> - *Risk factors*: full dilatation sections, malpresentations, prolonged second stage, intravenous Syntocinon™ prior to a decision to deliver by caesarean section, unsuccessful instrumental delivery, prolonged second stage, hyperstimulated uterus
> - *Warning signs*: see risk factors

MANAGEMENT

As soon as the diagnosis is made, manual replacement should be attempted. If unsuccessful, transfer the patient to the operating theatre for replacement of the uterus under anaesthetic. If unsuccessful, attempt hydrostatic replacement by running 2–3 L of warm saline via tubing into the vagina using your hands to create a seal around the vulva. This causes vagina vault and cervical ballooning, which allows the uterus and placenta to gradually reduce thus correcting the inversion. This is then confirmed manually and oxytocin is commenced once the uterus contracts in an attempt to maintain uterine contraction. If this is unsuccessful, surgical procedures including hysterectomy may be necessary.

UTERINE RUPTURE

Uterine rupture is a catastrophic event with significant associated maternal and fetal morbidity and mortality. It most commonly occurs in women who have previously delivered by caesarean section. In the UK, between April 2009 and April 2010, the estimated incidence of uterine rupture was 2 per 10,000 pregnancies overall. These rates increased to 21 and 3 per 10,000 pregnancies in women with a previous caesarean delivery planning vaginal or elective caesarean delivery, respectively. Two women with uterine rupture died (case fatality 1.3%, 95% CI 0.2–4.5). There were 18 perinatal deaths associated with uterine rupture among 145 infants (perinatal mortality 124 per 1,000 total births, 95% CI 75–189).

BOX 14.11: Uterine rupture: Prevention, risk factors and warning signs

- *Prevention*: reduce rates of primary caesarean section. Avoid vaginal delivery in women with previous myomectomies in which the endometrial cavity has been breached. Act with caution when inducing women with previous caesarean sections.
- *Risk factors*: previous myomectomies that have breached the endometrial cavity. The odds of rupture are increased in women who had two or more previous caesarean deliveries (adjusted odds ratio (aOR) 3.02, 95% CI 1.16–7.85), when it has been less than 12 months since the last caesarean delivery (aOR 3.12, 95% CI 1.62–6.02) and in labour induction and oxytocin use (aOR 3.92, 95% CI 1.00–15.33). The estimated incidence of uterine rupture was 2 per 10,000 pregnancies overall and 21 and 3 per 10,000 pregnancies in women with a previous caesarean delivery planning vaginal or elective caesarean delivery, respectively.
- *Warning signs*: maternal shock, fetal distress/ unable to auscultate fetal heart, unable to palpate any presenting part on vaginal examination, severe sudden abdominal pain.

BOX 14.12: Impacted head at caesarean section: Prevention, risk factors and warning signs

- *Prevention*: senior in-house supervision and help to deal with this emergency
- *Risk factors*: full dilatation sections, malpresentations, prolonged second stage, intravenous Syntocinon™ prior to a decision to deliver by caesarean section, unsuccessful instrumental delivery, prolonged second stage, hyperstimulated uterus
- *Warning signs*: see risk factors

clinician and for the parents. Many obstetricians first encounter impaction of the fetal head while in training, often at night without immediate access to senior help. No figures exist for the exact incidence rates but it could potentially affect as many as 20,000 births per year (there are 200,000 caesarean sections in the UK each year with approximately 10% at full dilation).

MANAGEMENT

An urgent laparotomy is required once uterine rupture is diagnosed. Vaginal examination should be performed and the fetus delivered by the quickest route possible. Assisted vaginal delivery is reasonable if the woman is fully dilated and safe vaginal delivery is possible. Regardless, an urgent laparotomy is then required to examine and repair the uterine rupture.

IMPACTED HEAD AT CAESAREAN SECTION

An impacted head at caesarean section can be an extremely stressful situation for the operating

MANAGEMENT

Full dilatation sections should have the obstetric consultant present in anticipation of this complication. Allow the uterus to relax before disimpacting the head. Disengagement of the head requires flexion and rotation of the head into the transverse position prior to delivery by lateral flexion. Forcing the head upwards risks trauma, including fractures to the fetal head and extension to the uterine angles, which can result in haemorrhage and damage to the viscera. If you are unable to flex and rotate the head, consider the use of a uterine relaxant such as glyceryl trinitrate spray or terbutaline, but beware the risk of post-partum haemorrhage following the use of uterorelaxant agents. Other options include having a senior assistant flex and rotate the head vaginally or the use of newer devices designed to release the vacuum that occurs between the fetal head and pelvis (e.g. C-Snorkel®). However, minimum evidence exists to support their use and extreme care must be taken to avoid iatrogenic trauma.

FURTHER READING

Knight M, Kenyon S, Brocklehurst P, Neilson J, Shakespeare J, Kurinczuk JJ (eds); MBRRACE-UK (2014). *Saving Lives, Improving Mothers' Care – Lessons learned to inform future maternity care from the UK and Ireland Confidential Enquiries into Maternal Deaths and Morbidity 2009–12*. National Perinatal Epidemiology Unit, University of Oxford.

National Institute for Health and Care Excellence (2010). *Hypertension in Pregnancy: Diagnosis and Management*. Clinical guideline [CG107]. http://www.nice.org.uk/guidance/cg107/resources/guidance-hypertension-in-pregnancy-pdf.

Paterson-Brown S, Howell C (2016). *Managing Obstetric Emergencies and Trauma. The MOET Course Manual*. Cambridge University Press.

RCOG (2009). Green-top guideline No 37a. Reducing the risk of thrombosis and embolism during pregnancy and the puerperium. https://www.rcog.org.uk/guidance/browse-all-guidance/green-top-guidelines/reducing-the-risk-of-thrombosis-and-embolism-during-pregnancy-and-the-puerperium-green-top-guideline-no-37a/.

RCOG (2009). Green-top guideline No 37b. The acute management of thrombosis and embolism during pregnancy and the puerpurium. https://www.rcog.org.uk/guidance/browse-all-guidance/green-top-guidelines/thrombosis-and-embolism-during-pregnancy-and-the-puerperium-acute-management-green-top-guideline-no-37b/.

RCOG (2009). Green-top Guideline No 52. Prevention and management of postpartum haemorrhage. https://www.rcog.org.uk/globalassets/documents/guidelines/gt52postpartumhaemorrhage0411.pdf.

RCOG (2011). Green-top guideline No 56. Maternal collapse in pregnancy and the puerperium. https://www.rcog.org.uk/guidance/browse-all-guidance/green-top-guidelines/maternal-collapse-in-pregnancy-and-the-puerperium-green-top-guideline-no-56/.

RCOG (2012). Green-top guideline No 64a. Bacterial sepsis in pregnancy. https://www.rcog.org.uk/globalassets/documents/guidelines/gtg_64a.pdf.

RCOG (2014). Green-top guideline No 50. Umbilical cord prolapse. https://www.rcog.org.uk/globalassets/documents/guidelines/gtg-50-umbilicalcord-prolapse-2014.pdf.

SELF-ASSESSMENT

For interactive SBAs and EMQs relating to this chapter, visit www.routledge.com/cw/mccarthy.

CASE HISTORY 1

Ms B is 39 weeks' gestation in her second pregnancy. Her first pregnancy was a term delivery, delivered 11 months previously by caesarean section at 5 cm dilated due to failure to progress. Ms B was induced due to FGR and has been on oxytocin for 4 hours and has made good progress. She is now 9 cm dilated when she develops severe constant lower abdominal pain over the area of her scar. The midwife looking after her labour records the fetal heart rate as 46 beats per minute and calls an emergency alert.

A What is the likely diagnosis?
B What risk factors does Ms B have for this complication?
C How would you manage this situation?

ANSWERS

A Ms B has likely ruptured her uterus due to the nature and location of the pain (constant and severe, worse above her scar) and the fetal bradycardia that has now occurred. Differential diagnosis includes fetal distress.

B Ms B has had a previous caesarean section and has been induced due to FGR. The use of oxytocin also increased the risk of uterine rupture. Ms B has also had a short interpregnancy interval (<12 months), which increases the risk of uterine rupture.

C Management involves calling for senior help (senior obstetrician, neonatal team, anaesthetic team), safe delivery of the fetus and repair of the rupture. Delivery of the fetus is by the safest quickest route. A vaginal examination should be performed and an assessment for vaginal delivery should be made. If vaginal delivery is possible, then this should be performed and an assessment should be undertaken for examination under anaesthetic and/or laparotomy. If vaginal delivery is not possible, the patient should be transferred to the operating theatre for category 1 caesarean section, examination under anaesthetic and laparotomy.

CASE HISTORY 2

Ms F is 30 minutes after a spontaneous vaginal delivery of a 4.7 kg baby boy. You are called to review her as the midwife noticed a 'large gush' of blood vaginally after she performed a routine palpitation of the uterine fundus, which she described as 'soft'. The midwife looking after her informs you on arrival that her heart rate is 110 beats per minute and her blood pressure is 80/40 mmHg.

A What is the likely diagnosis?
B What risk factor does Ms F have for this complication?
C What is the differential diagnosis?
D How would you manage this situation?

ANSWERS

A Ms B is suffering from a post-partum haemorrhage likely secondary to uterine atony. She is now developing signs of significant blood loss.
B Ms B has had a macrosomic baby, which increases her risk of uterine atony and post-partum haemorrhage.
C Tone, tissue, trauma and thrombin are the main causes of post-partum haemorrhage. Although the description sounds most like uterine atony, it is important to complete a thorough assessment and ensure there are not other contributing factors such as a high vaginal wall tear that will require specific management and repair.
D Management involves calling for senior help (senior obstetrician, neonatal team, anaesthetic team). As uterine atony is the most likely cause, uterine massage should be started to stimulate uterine contractions and empty the uterus of clot. Ensure intravenous access and that appropriate bloods tests are sent. Administer intravenous fluids and uterotonic agents assessing the response after each medication is administered (see **Figure 14.6** for stepwise management and further detail). Post-partum haemorrhage management is often practised now in simulation training.

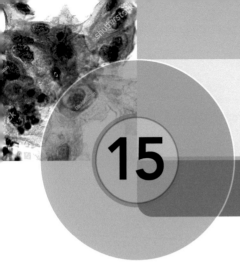

Puerperium

15

ANDREW D WEEKS

Learning Objectives
- Understand the physiological changes that occur in the normal puerperium.
- Understand the common disorders of the puerperium and how to manage them.
- Understand the process of breastfeeding and common disorders associated with it.
- Be able to recognize and manage common post-partum psychiatric disorders.

INTRODUCTION

The puerperium refers to the 6-week period following completion of the third stage of labour, when considerable adjustments occur before return to the pre-pregnant state. For those with complex medical problems, the early puerperium is especially dangerous, and most maternal deaths occur during this time (**Figure 15.1**). During this period of physiological change, the mother is also vulnerable to psychological disturbances, which may be aggravated by adverse social circumstances. Adequate understanding and support from the mother's partner and family are crucial. Difficulty in coping with the newborn infant occurs more frequently with the first baby, and vigilant surveillance is therefore necessary by the community midwife, general practitioner (GP) and health visitor.

PHYSIOLOGICAL CHANGES

UTERINE INVOLUTION

Involution is the process by which the post-partum uterus, weighing about 1 kg, returns to its pre-pregnancy state of less than 100 g. Immediately after delivery, the uterine fundus lies about 4 cm below the umbilicus or, more accurately, 12 cm above the symphysis pubis. However, by 2 weeks, the uterus becomes no longer palpable above the symphysis (**Figure 15.2**). Involution occurs by a process of autolysis, whereby muscle cells diminish in size as a result of enzymatic digestion of cytoplasm. This has virtually no effect on the number of muscle cells, and the excess protein produced from autolysis is absorbed into the bloodstream and excreted in the urine. Involution appears to be accelerated by the

10.1201/9781003196112-15

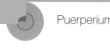

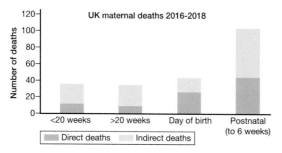

Figure 15.1 Timing of maternal deaths in the UK, 2016–2018.

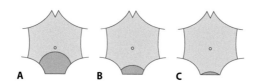

Figure 15.2 Involution of the uterus. (**A**) Day 1: 18-week-sized uterus (just below the umbilicus). (**B**) Day 7: 14-week-sized uterus. (**C**) Day 14: 12-week-sized uterus. The uterus is larger following caesarean section and in multiparous women.

release of oxytocin in women who are breastfeeding, as the uterus is smaller than in those who are bottle feeding. A delay in involution in the absence of any other signs or symptoms (e.g. bleeding) is of no clinical significance.

BOX 15.1: Causes of a high postnatal uterus

- Full bladder
- Loaded rectum
- Retained products of conception (or clots)
- Broad ligament haematoma (uterus is high and pushed laterally)
- Uterine infection
- Fibroids

GENITAL TRACT CHANGES

Following delivery of the placenta, the lower segment of the uterus and the cervix appear flabby and there may be small cervical lacerations. In the first few days, the cervix can readily admit two fingers; by the end of the first week it should become increasingly difficult to pass more than one finger, and certainly

by the end of the second week the internal os should be closed. However, the external os can remain open permanently, giving a characteristic funnel shape to the parous cervix. Assessment of the postnatal cervix is important in diagnosing retained products of conception (see the section 'Secondary post-partum haemorrhage' later in this chapter).

LOCHIA

Lochia is postnatal blood-stained uterine discharge comprising blood and necrotic decidua. Only the superficial layer of decidua becomes necrotic and is sloughed off. The basal layer adjacent to the myometrium is involved in the regeneration of new endometrium and this regeneration is complete by the third week.

During the first few days after delivery, the lochia is red (lochia rubra) and this gradually changes to pink as the endometrium is formed. By the second week, the discharge becomes serous (lochia serosa) and then finally turns to a scanty yellow-white discharge (lochia alba) that lasts for about 1 month. Persistent red lochia suggests delayed involution that is usually associated with infection or a retained piece of placental tissue (see the sections 'Secondary post-partum haemorrhage' and 'Genital tract infection/puerperal sepsis' later in this chapter).

KEY LEARNING POINT

Two weeks after birth, the lochia should no longer be red, the uterus should not be palpable above the symphysis pubis and pain from any perineal tears should be much improved or gone.

RECOVERY AFTER CHILDBIRTH

RECOVERY AFTER NORMAL BIRTH

Childbirth is a process of enormous significance in human lives, and with it comes massive physical and emotional changes. Although most parents will describe it as the best, most exciting experience of their lives, others will have bad outcomes and describe it as their worst. However, whatever the experience, there are very few who are not physically and emotionally drained in the first few weeks after childbirth. The combination of excitement, physical tiredness after labour and dealing with a demanding newborn makes this a time during which mothers (and fathers) often need a lot of support. Around the world, cultures have developed diverse ways of dealing with this. Traditionally, women from China and South India are confined to their homes for the first month postnatally, whereas traditional Sikh women are not allowed to cook for 40 days. Touch between men and women is prohibited while locia is being passed in some Orthodox Jewish couples and those from the Zulu tribe in South Africa. While some of these may seem strange in a modern world, these traditions recognize the enormity of what the woman had just been through and serve to provide new mothers with the chance to recover.

Alongside the psychological changes (see the section 'Psychiatric disorders' later in this chapter), the main physical effects are on the perineum, bladder and bowel.

PERINEAL PAIN

Perineal discomfort is a common problem for mothers. About 80% complain of pain in the first 3 days after delivery, with a quarter continuing to suffer discomfort at day 10. Discomfort is greatest in women who sustain spontaneous tears or have an episiotomy, especially following instrumental delivery. A number of non-pharmacological and pharmacological therapies have been used with varying degrees of success. However, local cooling (with crushed ice, witch hazel or tap water) and topical anaesthetics, such as 5% lignocaine gel, provide short-term symptomatic relief. Effective analgesia following perineal trauma can be achieved with regular paracetamol. If necessary, diclofenac given rectally or orally may also be added. Codeine derivatives are best avoided, as they cause constipation in the mother and drowsiness in some breastfed babies.

The perineum should be kept clean with daily cleaning or showering using tap water only, frequent changing of sanitary pads and handwashing before and after this (National Institute for Health and Care Excellence (NICE) 2021). Infections of the perineum are surprisingly uncommon considering the risk of bacterial contamination during delivery. However, all women should be asked about perineal pain, discharge, swelling and wound breakdown at postnatal visits – women with sutures or symptoms should also be examined (NICE 2021). Signs of infection (redness, pain, swelling and heat), especially with a raised temperature, must be taken seriously. Swabs for microbiological culture should be taken from the infected perineum, and broad-spectrum antibiotics (see the section 'Genital tract infection/puerperal sepsis' later in this chapter) should be commenced. If there is a collection of pus, drainage should be encouraged by removal of any skin sutures; otherwise, infection can spread, with increasing morbidity and a poor anatomical result.

Spontaneous opening of repaired perineal tears and episiotomies is usually the result of secondary infection. Surgical repair should never be attempted in the presence of infection. The wound should be irrigated twice daily and healing allowed to occur by secondary intention. If there is a large, gaping wound, secondary repair should be performed only when the infection has cleared, there is no cellulitis or exudate present, and healthy granulation tissue can be seen.

BLADDER FUNCTION

Voiding difficulties and overdistension of the bladder are not uncommon after childbirth, especially if regional anaesthesia (epidural/spinal) has been used. It is now known that after epidural anaesthesia the bladder may take up to 8 hours to regain normal sensation. During this time, about 1 litre of urine may be produced. Therefore, if urinary retention occurs, considerable damage may be inflicted on the detrusor muscle. Overstretching of the detrusor muscle can dampen bladder sensation and make the bladder hypocontractile, particularly with fibrous replacement of smooth muscle. In this situation, overflow incontinence of small amounts of urine may erroneously be assumed to be normal voiding. Fluid loading prior to epidural analgesia, the antidiuretic effect of high concentrations of oxytocin during labour, increased post-partum diuresis (particularly in the presence of peripheral oedema) and increased fluid intake by breastfeeding mothers all contribute to increased urine production in the puerperium. Therefore, an intake/output chart alone may not detect incomplete emptying of the bladder.

Women who have undergone a traumatic delivery, such as a difficult instrumental delivery, or who have suffered multiple/extended lacerations or a vulvovaginal haematoma may find it difficult to void because of pain or periurethral oedema. Other causes of pain, such as prolapsed haemorrhoids, anal fissures, abdominal wound haematoma or even stool impaction of the rectum may interfere with voiding. The midwife needs to be particularly vigilant after an epidural or spinal anaesthetic to avoid bladder distension. A distended bladder either would be palpable as a suprapubic cystic mass or may displace the uterus laterally or upwards, thereby increasing the height of the uterine fundus.

A formal assessment of bladder function is best made 6 hours postnatally, at which time the woman should have passed at least 300 mL of urine. If, after another attempt, they have passed less than that (or none at all), then a small intermittent catheter can be inserted, which should drain less than 150 mL. Those with more than this need close observation, but if there is over 1 litre of urine in the bladder then an indwelling catheter is left in for 48 hours to allow periurethral swelling to settle.

To minimize the risk of overdistension of the bladder in women who have had a spinal anaesthetic (for caesarean section or manual removal of the placenta), a urinary catheter is left in the bladder for at least 12 hours until the woman is mobile.

Although vaginal delivery is strongly implicated in the long-term development of urinary stress incontinence, it rarely poses a problem in the early puerperium. Therefore, any incontinence should be investigated to exclude a vesicovaginal, urethrovaginal or, rarely, ureterovaginal fistula. Obstetric fistulae are rare in the UK, but are a source of considerable morbidity in developing countries as a complication of obstructed labour. Prolonged pressure of the fetal head on the bladder or urethra causes pressure necrosis, and incontinence follows in the second week when the slough separates. Small fistulae may close spontaneously after a few weeks of free bladder drainage; large fistulae will require surgical repair by a specialist.

KEY LEARNING POINT

To prevent overdistension of the postnatal bladder, check that a woman has passed at least 300 mL in the first 6 hours after giving birth. If they haven't, then use a catheter or ultrasound to check that less than 150 mL remains in the bladder after voiding.

BOWEL FUNCTION

Constipation is a common problem in the early puerperium as a result of an interruption in the normal diet, intra-partum dehydration and opiate use. Advice on adequate fluid intake and increase in fibre intake may be all that is necessary. However, constipation may also be the result of fear of evacuation due to pain from a sutured perineum, prolapsed haemorrhoids or anal fissures. Avoidance of constipation and straining is of utmost importance in women who have sustained a third- or fourth-degree tear. A large, hard stool in this situation could disrupt the repaired anal sphincter and cause anal incontinence. It is therefore important to ensure that these women are prescribed lactulose and ispaghula husk or methylcellulose immediately after the repair, for a period of 2 weeks.

The high prevalence of anal incontinence and faecal urgency following childbirth has only recently been recognized. One prospective study using anal endosonography at 6 weeks following vaginal birth identified evidence of occult anal sphincter trauma in a third of primiparous women (only 13% were symptomatic) and in a remarkable 80% of those who had undergone forceps delivery. Larger, retrospective, short-term studies of parous women indicate a symptom prevalence of between 6% and 10%. Long-term anal incontinence following primary repair of a third- or fourth-degree tear occurs in 5% of women, and anovaginal/rectovaginal fistulae occur in 2–4% of these women (**Figure 15.3**). It is therefore important to consider a fistula as a cause of anal incontinence in the post-partum period, particularly if the woman complains of passing wind or stool per vagina. Approximately 50% of small anovaginal fistulae will close spontaneously over a period of 6 months, but larger fistulae will require formal repair.

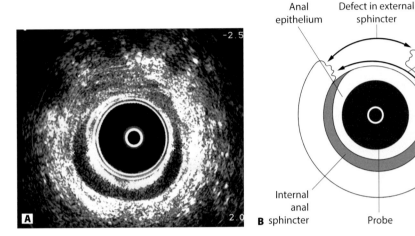

Figure 15.3 (**A**) Transanal ultrasound showing the anal mucosa and anterior disruption of the internal anal sphincter (dark band) following a third-degree tear at delivery. (**B**) Diagrammatic representation of (**A**).

PELVIC FLOOR EXERCISES

It is a widespread belief that pelvic floor exercises tone up the muscles of the pelvic floor and should therefore be advocated in the post-partum period. However, large randomized trials to evaluate their benefit in preventing genital prolapse, urinary incontinence or anal incontinence are lacking. There is also no evidence that antenatal exercises prevent incontinence or prolapse. However, as general exercise is known to strengthen striated muscle and as pelvic floor exercises are unlikely to be harmful, women are still taught postnatal exercises. This should also serve to cultivate a feeling of pelvic floor awareness, so that women with pelvic floor dysfunction seek medical help sooner.

RECOVERY FROM CAESAREAN SECTION

Many women now deliver their baby by caesarean section. Although this reduces the risk of pelvic floor problems, it increases the risk of other complications including infection (wound, urine and chest), anaemia and thromboembolism. The infective risks are discussed in the section 'Genital tract infection/ puerperal sepsis' later in this chapter, but are reduced by routine antibiotics at the time of caesarean section and careful wound care. The wound should be covered by a sterile dressing in theatre, which is removed after 24 hours. Women are advised to gently clean and dry the wound daily with tap water. Sutures or staples are removed on the fifth day.

Anaemia is common post-operatively and, given the inaccuracy of blood loss estimation, all women should have their haemoglobin levels measured post-operatively (ideally on day 2 or 3). Asymptomatic women with mild to moderate anaemia (haemoglobin >7 g/dL) can be treated with iron tablets, while the post-operative recovery of those with severe anaemia will be helped greatly by an iron infusion or blood transfusion.

The combination of abdominal surgery, pre-operative bed rest and physiological changes in clotting makes women who have had a caesarean section particularly prone to thromboembolism. Other risk factors include thrombophilias, immobility, previous thromboembolism, pre-eclampsia, post-partum haemorrhage (PPH), obesity, multiple pregnancy and smoking. Early mobilization and good hydration are important for all women, with 1–6 weeks of low-molecular-weight heparin given to those with multiple risk factors. In the UK, early mobilization is now encouraged, with low-risk women being discharged from hospital on day 1 or 2 following caesarean section. The changes discussed here have contributed to a decrease in thromboembolism deaths in the UK from a peak of 2.2 per 100,000 births in 1994–1996 to 0.92 per 100,000 in 2017–2019.

After the first few days, women who have undergone caesarean section should not have routine bed rest but should slowly increase their activity levels aided by oral analgesia as required. They can resume activities such as carrying heavy items, formal exercise, sexual intercourse and driving once they have returned to their pre-caesarean section strength with no physical restrictions or pain.

POSTNATAL VISITS

The degree of care provided by the health service varies from country to country. In the UK, a mother who has delivered in hospital may be discharged within 6 hours of an uncomplicated birth, although they may request to stay longer. Globally, however, the World Health Organization (WHO) recommends that women who give birth in a facility stay for at least 24 hours for monitoring before discharge (**Table 15.1**).

Traditionally, a midwife would visit the mother and newborn daily for a minimum of 10 days after delivery, with the health visitor taking on continuing care for up to 4 weeks. However, postnatal care is generally now a demand-led service for low-risk women, with

only one routine midwifery visit before care is handed over to the health visitor. More frequent visits will be required for high-risk women, for those with difficult social circumstances or if an abnormality such as hypertension or a pyrexia has been detected.

Table 15.1 Minimum postnatal care package recommendations by NICE (2021) and WHO (2013)

NICE guidelines	WHO guidelines
Discharged home at 6 hours after facility birth	Minimum 24-hour stay after facility birth
First postnatal visit within 36 hours by midwife	Home visit by health worker within 24 hours after home birth
Visit by health visitor in first 7 days if not visited antenatally	Home visit at day 2 or 3 by health worker
Health visitor home visit at 7–14 days	Home visit at 7–14 days by health worker
General practitioner postnatal review at 6–8 weeks	Postnatal review at 6 weeks with health worker

Additional visits or stays in the facility are arranged for those with complications or additional needs.
Source: NICE, National Institute for Health and Care Excellence; WHO, World Health Organization.

BOX 15.2: Maternal health components of postnatal care visits

Postnatal assessments of physical health (NICE 2021)
- Infection-related symptoms
- Nipple and breast discomfort
- Pain
- Symptoms of thromboembolism
- Vaginal discharge and bleeding
- Symptoms of anaemia
- Bladder function
- Symptoms of pre-eclampsia
- Bowel function
- Healing of any wounds (perineal or caesarean section)
- Examination to include temperature, pulse, pallor and wounds
- Test blood pressure and urine for protein

Topics for postnatal discussion (NICE 2021)
- The postnatal period and what to expect
- Postnatal mental health problems and how to seek help
- Danger signs and how to seek help
- Pelvic floor exercises
- Fatigue
- Diet, physical activity, smoking, alcohol and drug use
- Sexual intercourse and contraception
- Domestic violence

Additional topics in low- or middle-income settings (WHO 2013)
- Importance of birth spacing
- Hygiene and handwashing
- Safer sex and condoms
- Importance of bed nets at night in malaria-endemic areas
- Early mobilization, adopting gentle exercise with plenty of rest
- Routine oral iron and folate supplements

Additional topics on infant care and breastfeeding are covered in the relevant sections in this chapter.

At each visit, women should be specifically asked about their recovery, including bowel and bladder function, fatigue, headache and perineum (see **Box 15.2**, 'Maternal health components of postnatal care visits'). Further questions will cover breastfeeding and the health of the newborn (see **Chapter 16**). During this time, it is crucial that women are also provided with information about danger signs (Table 15.2) and given emotional support. They should also be provided with contact details of where they can get information. Mothers who are not rubella immune should be offered immunization.

Table 15.2 Signs and symptoms of potentially serious postnatal conditions for which women should seek immediate medical advice

Signs and symptoms	Condition
Sudden or very heavy vaginal bleeding, persistent or increased vaginal bleeding, or passage of clots, placental tissue or membranes*	Retained placental tissue or endometritis
Abdominal, pelvic or perineal pain, fever, shivering or vaginal discharge with an unpleasant smell	Infection
Leg swelling and tenderness or shortness of breath	Venous thromboembolism
Chest pain	Venous thromboembolism or cardiac problems
Persistent or severe headache	Hypertension, pre-eclampsia, postdural-puncture headache, migraine, intracranial pathology or infection
Worsening reddening and swelling of breasts persisting for more than 24 hours despite self-management	Mastitis

Source: Based on NICE (2021).
* NICE guidelines recommend taking extra care if women are anaemic or have a booking weight of under 50 kg (NICE 2021). NICE, National Institute for Health and Care Excellence; WHO, World Health Organization.

The only routine tests to be performed at every postnatal visit are the maternal blood pressure, pulse, temperature and urinalysis. Other maternal examinations and observations should be determined by the mother's condition and symptoms (see Table 15.2). For example, those with offensive vaginal loss or signs of infection will require pulse and temperature assessments along with an assessment of uterine involution. Those who have had a PPH or who have abnormal vaginal bleeding will require an assessment of uterine involution along with pulse and blood pressure. For women with antenatal anaemia, complicated deliveries or PPH, the haemoglobin level should be checked between day 1 and day 3 and iron should be offered to those who are anaemic. Women who are particularly symptomatic or who have a haemoglobin level of <7 g/dL should be offered an iron infusion or blood transfusion.

At 2 weeks postnatally, women should be specifically asked about the resolution of the 'baby blues' (see the section 'Pathophysiology of post-partum affective disorders' later in this chapter).

A formal postnatal examination is generally carried out at about 6 weeks' post-partum by the GP, or by the obstetrician if delivery was complicated. The examination includes an assessment of the woman's mental and physical health (see Table 15.3), as well as the progress of the baby. In particular, direct questions should be asked about urinary, bowel and sexual function. Incontinence and dyspareunia are embarrassing issues that women do not readily discuss. Weight, urine analysis and blood pressure are checked and an examination is performed as required. If a cervical smear is due, it can be taken, although it is preferable to wait until 3 months' post-partum. Contraception, pelvic floor exercises and infant immunizations are also discussed.

PUERPERAL DISORDERS

HYPERTENSION

During pregnancy, women with hypertension are carefully managed with monitoring, antihypertensives and timed delivery to prevent complications. After childbirth, however, they often receive less attention, even though they remain at significant

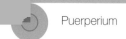

Table 15.3 Diagnosis and management of puerperal pyrexia

Symptoms	Diagnosis	Specific investigations	Management
Cough Purulent sputum Dyspnoea	Pneumonia	Sputum M, C & S Chest X-ray	Physiotherapy Antibiotics
Sore throat Cervical lymphadenopathy	Tonsillitis	Throat swab	Antibiotics
Headaches Neck stiffness (epidural/ spinal anaesthetic)	Meningitis	Lumbar puncture	Antibiotics
Dysuria Loin pain and tenderness	Pyelonephritis	Urine M, C & S	Antibiotics Increased fluid intake
Secondary PPH Tender bulky uterus	Endometritis or retained placental tissue	Clinical diagnosis with or without pelvic ultrasound	Antibiotics and/or uterine evacuation
Pelvic/calf pain/tenderness	Deep vein thrombosis	Doppler/venogram of legs	Low-molecular-weight heparin
Chest pain Dyspnoea	Pulmonary embolism	Chest X-ray and blood gases, lung perfusion scan, angiogram	Low-molecular-weight heparin
Painful engorged breasts	Mastitis or breast abscess	Clinical examination M, C & S of expressed milk	Express milk Antibiotics Incision and drainage

M, C & S, microscopy, culture and sensitivity; PPH, post-partum haemorrhage.

risk for the first week. Nearly half of all eclamptic fits occur postnatally, and it is the highest risk time for fluid overload. Those with severe pre-eclampsia should be managed for the first 24 hours on a high-dependency unit until their blood pressure is controlled and they achieve a good diuresis (see **Chapter 9**). Those with mild or moderate pre-eclampsia are managed on a postnatal ward until stable. They should continue any antenatally prescribed antihypertensives with the aim of keeping their blood pressure under 150/100 mmHg. Labetalol or slow-release nifedipine are good choices for this, and are commonly needed for 1–2 weeks postnatally. First-line therapy for new-onset postnatal hypertension is nifedipine or amlodipine (if of African origin) or enalapril (if of European origin). For more control, these can be combined or atenolol or labetalol can be added. At home, the blood pressure is measured every 2 days and the dosage halved when it is <140/90 mmHg. Those who are still on antihypertensives 6 weeks postnatally should be referred for specialist assessment. Women should be informed that the recurrence risk of pre-eclampsia is around 15% (higher still if it was early onset) and that their long-term risk of developing cardiovascular disease is doubled.

SECONDARY POST-PARTUM HAEMORRHAGE

Secondary PPH is defined as fresh bleeding from the genital tract between 24 hours and 6 weeks after delivery (see **Chapter 14**). The most common time for secondary PPH is between days 7 and 14. The cause is usually either endometritis or retained placental tissue, and it is often very difficult to distinguish between them. Classically, women with endometritis have constant low abdominal pain and a tender uterus with a closed internal os. In contrast, women with retained products of conception have crampy low abdominal pain and a uterus larger than appropriate (see **Figure 15.2**) with an open internal os. There is often a history of a prolonged third stage of labour or sometimes the passage of bits of placental tissue or membranes. Both endometritis and retained products may have symptoms and signs of infection with low-grade fever, pungent lochia and uterine tenderness. Those bleeding heavily will require circulatory support with fluids or blood along with strong oxytocics (e.g. ergometrine) and uterine evacuation. Antibiotics should be given if placental tissue is found, even without evidence of overt infection. If blood loss is not excessive, the use of pelvic ultrasound to exclude retained products is sometimes used, but is only helpful if the uterus is seen to be empty. Debris, clots and fluid are commonly found even within the normal post-partum uterus and their presence does not mean that there is retained placental tissue. In the absence of a clear diagnosis, expectant management with empirical antibiotics is often used. Other causes of secondary PPH include hormonal contraception, bleeding disorders (e.g. von Willebrand disease) and, occasionally, choriocarcinoma.

OBSTETRIC PALSY

Obstetric palsy, or traumatic neuritis, is a condition in which one or both lower limbs develop signs of a motor and/or sensory neuropathy following delivery. Presenting features include sciatic pain, foot-drop, paraesthesia, hypoaesthesia and muscle wasting. The mechanism of injury is proximal nerve damage when the lumbosacral plexus and nerve tracks are stretched and compressed by the fetal head as they cross the pelvic brim. It is almost always associated with prolonged or obstructed labour and is now very rare following modern labour management. If obstetric paralysis develops following a normal labour, then epidural complications and/or herniation of lumbosacral discs should be excluded, particularly if the woman has been in an exaggerated lithotomy position for instrumental delivery. Peroneal nerve palsy can occur when the nerve is compressed between the head of the fibula and the lithotomy pole, resulting in unilateral foot-drop. The development of urinary and faecal incontinence is most likely due to structural damage to the anal sphincter muscle and supporting fascia.

SYMPHYSIS PUBIS DIASTASIS

Spontaneous separation of the symphysis pubis occurs in at least 1 in 800 vaginal deliveries. It is usually noticed after delivery and has been associated with forceps delivery, a rapid second stage of labour or severe abduction of the thighs during delivery. Common signs and symptoms include symphyseal pain aggravated by weight-bearing and walking, a waddling gait, pubic tenderness and a palpable interpubic gap. Treatment includes bed rest, anti-inflammatory agents, physiotherapy and a pelvic corset to provide support and stability.

THROMBOEMBOLISM

The risk of thromboembolic disease rises fivefold during pregnancy and the puerperium. The majority of fatal thromboembolisms occur in the puerperium and are more common after caesarean section. Those at high risk may be given prophylactic heparin injections. If deep vein thrombosis or pulmonary embolism is suspected, full anticoagulant therapy should be commenced and a lower limb compression ultrasound and/or lung scan should be carried out within 24–48 hours (see **Chapters 6** and **14**).

PUERPERAL PYREXIA

Significant puerperal pyrexia is defined as a temperature of 38°C or higher on any 2 of the first 10 days post-partum, excluding the first 24 hours. A mildly elevated temperature is not uncommon in the first 24 hours, but any pyrexia associated with tachycardia merits investigation. In about 80% of women who develop a temperature in the first 24 hours following a vaginal delivery, no obvious evidence of infection can be identified. The reverse holds true for women delivering by caesarean section, when a wound infection should be considered. Common sites associated with puerperal pyrexia include chest, throat, breasts, urinary tract, pelvic organs, caesarean or perineal wounds, and legs (**Table 15.3**).

CHEST COMPLICATIONS

Chest complications are most likely to appear in the first 24 hours after delivery, particularly after general anaesthesia. Atelectasis may be associated with fever and can be prevented by early and regular chest physiotherapy. Aspiration pneumonia (Mendelson syndrome) must be suspected if there is a spiking temperature associated with wheezing, dyspnoea or evidence of hypoxia following a general anaesthetic.

GENITAL TRACT INFECTION/ PUERPERAL SEPSIS

Genital tract infection following delivery is referred to as puerperal sepsis and is synonymous with older descriptions of puerperal fever, milk fever and child-bed fever. It was not realized until the mid-19th century that the high maternal mortality and morbidity in the UK was due to poor hygiene; the establishment of lying-in hospitals and overcrowding perpetuated the condition to epidemic proportions. Until 1937, puerperal sepsis was the major cause of maternal mortality. The discovery of sulphonamides in 1935 and improved hygiene at the time of birth resulted in a dramatic fall in maternal mortality. However, surveys continue to show that, around the world, sepsis deaths are still common, accounting for around 10% of all maternal deaths.

AETIOLOGY

A mixed flora with low virulence normally colonizes the vagina. Puerperal infection is usually polymicrobial and involves contaminants from the bowel that colonize the perineum and lower genital tract (see **Box 15.3**, 'Organisms commonly associated with puerperal genital infection'). Following delivery, natural barriers to infection are temporarily removed and therefore organisms with a pathogenic potential can ascend from the lower genital tract into the uterine cavity. Placental separation exposes a large raw area equivalent to an open wound, and retained products of conception and blood clots within the uterus can provide an excellent culture medium for infection. Furthermore, vaginal delivery is commonly associated with lacerations of the genital tract (uterus, cervix and vagina). Although these lacerations may not need surgical repair, they can become a focus for infection similar to iatrogenic wounds, such as caesarean section and episiotomy.

BOX 15.3: Organisms commonly associated with puerperal genital infection

Aerobes
- Gram-positive:
  - beta-haemolytic *Streptococcus*, groups A, B and D
  - *Staphylococcus epidermidis* and *S. aureus*
  - enterococci – *Streptococcus faecalis*
- Gram-negative:
  - *Escherichia coli*
  - *Haemophilus influenzae*
  - *Klebsiella pneumoniae*
  - *Pseudomonas aeruginosa*
  - *Proteus mirabilis*
- Gram-variable:
  - *Gardenella vaginalis*

Anaerobes
- *Peptococcus* sp.
- *Peptostreptococcus* sp.
- *Bacteroides* sp. – *B. fragilis*, *B. bivius* and *B. disiens*
- *Fusobacterium* sp.

Miscellaneous
- *Chlamydia trachomatis*
- *Mycoplasma hominis*
- *Ureaplasma urealyticum*

BOX 15.4: Common risk factors for puerperal infection

- Underlying conditions:
  - obesity
  - diabetes
  - human immunodeficiency virus (HIV)
- Antenatal:
  - chorioamnionitis
  - prolonged rupture of membranes
  - cervical cerclage for cervical incompetence
- Intra-partum:
  - prolonged labour
  - multiple vaginal examinations
  - instrumental delivery
  - caesarean section
  - manual removal of the placenta
  - retained products of conception

PREVENTION

Increased awareness of the principles of general hygiene, a good surgical approach and the use of aseptic techniques have all contributed to the decline in severe puerperal sepsis. Unfortunately, although it is over 150 years since the Hungarian obstetrician Ignaz Semelweiss identified the importance of hand-washing for preventing spread of infection between postnatal women, poor attention to hand-washing remains a significant problem. The arrival of alcohol-based hand rubs has facilitated the process: every clinician should use them regularly in clinical areas, at least between every patient contact. The risk of postnatal infection is higher following caesarean section, preterm pre-labour rupture of membranes, operative vaginal births, manual removal of placenta or third-degree tears, but can be prevented by routine prophylactic antibiotics. For caesarean sections, a single intraoperative dose of antibiotics (penicillin or first-generation cephalosporin) is given before the skin incision. Antibiotic prophylaxis should also be used for those with group B *Streptococcus* colonization. Puerperal parametritis develops in a third of women who had a pre-existing C. *trachomatis* infection, but presentation is usually delayed. The risk of postnatal infection can be further reduced by vaginal cleansing with chlorhexidine or povidone-iodine prior to emergency caesarean section. The problem of resistant bacteria (e.g. methicillin-resistant S. *aureus* [MRSA]) has led some units to routinely screen all women admitted electively to the hospital so that those carrying the resistant bacteria can be barrier nursed to prevent their spread.

CLINICAL PRESENTATION

There are a number of factors that determine the clinical course and severity of the infection, namely the general health and resistance of the woman, the virulence of the offending organism, the presence of haematoma or retained products of conception, the timing of antibiotic therapy and associated risk factors. The common methods of spread of puerperal infection are as follows:

- An ascending infection from the lower genital tract or primary infection of the placental site may spread via the fallopian tubes to the ovaries, giving rise to a salpingo-oophoritis and pelvic peritonitis. This could progress to a generalized peritonitis and the development of pelvic abscesses.
- Infection may spread directly into the myometrium and the parametrium, giving rise to an endometritis or parametritis, also referred to as pelvic cellulitis. Pelvic peritonitis and abscesses may also occur.
- Infection may spread to distant sites via lymphatics and blood vessels. Infection from the uterus can be carried by uterine vessels into the inferior vena cava via the iliac vessels or, directly, via the ovarian vessels. This could give rise to a septic thrombophlebitis, pulmonary infections or generalized septicaemia and endotoxic shock.

In contrast with pelvic inflammatory disease unrelated to pregnancy, tubal involvement in puerperal sepsis is in the form of peri-salpingitis, which,

Table 15.4 Investigations for puerperal genital infections

Investigations	Abnormalities
Full blood count	Anaemia, leucocytosis and thrombocytopaenia
Urea and electrolytes	Fluid and electrolyte imbalance
Culture of blood, sputum or breast milk or swabs from high vagina, wound or throat	Bacterial or viral culture
Chest X-ray	Evidence of infection
Pelvic ultrasound	Retained products and pelvic abscess
Clotting screen (haemorrhage or shock)	Disseminated intravascular coagulation
Blood lactate	Lactic acid ≥2 mmol/L (can be raised immediately after birth so serial samples are useful)
Blood gas (arterial if respiratory effects)	Acidosis and hypoxia (shock), hypoglycaemia and lactic acidosis

BOX 15.5: Symptoms of puerperal pelvic infection

- Malaise, headache, fever and rigors
- Abdominal discomfort, vomiting and diarrhoea
- Offensive lochia
- Secondary PPH

BOX 15.6: Signs of puerperal pelvic infection

- Pyrexia and tachycardia
- Uterus – boggy, tender and larger
- Infected wounds – caesarean/perineal
- Peritonism
- Paralytic ileus
- Indurated adnexae (parametritis)
- Bogginess in pelvis (abscess)

Table 15.5 Risk stratification for suspected sepsis

Moderate- to high-risk criteria	Severe sepsis
Patient or family reports new onset of altered behaviour or mental state	Objective evidence of new altered mental state
Respiratory rate: 21–24 breaths per minute (counted over 60 seconds)	Respiratory rate ≥25 breaths per minute (counted over 60 seconds), or need for oxygen to keep O_2 saturation >92%.
Systolic blood pressure: 91–100 mmHg	Systolic blood pressure: ≤90 mmHg (or >40 mmHg below normal)
Heart rate: 100–130 beats per minute or new onset arrhythmia	Heart rate: >130 beats per minute
Not passed urine in past 12–18 hours (or urine output 0.5–1 mL/kg if catheterized)	Not passed urine in past 18 hours (or urine output <0.5 mL/kg if catheterized)
Signs of potential infection at surgical site	Skin mottled or ashen, cyanosis and non-blanching skin rash
	Tympanic temperature: <36°C

Source: Based on National Institute for Health and Care Excellence (NICE) 2017. If there are any criteria for severe sepsis, emergency investigation and treatment is needed. If any moderate- to high-risk criteria are identified, urgent clinical review is needed within an hour.

rarely, causes tubal occlusion and consequent infertility. Tubo-ovarian abscesses are also a rare complication of puerperal sepsis. Investigations for puerperal genital infections are shown in **Table 15.4**.

MANAGEMENT

Mild to moderate infections can be treated with a broad-spectrum antibiotic (e.g. co-amoxiclav or a cephalosporin, such as cefalexin, plus metronidazole). Depending on the severity, the first few doses should be given intravenously.

With severe infections, there is a release of inflammatory and vasoactive mediators in response to the endotoxins produced during bacteriolysis. The resultant local vasodilatation causes circulatory embarrassment and hence poor tissue perfusion. This phenomenon is known as septicaemic, septic or endotoxic shock, and the features are shown in **Table 15.5**. Delay in appropriate management could be fatal and *immediate* high-dose, broad-spectrum antibiotics and resuscitation with intravenous fluids must be provided on a high-dependency unit. Close liaison with microbiologists and internal medicine specialists is vital.

Necrotizing fasciitis is a rare but frequently fatal infection of the skin, fascia and muscle. It can originate in perineal tears, episiotomies and caesarean section wounds. Perineal infections extend rapidly to involve the buttocks, thighs and lower abdominal wall. A variety of bacteria can be involved, but anaerobes predominate and *Clostridium perfringens* is usually identified. In addition to general signs of infection, there is extensive necrosis, crepitus and inflammation. As well as the measures usually taken to manage septic shock, wide debridement of necrotic tissue under general anaesthesia is absolutely essential to avoid mortality. Split-thickness skin grafts may be necessary at a later date.

BOX 15.7: Sepsis management (actions to be completed within an hour)

- Administer oxygen (aim for oxygen saturation of 94–98%)
- Take blood for culture (also for full blood count, C-reactive protein, urea and electrolytes, liver function tests and coagulation)
- Check lactate (if ≥2 mmol/L, repeat after fluid challenge)
- Give intravenous fluids (if hypotensive or lactate >2, give 500 mL over 15 minutes)
- Give intravenous antibiotics within 1 hour
- Measure urine output accurately (insert catheter, use fluid balance chart)
- Identify source (cultures, chest X-ray and electrocardiogram as indicated)

PSYCHIATRIC DISORDERS

Although the incidence of mild mental health problems is not significantly different during pregnancy, the risk of bipolar or severe depressive illness is greatly increased post-partum and this period represents the highest risk period in a woman's life for the development of a psychiatric disorder. Furthermore, women with previous serious mental health problems are at high risk of a recurrence during both the antepartum and post-partum periods. A multidisciplinary approach, supervised by specialist perinatal mental health teams, is vital to optimize care, limit morbidity and help prevent the tragic cases of suicide detailed in the maternal mortality reports. The problems of substance and alcohol misuse during pregnancy overlap significantly with mental health issues, and coordination is required between specialist services and providers of maternity care.

The impact of psychiatric disease in pregnancy has been emphasized repeatedly by the UK Confidential Enquiries into Maternal Deaths (of Mothers and Babies, Reducing Risk through Audits and Confidential Enquiries across the UK [MBRRACE-UK]). The 2021 report *Saving Lives: Improving Mothers' Care* covers 2017–2019 and reports on 191 deaths, 10 (5%) of which

were from suicide. Suicide during pregnancy is unusually violent (shootings, hangings) in contrast with suicide attempts in younger women, which commonly take the form of overdose and are less frequently successful. This emphasizes the severity of mental health problems occurring after delivery, when most maternal suicides take place.

PATHOPHYSIOLOGY OF POST-PARTUM AFFECTIVE DISORDERS

Psychosocial factors play a major role in the aetiology of non-psychotic mild and moderate post-partum depressive illness. This is in contrast with puerperal psychosis and severe post-partum depressive illness, in which other factors (e.g. family history) predominate, suggesting a biological aetiology.

The constancy of incidence across cultures and the temporal relationship with childbirth would tend to suggest a neuroendocrine basis for the more severe conditions. Changes in cortisol, oxytocin, endorphins, thyroxine, progesterone and oestrogen have all been implicated in the causation. Comparable dramatic changes in steroidal hormones outside the post-partum period have a well-known association with affective psychoses and mood disorders. A plausible theory is that the sudden fall in oestrogen post-partum triggers a hypersensitivity of certain dopamine receptors in a predisposed group of women and may be responsible for the severe mood disturbance that follows. The occurrence and the severity of the 'postnatal blues' are thought to be related to both the absolute level of progesterone and the relative drop from a prepartum level. However, there is no clear association between the 'post-partum blues' and affective psychoses and there is no evidence to implicate progesterone in the aetiology of puerperal psychosis or severe postnatal depression.

Depression is a characteristic feature of hypothyroidism, which may occur as a consequence of post-partum thyroiditis. The other features of hypothyroidism may be missed, and checking thyroid function is important in women with milder depressive symptoms in the first year following childbirth, as correction with thyroid supplements may elevate the mood.

NORMAL EMOTIONAL AND PSYCHOLOGICAL CHANGES DURING PREGNANCY

Diagnosing mental illness in pregnancy is complicated by the wide variety of 'normal' emotional and behavioural changes that may occur.

POSTNATAL

- The 'pinks': for the first 24–48 hours following delivery, it is very common for women to experience an elevation of mood, a feeling of excitement, some overactivity and difficulty sleeping.
- The 'blues': as many as 80% of women may experience the 'postnatal blues' in the first 2 weeks after delivery. Fatigue, short temper, difficulty sleeping, depressed mood and tearfulness are common but usually mild, and resolve spontaneously in the majority of cases. The following psychological disruptions should not be considered normal and require further assessment:
  - panic attacks
  - episodes of low mood of prolonged duration (>2 weeks)
  - low self-esteem
  - guilt or hopelessness
  - suicidal thoughts
  - thoughts of (or actual) self-harm – these are very unusual in pregnancy or early post-partum and should always prompt referral
  - any mood changes that disrupt normal social functioning
  - 'biological' symptoms (e.g. poor appetite, early wakening)
  - change in 'affect'

SCREENING FOR MENTAL HEALTH PROBLEMS DURING AND AFTER PREGNANCY

NICE Clinical Guideline No 45, *Antenatal and Postnatal Mental Health*, sets out screening questions that all postnatal women should be asked (see

Box 15.8, 'NICE screening questions for mental health problems during and after pregnancy'). If the answers to these questions raise concerns, then the woman should be referred back to her GP, to her own psychiatrist (if she has one) or to a specialist perinatal mental health team depending on the severity of the symptoms or previous history.

> **BOX 15.8: NICE screening questions for mental health problems during and after pregnancy**
>
> All women should be asked the following at booking and in the postnatal period:
> "During the past month, have you often been bothered by:
> - feeling down, depressed or hopeless?
> - having little interest or pleasure in doing things?"

POST-PARTUM (NON-PSYCHOTIC) DEPRESSIVE ILLNESS

Between 10% and 15% of women will suffer with some form of depression in the first year after the delivery of their baby. At least 7% will satisfy the criteria for mild major depressive illness and many more could be described as having minor depression; 3–5% will suffer a severe major postnatal depressive episode. Without treatment, most women will recover spontaneously within 3–6 months; however, 1 in 10 will remain depressed at 1 year.

Women with a history of severe depression are at even higher risk. Those with a history of depression not related to pregnancy carry between a 1:3 and 1:5 risk of a major post-partum depressive illness, while the recurrence rate of postnatal depression is as high as 50%.

CLINICAL FEATURES

In contrast with puerperal psychosis, non-psychotic post-partum depression usually presents later in the postnatal period, most commonly around 6 weeks, with a more gradual onset. The 6-week postnatal check is an ideal opportunity to detect early post-partum non-psychotic depression, but the signs are often missed. NICE recommends that all women are asked about their mood at least twice in the postpartum period by midwives, obstetricians, health visitors or GPs, ideally at 6 weeks and 3–4 months after the birth (see **Box 15.8**, 'NICE screening questions for mental health problems during and after pregnancy'). Particular attention should be paid to the assessment of women with risk factors for postnatal depressive illness. Indeed, women deemed at highest risk should be under close surveillance by a specialist community psychiatric nurse, with early admission to the local mother-and-baby unit if there are signs of concern. Those who screen positive on the two questions in **Box 15.8** should receive a more detailed questionnaire, for example the 10-question Edinburgh Postnatal Depression Scale, which has been validated in multiple languages.

Severe postnatal affective disorders usually present earlier than milder forms and, in this group, biological risk factors may be more important than psychosocial factors.

Treatment options include:

- remedy of social factors
- non-directive counselling
- interpersonal psychotherapy
- cognitive–behavioural therapy
- drug therapy

The earlier the onset of the depression and the more severe it becomes, the more likely it is that formal psychiatric intervention will be needed. However, randomized trials have demonstrated the benefits of non-directive counselling from specially trained midwives and health visitors in the management of milder disorders. Even simple encouragement to join a local postnatal group may prevent social isolation and limit depression.

If pharmacotherapy is deemed necessary, tricyclic antidepressants or selective serotonin reuptake inhibitors (SSRIs) are appropriate. There is good evidence to support the safety of the former in breastfeeding, but less so for the latter. However, SSRIs in usual doses are probably safe.

There has been popularity in the past for treating postnatal depression with progestogens in the erroneous belief that the fall in progesterone levels postpartum is the cause of postnatal depression. There is no good evidence to support this, and it may even be harmful if the use of other effective treatments is delayed because of it. This practice should therefore be avoided. High-dose oestrogen regimes have been tried in research trials, but these are not used routinely.

Women with a past history of severe postnatal depressive illness may be candidates for some form of prophylactic treatment, and the help of a specialist in perinatal mental health care should be sought before delivery.

BOX 15.9: Risk factors for postnatal depressive illness

- Past history of psychiatric illness
- Depression during pregnancy
- Obstetric factors (e.g. caesarean section/fetal or neonatal loss)
- Social isolation and deprivation
- Poor relationships
- Recent adverse life events (bereavement/illness)
- Severe postnatal 'blues'

BOX 15.10: Symptoms of severe postnatal depressive disorder

- Early-morning wakening
- Poor appetite
- Diurnal mood variation (worse in the mornings)
- Low energy and libido
- Loss of enjoyment
- Lack of interest
- Impaired concentration
- Tearfulness
- Feelings of guilt and failure
- Anxiety
- Thoughts of self-harm/suicide
- Thoughts of harm to the baby

MBRRACE-UK 'red flag' presentations (require immediate referral)

- Recent significant change in mental state or emergence of new symptoms
- New thoughts or acts of violent self-harm
- New and persistent expressions of incompetency as a mother or estrangement from the infant

PUERPERAL PSYCHOSIS

This very severe disorder affects between 1:500 and 1:1,000 women after delivery. It rarely presents before the third post-partum day (most commonly the fifth), but it usually does so before 4 weeks. The onset is characteristically abrupt, with a rapidly changing clinical picture.

> **BOX 15.11: Risk factors for post-partum psychosis**
>
> - Previous history of puerperal psychosis
> - Previous history of severe non-post-partum depressive illness
> - Family history (first- or second-degree relative) of bipolar disorder/affective psychosis

> **BOX 15.12: Symptoms of puerperal psychosis**
>
> - Restless agitation
> - Insomnia
> - Perplexity/confusion
> - Fear/suspicion
> - Delusions/hallucinations
> - Failure to eat and drink
> - Thoughts of self-harm
> - Depressive symptoms (guilt, self-worthlessness, hopelessness)
> - Loss of insight

MANAGEMENT

Post-partum psychosis is a psychiatric emergency. The patient should be referred urgently to a psychiatrist and will usually require admission to a psychiatric unit. If possible, this should be a mother-and-baby unit under the supervision of a specialist perinatal mental healthcare team. These units prevent separation of the baby from the mother and this may help with bonding and the future relationship.

Treatments include:

- acute pharmacotherapy with benzodiazepines (e.g. lorazepam) and antipsychotics (e.g. chlorpromazine or haloperidol)
- lithium carbonate
- electroconvulsive therapy, particularly for severe depressive psychoses

Recovery usually occurs over 4–6 weeks, although treatment with antidepressants will be needed for at least 6 months. These women remain at high risk of pregnancy-related and non-pregnancy-related recurrences. The risk of recurrence in a future pregnancy is approximately 1 in 2, particularly if the next pregnancy occurs within 2 years of the one complicated by puerperal psychosis. Women with a previous history of puerperal psychosis should be considered for prophylactic lithium, started on the first post-partum day.

ANXIETY DISORDERS

Pregnancy, the anticipation of labour and the arrival of a new baby may all exacerbate an existing anxiety disorder. Cognitive–behavioural therapy may limit the need for drug treatment. Neonatal withdrawal effects are evident in the babies born to women who have used regular higher doses of benzodiazepines during pregnancy, and their use should be limited where possible. Breastfeeding may help to reduce the severity of the neonatal withdrawal (neonatal abstinence syndrome), as small amounts do reach breast milk.

BREASTS AND BREASTFEEDING

ANATOMY

The breasts are largely made up of glandular, adipose and connective tissue (**Figure 15.4**). They lie superficial to the pectoralis major, external oblique and serratus anterior muscles, extending between the second and sixth ribs from the sternum to the axilla. A pigmented area called the areola, which contains sebaceous glands, surrounds the nipple. During pregnancy, the areola becomes darker and the sebaceous glands become prominent (Montgomery's tubercles). The breast is comprised of 15–25 functional units arranged radially from the nipple and each unit is made up of a lactiferous duct, a mammary gland lobule and alveoli. The lactiferous ducts

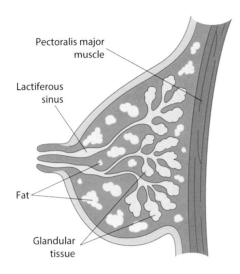

Pectoralis major muscle

Lactiferous sinus

Fat

Glandular tissue

Figure 15.4 The breast during lactation.

dilate to form a lactiferous sinus before converging to open in the nipple. Contractile myoepithelial cells surround the ducts as well as the alveoli.

PHYSIOLOGY

The human species is unique in that most of the breast development occurs at puberty and is therefore primed to produce milk within 2 weeks of hormonal stimulation. The control of mammary growth and development is not fully understood and many hormones may contribute to this process. In general, oestrogens stimulate proliferation of the lactiferous ducts (possibly with adrenal steroids and growth hormones), while progesterone is responsible for the development of the mammary lobules. During early pregnancy, lactiferous ducts and alveoli proliferate, while in later pregnancy the alveoli hypertrophy in preparation for secretory activity. The lactogenic hormones prolactin and human placental lactogen probably modulate these changes during pregnancy.

COLOSTRUM

Colostrum is a yellowish fluid secreted by the breast that can be expressed as early as the 16th week of pregnancy, but is replaced by milk during the second post-partum day. Colostrum has a high concentration of proteins but contains less sugar and fat than breast milk, although it contains large fat globules. The proteins are mainly in the form of globulins, particularly immunoglobulin A (IgA), which plays an important role in protection against infection. Colostrum is also believed to have a laxative effect, which may help empty the baby's bowel of meconium.

BREAST MILK

The major constituents of breast milk are lactose, protein, fat and water. However, the composition of breast milk is not constant; early lactation differs from late lactation, one feed differs from the next and the composition can even change during a feed. Compared with cow's milk, breast milk provides slightly more energy and has less protein but more fat and lactose. The major protein fractions are lactalbumin, lactoglobulin and caseinogen. Lactalbumin is the major protein in breast milk, whereas caseinogen forms 90% of the protein in cow's milk. The mineral content (particularly sodium) is much higher in cow's milk, which can therefore be dangerous if given to a baby who is dehydrated from gastroenteritis. In addition to IgA, breast milk contains small amounts of IgM and IgG and other factors such as lactoferrin, macrophages, complement and lysozymes. Although breast milk contains a lower concentration of iron, its absorption is better than from cow's milk or iron-supplemented infant formula (75%, 30% and 10%, respectively). The improved bioavailability may be related to lactoferrin, an iron-binding glycoprotein, which also inhibits bacterial growth. With the exception of vitamin K, all other vitamins are found in breast milk and therefore vitamin K is given to the baby to minimize the risk of haemorrhagic disease (see **Chapter 16**).

PROLACTIN

Prolactin is a long-chain polypeptide produced from the anterior pituitary; levels rise up to 20-fold during pregnancy and lactation. Peak levels of prolactin are reached within 45 minutes of suckling, but return to normal immediately after weaning and in non-breastfeeding mothers. The exact mechanism of action is not fully understood, but prolactin appears to have a direct action on the secretory cells to synthesize milk proteins. Prolactin is essential for lactation and it is hypothesized that nipple stimulation prevents the release of prolactin-inhibiting factor from the hypothalamus, thereby initiating the production of prolactin by the anterior pituitary. This theory is supported by the fact that lactation can be arrested with bromocriptine, a dopamine agonist that inhibits prolactin. A similar phenomenon occurs following pituitary necrosis (Sheehan syndrome) when prolactin production ceases.

OXYTOCIN

Once milk has been produced under the influence of prolactin, it has to be delivered to the infant. The milk-ejection or let-down reflex is initiated by suckling, which stimulates the pulsatile release of oxytocin from the posterior pituitary. Oxytocin contracts the myoepithelial cells surrounding the alveoli, as well as the myoepithelial cells lying longitudinally along the lactiferous ducts, thereby aiding the expulsion of milk. Oxytocin release can also be stimulated by visual, olfactory or auditory stimuli (e.g. hearing the baby cry), but can be inhibited by stress. Oxytocin can also stimulate uterine contractions, giving rise to the 'after pains' of childbirth.

BREASTFEEDING

Women who opt to breastfeed tend to decide before or very early in their pregnancy. This decision is usually based on previous experience, influence of family or friends, culture and custom. A new mother who is unprepared for breastfeeding may find it a frustrating task and turn to bottle feeding. There is now evidence to suggest that antenatal classes and literature on breastfeeding given antenatally may be beneficial.

The most common reasons mothers give for abandoning breastfeeding are inadequate milk production and sore and cracked nipples. Both of these problems can be overcome by correct positioning of the baby on the breast (**Figure 15.5**). The mouth should be placed over the nipple and areola so that suction created within the baby's mouth draws the breast tissue into a teat that extends as far back as the junction of the soft and hard palate. The tongue

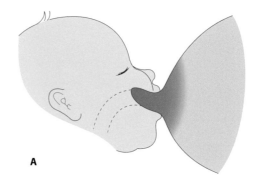

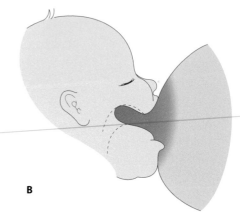

Figure 15.5 (**A**) Poor positioning for breastfeeding. (**B**) Good positioning.

applies peristaltic force to the underside of the teat against the support of the hard palate. In this way, there should be no to-and-fro movement of the teat in and out of the baby's mouth, thus minimizing friction. The mother should also be taught how to implement the rooting reflex. When the skin around the baby's mouth is touched, the mouth begins to gape. At this point, the mother should reposition the baby so that the lower rim of the baby's mouth fits well below the nipple, allowing a liberal mouthful of breast tissue. When the baby is properly attached, breastfeeding should be pain free. The use of creams and ointments for cracked nipples has not been shown to be beneficial and the use of a nipple shield merely reduces milk production.

Although no study has identified the threshold of the critical time limit for successful breastfeeding, early suckling appears to be beneficial. However, this should not be rushed and perhaps should be done initially under supervision when the mother is comfortable and in privacy.

There is no scientific evidence to justify a rigid breastfeeding schedule. Babies should be fed on demand and left on the breast until feeding finishes spontaneously. An imposed time limit on feeding can have a deleterious effect on calorie intake.

Supplementary feeds of formula, glucose or water are sometimes given to breastfed infants in the mistaken belief that the baby is still hungry or thirsty. This should be discouraged, as it increases the risk of total abandonment of breastfeeding.

Test-weighing infants before and after a feed to establish the quantity of milk intake has no role in healthy babies but is sometimes used by specialists to explore the reasons for poor weight gain.

When treating a breastfeeding woman, care needs to be taken to avoid drugs that can be passed onto the baby through the breast milk (see **Box 15.13**, 'Commonly used drugs in breastfeeding by mothers').

BOX 15.13: Commonly used drugs in breastfeeding by mothers

Breastfeeding contraindicated

- Aspirin (at doses of 300 mg or more)
- Amiodarone
- Lithium
- Anticancer drugs (antimetabolites)
- Radioactive substances (stop breastfeeding temporarily)

Continue breastfeeding with caution

Neonatal side effects possible (monitor baby closely):

- benzodiazepines (e.g. diazepam), psychiatric drugs and anticonvulsants
- carbimazole

Use alternative drug if possible:

- chloramphenicol, tetracyclines, metronidazole, ciprofloxacin

Monitor baby for jaundice:

- sulphonamides, dapsone, sulphamethoxazole/trimethoprim (cotrimoxazole), sulphadoxine/pyrimethamine

Use alternative drug (may inhibit lactation):

- oestrogens, including oestrogen-containing contraceptives, thiazide diuretics, regular ergometrine

Safe in usual dosage (monitor baby)

Most commonly used drugs:

- analgesics and antipyretics – short courses of paracetamol, low-dose aspirin, ibuprofen, heparin, occasional doses of morphine and pethidine
- antibiotics – ampicillin, amoxicillin, cloxacillin and other penicillins, erythromycin
- anti-tuberculosis drugs, anti-leprosy drugs (see dapsone above)
- antimalarials (except mefloquine, sulphadoxine/pyrimethamine), antihelminthics, antifungals
- bronchodilators (e.g. salbutamol), corticosteroids, antihistamines, antacids, drugs for diabetes, most antihypertensives, digoxin
- nutritional supplements of iodine, iron, vitamins

BOX 15.14: Advantages of breastfeeding

- Readily available at the right temperature and ideal nutritional value
- Cheaper than formula feed
- Has a contraceptive effect with associated amenorrhoea
- In the longer term it is associated with reduced:
  - necrotizing enterocolitis in preterm babies
  - childhood infective illnesses, especially gastroenteritis
  - atopic illnesses (e.g. eczema and asthma)
  - juvenile diabetes
  - childhood cancer, especially lymphoma
  - premenopausal breast cancer

NON-BREASTFEEDING MOTHERS

There are various reasons why a woman may not breastfeed, ranging from a choice based on personal preference to the tragedy of a stillbirth. Previously, all women infected with HIV were discouraged from breastfeeding due to the presence of HIV in breast milk. However, it is now clear that the highest risk of transmission from the mother to the child is from mixed breast- and bottle feeding. Furthermore, in resource-poor settings, child mortality is increased by not breastfeeding. Therefore, while HIV-positive women in resource-rich settings are advised not to breastfeed, WHO recommends that women in low-resource settings take antiretroviral medication and exclusively breastfeed.

Non-breastfeeding mothers may suffer considerable engorgement and breast pain. Dopamine receptor stimulants, such as bromocriptine and cabergoline, inhibit prolactin and thus suppress lactation. However, both commonly cause drowsiness, hypotension, headache and gastrointestinal side effects. Furthermore, fluid restriction and a tight brassiere have been shown to be as effective as bromocriptine usage by the second week and therefore this is the method of choice for the suppression of lactation.

BREAST DISORDERS

BLOOD-STAINED NIPPLE DISCHARGE

Blood-stained nipple discharge of pregnancy ('rusty pipe syndrome') is typically bilateral and believed to be due to epithelial proliferation. It usually occurs in late pregnancy or early breastfeeding and lasts for up to 1 week. As the condition is self-limiting, no investigation or treatment is necessary, and the woman should be reassured.

PAINFUL NIPPLES

Nipples become very sensitive during late pregnancy and in the first week of breastfeeding. 'Sensitive nipples' can cause marked discomfort during the first minute of breastfeeding, but it settles spontaneously. 'Painful nipples', however, occur after the first week of feeding and worsen during feeds. A common cause of this is cracked nipples (small fissures in the nipple) and this is associated with an increased risk of breast abscess. The cause is usually poor positioning of the baby on the breast, although thrush (candidiasis) may also cause soreness. The treatment is to correct the underlying problem, but may also require local antibiotic ointment, analgesics or even resting the affected nipple. The milk can be expressed during this time and the breastfeeding restarted once the nipples have healed.

GALACTOCELE

A galactocele (or lactocele) is a sterile, milk-filled retention cyst of the mammary ducts following blockage by thickened secretions. It is identified as a fluctuant swelling with minimal pain and inflammation. It usually resolves spontaneously assisted by massage of the breast towards the nipple, but may also be aspirated; with increasing discomfort, surgical excision may become necessary.

BREAST ENGORGEMENT

Engorgement of the breasts usually begins by the second or third post-partum day and if breastfeeding has not been effectively established, the overdistended and engorged breasts can be very uncomfortable. Breast engorgement results in a puerperal fever of up to 39°C in around 15% of women. Although the fever rarely lasts more than 16 hours, other infective causes must be excluded. A number of remedies for the treatment of breast engorgement, such as manual expression, firm support, cabbage leaves, ice bags and electric breast can all be effective, but allowing the baby easy access to the breast is the most effective method of treatment and prevention.

MASTITIS

Inflammation of the breast is not always due to an infective process. Mastitis is commonly related to breastfeeding problems and occurs when a blocked duct obstructs the flow of milk and distends the alveoli. If this pressure persists, the milk extravasates into the perilobular tissue, initiating an inflammatory process. The affected segment of the breast is painful and appears red and oedematous. The woman also experiences flu-like symptoms with a tachycardia and pyrexia. In contrast with breast engorgement, the pyrexia with infective mastitis develops later (typically the third to fourth post-partum week) and persists for longer. The most common infecting organism is *S. aureus*, which is found in 40% of women with mastitis.

Other bacteria include coagulase-negative staphylococci and *Streptococcus viridans*. Early localized mastitis can be managed with massage of the breast (towards the nipple) and analgesia. If the mastitis worsens, then a sample of the milk should be taken for microbiological culture and flucloxacillin commenced while awaiting sensitivity results. Breastfeeding should be continued during this process. About 10% of women with mastitis develop a breast abscess (diagnosed using ultrasound). Treatment is by a radial surgical incision and drainage under general anaesthesia.

CONTRACEPTION

The exact mechanism of lactational amenorrhoea is poorly understood, but the most plausible hypothesis is that during lactation there is inhibition of the normal pulsatile release of luteinizing hormone from the anterior pituitary. Breastfeeding therefore provides a contraceptive effect, but it is not totally reliable, as up to 10% of women conceive while breastfeeding. However, it has recently been shown that a mother who is still in the phase of post-partum amenorrhoea while fully breastfeeding their baby has a less than 2% chance of conceiving in the first 6 months. Although this is comparable to some other forms of contraception (see *Gynaecology by Ten Teachers*), most women with good access to healthcare use some sort of additional contraception, such as barrier methods.

An intrauterine contraceptive device may be inserted immediately postnatally or at the time of a caesarean section, but the expulsion rate is doubled to 10% and there is a high rate of perforation on insertion (~1%). It is ideal therefore to wait for 4–8 weeks to allow for involution.

The combined oral contraceptive pill enhances the risk of thrombosis in the early puerperium and can have an adverse effect on the quality and constituents of breast milk. Its use is therefore restricted to non-breastfeeding women at low risk of thrombosis. In others, the progesterone-only pill (the minipill) is preferable. Both should be commenced about day 21 following delivery. Injectable contraception, such as depot medroxyprogesterone acetate (Depo-Provera™) given 3-monthly or norethisterone enantate (Noristerat™) given 2-monthly, is also very effective. Injectable contraception can be given within 48 hours of delivery for convenience, but it can cause breakthrough bleeding and therefore should preferably be given 5–6 weeks post-partum.

Sterilization can be offered to mothers who are certain that they have completed their family. Tubal ligation can be performed during caesarean section or by the open method (mini-laparotomy) in the first few post-partum days. However, it is better delayed until after 6 weeks post-partum, when it can be done by laparoscopy. This allows the mother to spend more time in comfort with their newborn baby and, furthermore, laparoscopic clip sterilization is less traumatic and associated with a lower failure rate.

Women who are not breastfeeding should commence the pill 3 weeks after delivery, as ovulation can occur by 4–6 weeks post-partum.

PERINATAL DEATH

Bereavement counselling following perinatal death requires special expertise and is best left to a senior clinician and a trained bereavement counsellor. Inappropriate management of this traumatic period can have a devastating effect on the woman's emotional and marital life. Effective communication and support are crucial and women should be encouraged to contact organizations such as the Stillbirth and Neonatal Death Society (SANDS).

> **BOX 15.15: Useful definitions for describing perinatal death**
>
> - *Stillbirth*: a baby born with no signs of life
> - *Perinatal death*: stillbirth >24 weeks' gestation or death within 7 days of birth
> - *Live birth*: any baby that shows signs of life irrespective of gestation

The grieving process can be facilitated by practices such as seeing and holding the dead baby, naming the baby and taking hand-/footprints and photographs. Coming to terms with the perinatal death of a twin is more complicated because the mother has to mourn one baby and celebrate the arrival of the other.

A post-mortem is the most important diagnostic test, even though there may be no positive findings. Couples who decline a post-mortem may do so because of religious reasons or because of anxieties about the invasive techniques. In this situation, a partial post-mortem should be discussed, whereby an autopsy of a single organ or a tissue biopsy can be performed. A full-body X-ray or, preferably,

Table 15.6 Investigations into perinatal death

Investigations	Reason
For all perinatal deaths unless cause clearly known	
Full blood count	Anaemia, leucocytosis
HbA1c	Undiagnosed diabetes
Thyroid function tests	Undiagnosed hypothyroidism
Virology, infection screen	Cytomegalovirus, parvovirus, toxoplasmosis
Autoantibody screen (anticardiolipin, lupus anticoagulant and anti-beta-2 glycoprotein-1 antibodies)	Anti-phospholipid syndrome, systemic lupus erythematosus
Thrombophilia screen (do at least 6 weeks postnatally)	Thrombophilias
Swab from baby's axilla	Fetal infection/chorioamnionitis
Placental swab for culture (from maternal side only)	Infections such as *Listeria monocytogenes*
Placental pathology	Evidence of infection or vasculopathy
Post-mortem or full-body X-ray or MRI	To identify congenital defects
Selective investigations (only if clinical indication)	
Urine for cocaine metabolites	If maternal substance abuse is suspected
Kleihauer test	If abruption is suspected
Red cell antibodies (including anti Ro and La)	In cases of fetal hydrops or haemolytic disease
Maternal alloimmune antiplatelet antibodies	If intracranial haemorrhage is found at post-mortem
Chromosomal analysis of umbilical cord	If fetal abnormality is suspected

HbA1c, glycated haemoglobin; MRI, magnetic resonance imaging.

magnetic resonance imaging may be useful in some cases (**Table 15.6**).

If the baby was stillborn, a stillbirth certificate should be completed by the attending doctor; otherwise, the paediatrician should complete the certificate. The certificate should be given to the parents to register the death with the Registrar of Births and Deaths. Funeral arrangements can be made privately or by the hospital.

Every mother who has lost a baby should have the 6-week postnatal visit at hospital to discuss the underlying cause and to plan for the future.

KEY LEARNING POINTS

- The puerperium refers to the 6-week period following childbirth.
- Care during this transition period is crucial as the woman returns to her pre-pregnant state.
- Perineal discomfort is a major complaint following vaginal delivery and therefore adequate analgesia should be prescribed.
- All women should be screened for depression at least twice in the post-partum period.
- Common disorders include puerperal sepsis, thromboembolism and bowel and bladder dysfunction.

FURTHER READING

Knight M, Bunch K, Tuffnell D, Patel R, Shakespeare J, Kotnis R, Kenyon S, Kurinczuk JJ (eds.); MBRRACE-UK (2021). *Saving Lives, Improving Mothers' Care – CORE report lessons learned to inform maternity care from the UK and Ireland Confidential Enquiries into Maternal Deaths and Morbidity 2017–19*. National Perinatal Epidemiology Unit, University of Oxford.

NICE (2021). *Postnatal Care*. NICE guideline [NG194].

NICE (2016). *Sepsis: Recognition, Diagnosis and Early Management*. NICE guideline [NG51]. Last updated: 13 September 2017.

NICE (2014). *Antenatal and Postnatal Mental Health: Clinical Management and Service Guidance*. Clinical guideline [CG192]. Last updated: 11 February 2020.

WHO (2015). *WHO Recommendations for Prevention and Treatment of Maternal Peripartum Infections*. WHO Press.

WHO (2014). *WHO Recommendations on Postnatal Care of the Mother and New-born*. WHO Press.

SELF-ASSESSMENT

For interactive SBAs and EMQs relating to this chapter, visit www.routledge.com/cw/mccarthy.

CASE HISTORY 1

An 18-year-old woman with a body mass index of 35 who had a forceps delivery after a prolonged second stage of labour 10 days previously presents with heavy, fresh vaginal bleeding and clots. She feels unwell and complains of abdominal cramps. On examination, she has a temperature of 38.2°C and there is mild suprapubic tenderness. Vaginal examination reveals blood clots, but no products of conception. The cervix admits one finger and the uterus is tender and measures 16 weeks in size. A review of the delivery notes reveals that the placenta was delivered complete, but the membranes were noted to be ragged.

A What is the most likely diagnosis?

B What are the key features that suggest retained products of conception?

C How should the patient be managed?

ANSWERS

A Secondary PPH due to infected retained products of conception.

B Secondary PPH. Enlarged uterus. Open cervical os.

C Blood cultures. Intravenous broad-spectrum antibiotics (e.g. cephalosporin and metronidazole). Surgical evacuation of the retained products.

CASE HISTORY 2

A recent Eastern European immigrant to the UK, with minimal English, was seen by her GP at 12 weeks' gestation. The only history of note was that her father had suffered a long-standing psychiatric illness that the woman believed to be 'schizophrenia'. He died when she was young in a road traffic accident. Her pregnancy proceeded without complication, and she went home on the second postnatal day following a normal delivery at term.

Within a couple of weeks, her partner reported to the community midwife that he had concerns about her mood. She seemed agitated, fearful and unduly concerned about the well-being of the baby and she refused any help offered by him. The GP saw her, without an interpreter, and diagnosed 'postnatal depression'. He commenced tricyclic antidepressants. However, 1 week later, she became frankly delusional and believed that her partner was trying to kill the baby. She was hardly sleeping and eating very little, but was continuing to breastfeed her baby.

A What is the most likely diagnosis?

B How should this be managed?

C How should her breastfeeding be managed?

D In retrospect, how should the pregnancy have been managed?

ANSWERS

A The most likely diagnosis is puerperal psychosis.

B She should be admitted to a regional mother-and-baby unit with her newborn where she can receive multidisciplinary care from the specialist medical, nursing and midwifery staff. The antidepressants should be stopped and she should be treated with benzodiazepines and antipsychotics (e.g. trifluoperazine).

C She should be encouraged to continue breastfeeding but the baby should be monitored for side effects.

D Ideally, the woman should have been seen with an interpreter and asked to explore the nature of her family history. This would have revealed that her father suffered from schizophrenia. If this had been known, then it could have prompted review by a specialist in perinatal mental health, leading to regular postnatal review by a community psychiatric nurse being organized. This might have led to earlier intervention and prevented her deterioration to such a severe state.

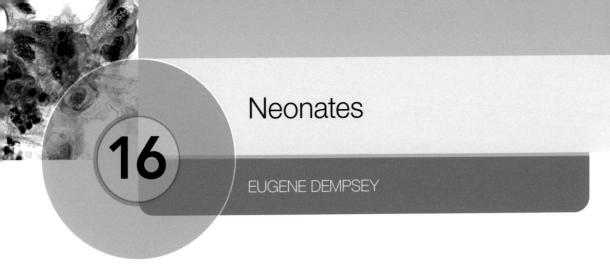

Neonates

16

EUGENE DEMPSEY

Learning Objectives
- Understand and be able to describe the unique features of newborn babies and the transition to extrauterine life.
- For common neonatal problems, be able to describe:
  - key features from an obstetric point of view
  - urgent action in the delivery room or soon afterwards
  - important messages for parents
- Describe key points relevant to postnatal management that need to be communicated by professionals involved in antenatal care.

INTRODUCTION

The word neonatology was first coined in 1960 and, needless to say, significant advances in neonatal care have occurred over the last 60 years. Mortality for babies delivered at 1 kg in the 1960s was 95%, whereas today survival for these infants is 95%. This significant improvement has come about thanks to the ongoing collaboration between neonatologists, obstetricians and midwives working hand in hand to ensure the best outcome for newborn infants and their families.

This chapter is about newborn infants and is directed primarily at an obstetrical audience. Areas in which neonatal care and obstetrical care are intertwined are addressed. Central to this relationship is our understanding of neonatal transition and how aberrations in this process can result in adverse outcomes for the newborn. This chapter provides an insight into caring for sick term newborn infants, in particular with conditions such as pulmonary hypertension and neonatal encephalopathy. It gives a general overview of some of the more common neonatal conditions encountered during the first days of life. Caring for preterm infants, and in particular those delivered at the cusp of viability, is an area in which discussions between neonatologists and obstetricians are crucial to ensure the best possible outcome.

10.1201/9781003196112-16

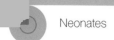

An overview of the key challenges, both antenatally and postnatally, is presented in this chapter. Finally, the importance of ongoing communication between the various specialities, along with communication with the newborn infant's family, is addressed.

NEWBORN TRANSITION

The transition to extrauterine existence is a highly complex process. The fetal lungs are liquid filled, pulmonary blood flow is very low and no gas exchange occurs. Oxygenated blood is provided by the placenta: this travels via the umbilical vein to the ductus venosus into the right atrium, preferentially across the patent foramen ovale into the left atrium and ventricle, providing oxygenated blood to the brain and heart via the carotid and coronary vessels. When babies are born and the cord is clamped, significant alterations occur. Now, the infant has to derive oxygenated blood from the lungs. Therefore, lung fluid must be cleared at birth to permit gas exchange. This highlights the importance of lung aeration as the key component in newborn resuscitation/stabilization. Three phases of respiratory adaptation have been described:

1. airway liquid clearance
2. lung fluid within the interstitial tissue compartment
3. gas exchange

The first phase, airway liquid clearance, occurs to some extent with advancing gestation and is stimulated by labour. Hormones such as cortisol and adrenaline enhance the in utero absorption of lung fluid. A small amount of fluid is lost during delivery secondary to fetal spinal flexion, which results in the 'squeezing' out of fluid out via the mouth and nose at delivery. The greatest removal of lung fluid occurs with the onset of breathing when the clearance of lung fluid occurs from the proximal to the distal airways. The second phase of clearance is characterised by the presence of this lung fluid within the interstitial tissue compartment. This fluid can re-enter the alveoli depending on the variation in pressure gradients generated with respiration and, as such, serves as the basis for transient tachypnoea of the newborn, one of the most common breathing

difficulties encountered in term newborn infants (which will be discussed in the section 'Commonly encountered neonatal problems in the term infant' later in this chapter). Fluid clearance occurs via the lymph system in the subsequent hours. Grunting, the process of partially closing the glottis to increase intra-alveolar pressure, contributes to a reduction in this cycle of the re-entry of fluid. The final phase is characterized by gas exchange. Surfactant production increases with advancing gestational age and is augmented by labour, thus increasing the amount of surfactant in the lung fluid.

The cardiovascular changes that take place following delivery involve primarily reorganizing the systemic and pulmonary circulations. Lung aeration results in a decrease in pulmonary vascular resistance, an increase in pulmonary blood flow and, as a result, an increase in the volume of blood contained in the left ventricle. The timing of cord clamping is critical here. Immediate clamping results in an increase in systemic vascular resistance and a reduction in blood return via the umbilical vein to the right atrium, pulmonary bed and ultimately left ventricle. In this situation, the left ventricle has decreased volume and has to pump against increased resistance and thus cardiovascular compromise can occur. The timing of cord clamping is thus essential and, in essence, needs to occur at least following initiation of spontaneous breathing or following adequate ventilation. It is apparent that lung aeration is the critical element of adaption, reaffirming the importance of effective ventilation as the mainstay of newborn stabilization. These factors highlight the importance of understanding adaptation and the implications for practice for both obstetricians and neonatologists at the time of delivery. Communication between both groups of professionals at this time is critical to ensuring optimal adaptation. **Figure 16.1** depicts an example of delayed cord clamping.

NEWBORN RESUSCITATION TRAINING PROGRAMMES AND SIMULATION

Newborn adaptation is a complex process, as previously discussed. What is interesting is that the majority of infants will transition with minimal input required. However, when it is required, it is essential

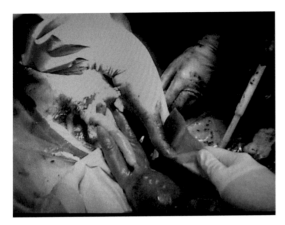

Figure 16.1 Delayed cord clamping following the delivery of the baby. The baby is dried, stimulated and allowed to rest on the mother's draped legs.

that appropriately trained personnel are present and provide the necessary support. Numerous newborn resuscitation training programmes exist. The purpose of standardized neonatal resuscitation training programmes is to translate the science of resuscitation into training, allowing transfer of the knowledge and skills of resuscitation to the participant, with the ultimate goal being to improve outcome.

Newborn Life Support (NLS) is the training programme used in the UK and all personnel involved in newborn care are expected to be trained in this programme. The key element of all programmes is effective mask ventilation to inflate the lungs and facilitate transition, as described previously (i.e. highlighting the importance of lung aeration). A recent meta-analysis found that neonatal resuscitation training programmes in low- and middle-income countries reduced early neonatal mortality, but the effect of these programmes on birth asphyxia and neurodevelopmental outcomes is yet to be determined.

Simulation is a really important element of newborn resuscitation training. Professor DM Gaba, in his article 'The future vision of simulation in healthcare' (*Quality and Safety in Health Care*, 2004), states that simulation is a technique – not a technology – 'to replace or amplify real experiences with guided experiences that evoke or replicate substantial aspects of the real world in a fully interactive manner'. Simulation locations do not necessarily need to be high fidelity. Every centre caring for newborn infants should strive to ensure access to neonatal

mannequins – the necessary essential equipment to replicate real-world scenarios – and have appropriate time set aside to ensure that standardized frequent training occurs. Joint sessions including obstetrical and neonatal personnel should occur frequently to address emergency scenarios such as shoulder dystocia, placental abruption and extreme preterm deliveries, as well as the management of extreme preterm infants receiving delayed cord clamping. Infrequent interventions such as chest compressions and adrenaline administration highlight the importance of adequate simulation training. Frequent on-site mock code scenarios/simulation sessions should include this important aspect of resuscitation care, as these low-occurrence events are very high-stress situations for all involved.

KEY LEARNING POINTS

- The majority of term newborn infants transition to extrauterine life without any support required.
- Respiratory adaptation includes three phases: airway fluid clearance, interstitial fluid clearance and effective gas exchange.
- Lung aeration is the key to successful transition, resulting in a reduction in pulmonary vascular resistance and an increase in pulmonary blood flow.
- Personnel trained in newborn resuscitation should be readily available.

ROUTINE NEWBORN CARE

The vast majority of term babies are managed on the postnatal ward and do not require admission to the special care baby unit (SCBU) or the neonatal intensive care unit (NICU). They should all have a routine newborn assessment. Similar to antenatal care, postnatal care is based on a risk assessment and stratification into groups that are used to guide management, with movement between groups very important if the baby's needs change.

Routine care is conducted by mothers, with contact by maternity staff members to support feeding, advise mothers (e.g. if it is their first baby), anticipate social problems and detect issues such as jaundice or hypoglycaemia.

Targeted care is aimed at babies at risk of conditions such as infection or hypoglycaemia. Neonates who have risk factors for infection may be safely observed rather than given antibiotics. Babies at risk of hypoglycaemia because of conditions such as fetal growth restriction or maternal diabetes have pre-feed estimations of blood glucose. These issues are dealt with in greater detail in the section 'Commonly encountered neonatal problems in the term infant' later in this chapter.

NEWBORN EXAMINATION

Every newborn infant should have a full, detailed newborn examination prior to discharge. This is typically performed by a medical doctor but in many institutions can be performed by advanced nurse practitioners, neonatal nurses or midwives specifically trained in this area. A structured approach to the examination is critical. While a detailed description of the examination is beyond the scope of this chapter, a full head-to-toe assessment is typically performed with the parents present. The examination can occur in the crib or on the mother's bed. Expose the newborn with the nappy left in situ.

Begin by palpating the suture lines of the skull, noting any caput or cephalohematomas. Subgaleal haemorrhages are rare but can be significant. The head circumference, weight and length should be plotted appropriately for the particular gestational age. Undertake fundoscopy to ensure bilateral red reflexes are present, review the palate by inspection and palpation, and note ear position; this completes examination of the face. Crepitus over the clavicular area may represent a clavicular fracture; inspect the chest for symmetry and respiratory rate, palpate for any heaves or thrills and then auscultate for heart sounds, any added sounds and the presence of any murmurs.

The liver edge is typically palpable and the tip of a spleen may be palpable in up to 10% of all newborns. An easily palpable spleen is abnormal. In the groin area, check for any hernia, palpate the femoral pulses and check for the presence of testes in boys. Ensure the anal margin is normal and note any sacral dimples. Typical foot anomalies include a calcaneovalgus deformity or postural talipes. Fixed talipes requires orthopaedic intervention. Complete the exam by performing a standard neurological exam, including an assessment of tone by 'pulling the baby to sit' holding the baby in vertical and ventral suspension and determining the presence of a number of primitive reflexes. I typically finish by assessing the hips.

HIP SCREENING

The hips should be abducted and adducted in order to elicit dislocated or dislocatable hips. If the hips are dislocated or dislocatable, the baby is referred for orthopaedic management. Developmental dysplasia of the hip (DDH) occurs in 1–2 per 1,000 live births, with up to 20 per 1,000 live births having unstable hips. Untreated DDH leads to abnormal gait, limp and early onset of hip osteoarthrosis, requiring early hip replacement. Treatment of DDH is effective with a harness in most infants. Neonatal screening for DDH is well established. Risk factors include first-born female infants, a positive family history and breech presentation.

When the neonatal screen for DDH is positive, the baby is referred for ultrasound and orthopaedic assessment. If DDH is confirmed, the initial treatment is with a Pavlik harness that holds the legs in the best position to support the growth of the acetabulum. The harness is used for up to 12 weeks and in a very high percentage of cases (approximately 95%) no further intervention is required. If the harness does not solve the problem, then surgical approaches are likely to be required. Many babies have stable joints but are found to have a 'clicky hip'. This is not abnormal but can be associated with an unstable joint, so babies with clicky hips are also referred for a hip ultrasound and orthopaedic review.

HEARING SCREENING

Some cases of permanent hearing loss can be detected in the newborn period, and this allows early provision for the child and family. In high-income settings, screening should be done with objective tests. In the UK, newborn hearing screening is conducted with otoacoustic emissions. Screen failure or an uncertain response leads to an automated auditory brainstem response test. In income-constrained settings, questionnaires or behavioural testing can be used in a targeted or unselected way but need to be piloted and linked to educational and other support.

NEWBORN BLOOD SPOT TESTING

In the UK, the newborn blood test is done about 5 days after birth. The diseases screened for are sickle cell disease, cystic fibrosis, congenital hypothyroidism and six metabolic conditions: phenylketonuria (PKU), medium-chain acyl-CoA dehydrogenase deficiency (MCADD), maple syrup urine disease (MSUD), isovaleric acidaemia (IVA), glutaric aciduria type 1 (GA1) and homocystinuria (pyridoxine unresponsive) (HCU).

⊙⊶ KEY LEARNING POINTS

- The majority of newborn infants can be managed on the postnatal ward and do not require admission to the SCBU.
- Newborn screening includes physical examination, newborn hearing screening and newborn blood spot.
- Newborn blood spot testing screens for nine inherited conditions in the UK.

COMMONLY ENCOUNTERED NEONATAL PROBLEMS IN THE TERM INFANT

TRANSIENT TACHYPNOEA OF THE NEWBORN

Transient tachypnoea of the newborn is one of the most common reasons for admission to the newborn nursery. It is caused by inadequate lung fluid clearance and is much more common following elective caesarean section. It is more common in infants delivered at 37/38 weeks than those delivered at 39 weeks. It is characterized by tachypnoea, grunting, sternal recession and, at times, an oxygen requirement. The pathophysiology is described in the section 'Newborn transition' earlier in this chapter. For a small, but not insignificant, number, more advanced respiratory support is required, including the provision of high-flow nasal cannula, nasal continuous positive airway pressure (CPAP) or occasionally mechanical ventilation. An awareness of this risk is important for both obstetricians and

families when deciding on the timing of elective delivery. Standard management includes admission to the SCBU, administration of respiratory support as outlined earlier and intravenous fluids or nasogastric tube feeding if not too distressed. Reassurance should be given to the parents that the symptoms should settle over the first 24 hours, but that, for a minority of infants, they may get worse before they get better. Occasional complications can arise such as a pneumothorax, which may require needle aspiration or the placement of a pigtail catheter. This is a difficult procedure to learn, and training should occur in a simulation setting. Only when a trainee is deemed competent in the simulation setting should this procedure be undertaken.

HYPOGLYCAEMIA

The newborn baby needs to adapt from a continuous infusion of maternal glucose via the placenta to intermittent feeds when delivered. Healthy term babies can cope with gaps between feeds because they have enough glycogen stores and the endocrine milieu will mobilize these stores. Therefore, glucose concentrations are not measured in healthy babies born at term unless there are certain risk factors.

If babies are at risk of not being able to cope with intermittent feeds, they are screened by measuring blood glucose before feeds. This means that there is a need for clear communication about risk factors from the antenatal team to the postnatal team. As noted previously, some babies become hypoglycaemic and some of them become symptomatic. Most of these have risk factors. Therefore, targeted monitoring should occur in those infants deemed to have risk factors. **Box 16.1**, 'Causes of hypoglycaemia', outlines some of the conditions that require glucose screening.

Pre-feed glucose is the important measurement. Post-feed measurements have limited value because of inconsistencies in absorption. Severe hypoglycaemia can cause brain injury, so it is an emergency and needs prompt intervention. Prolonged neonatal hypoglycaemia damages the brain and is largely avoidable. Hypoglycaemia can present in many ways and so a blood sugar test is always warranted if there is a clinical concern. As with any unwell newborn, it is standard practice to check the blood sugar.

BOX 16.1: Causes of hypoglycaemia

Transient hypoglycaemia associated with neonatal causes:

- prematurity
- low birthweight
- fetal growth restriction
- postmature
- perinatal stress
- hypothermia
- infection
- polycythaemia

Transient hypoglycaemia associated with maternal causes:

- maternal medications (e.g. propranolol)
- maternal conditions (e.g. gestational diabetes)

Persistent hypoglycaemia:

- hyperinsulinism
- inborn errors of metabolism
- endocrine disorders

Most causes of hypoglycaemia are transient and will respond to appropriate medical therapy, including intravenous dextrose infusions and feeding. There are rare situations in which the sugar can be persistently low and, in these situations, other causes need to be considered, such as hyperinsulinism or underlying endocrine problems.

JAUNDICE

In the days after birth, the production of bilirubin is often more than the liver enzymes can handle. This leads to an increase in the circulating concentrations of unconjugated bilirubin. This can present as jaundice and is a concern because very high concentrations of unconjugated bilirubin are neurotoxic. The liver enzymes are induced over the first 3–4 days after birth. Breastfed babies take longer to induce their enzymes, but this does not cause harm. Pathological jaundice is a sign of a departure from the expected normal adaptation. Visible jaundice within 24 hours of birth is most often pathological and is usually due to infection or haemolysis and needs prompt assessment.

The management of neonatal jaundice involves strong overlap between maternity and neonatal services. Antenatal information about conditions that lead to jaundice is invaluable for starting treatment promptly. Postnatal management can usually be conducted on the postnatal wards, keeping the mother with the baby.

The management of neonatal jaundice involves well-established pathways that include escalations of therapy guided by bilirubin measurements. Treatment of jaundice is based on phototherapy (**Figure 16.2**), which uses light in the visible spectrum to conduct a photoisomerization of bilirubin to safe isomers, some of which are excreted rapidly. This is administered by the projection of light onto the neonate's skin. Light in the wavelength of 460–490 nm triggers an isomeric change in the bilirubin molecule, making it more water soluble, and increases the proportion excreted in the urine. The key to successful phototherapy is adequate exposure. Inappropriate positioning of the light source can lead to non-uniform illumination of exposed skin. Positioning the infant within the recommended distance of the light source and in an optimal position within the incubator/cot to maximize exposure are important considerations that may often be overlooked during treatment. If overhead lights are used, then the eyes should be protected. Phototherapy can be interrupted for breastfeeding unless there is a high likelihood of exchange transfusion.

If phototherapy does not prevent the concentrations of bilirubin from climbing to levels associated with brain injury, then exchange transfusion may be indicated. Exchange transfusion involves

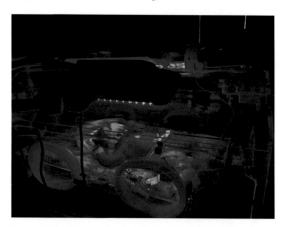

Figure 16.2 Neonate undergoing phototherapy.

withdrawing a small aliquot of blood from the baby and replacing it with a small aliquot of cross-matched blood. This is repeated every 5 minutes, typically over 3–4 hours. The aim is to replace twice the baby's circulating volume (140 mL/kg). If there is evidence of active alloimmune disease (e.g. rhesus or ABO incompatibility) on direct antiglobulin testing, then immunoglobulin during phototherapy may reduce the need for exchange transfusion.

Causes of neonatal jaundice include abnormalities of red cell enzymes or structure, extravasated blood (e.g. cephalohematoma), increased enterohepatic circulation and endocrine conditions such as hypothyroidism. Prolonged jaundice is not uncommon in solely breastfed infants and can be present up to 8 weeks. However, investigations are required to rule out other potential causes and, ultimately, prolonged jaundice secondary to breast milk is a diagnosis of exclusion.

Conjugated bilirubin is not neurotoxic. High circulating concentrations of conjugated bilirubin reflect problems excreting bile. This can be due to an obstruction. In term babies, this can relate to the rare but important condition of biliary atresia. In preterm babies, obstructive jaundice is often related to parenteral nutrition. In all age groups, conjugated or prolonged jaundice has an extensive differential diagnosis that requires detailed evaluation.

HEART MURMURS

Murmurs are very common in newborn infants, especially when they are examined within the first day of life. The majority of these are innocent in nature and often reflect transitional adaptation such as mild tricuspid regurgitation or a patent ductus arteriosus. They are often short, soft and systolic in their nature. Loud harsh systolic murmurs are often muscular ventricular septal defects, but clinical diagnosis can be difficult. It is important to listen for the quality of the heart sounds, the quality of the murmur, the location of the murmur and the presence of any parasternal heaves. Palpation of the femoral and brachial pulses are important. Locating the femoral pulses at times can be challenging, so it is important to have the baby settled for this element of the examination. Truly absent or diminished femoral pulses are often associated with

coarctation of the aorta. Diminished femoral and brachial pulses are often associated with hypoplastic left heart syndrome. Universal pulse oximetry screening is used in many countries to help identify cyanotic heart disease. Currently, it is not part of the UK screening programme. An echocardiogram is essential if there is clinical concern relating to the cardiac evaluation.

HYPOSPADIAS

Hypospadias occurs in 1 in 300 boys. It typically involves an abnormally placed urinary meatus, chordee (bend) of the penis and a retracted foreskin. Surgical correction takes place typically around 1 year after birth. It is important to advise the parents to avoid circumcision, because the foreskin is used during the operation.

Hypospadias may rarely be part of ambiguous genitalia. If a baby has ambiguous genitalia, it is important to share concerns with the family, to avoid assigning a sex and to arrange urgent review by a skilled multidisciplinary team (including paediatric endocrinologists, surgeons and radiologists). This can be a very traumatic event for parents, so psychosocial support is essential.

CLEFT LIP AND PALATE

In the UK, the care of babies with cleft lip or palate is centralized into 11 networks (nine in England and Wales, one each in Scotland and Northern Ireland). The immediate management is based on individualized assessment of the baby's feeding abilities. Many children with cleft lip or palate need adaptations to the feeding process, for example by giving expressed breast milk using a flexible teat. Corrective surgery is not urgent and is usually done several months after birth. Cleft lip is usually repaired around 4 months and cleft palate around 9 months.

SUSPECTED INFECTIONS

In newborn babies, several risk factors and signs of infection can be seen. The problem is that these signs are common and often non-specific (poor feeding and mild respiratory distress) and, while

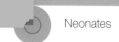

proven infection is rare, it can have devastating consequences. Thus, any suspected infection requires prompt treatment. Aggressive treatment is continued if there is a proven infection or if clinical condition is poor. For example, treatment for suspected infection can be stopped after 24–36 hours if the baby is well, blood cultures are negative and two measurements of C-reactive protein are less than 10 mg/L. A key to managing suspected and proven infection is antimicrobial stewardship in the neonatal unit. It is important that centres have established a multidisciplinary team that focuses on antibiotic usage. Widespread antibiotic usage brings its own unwanted side effects, including antibiotic resistance and impacts on the developing intestinal microbiome (see the section 'Prematurity' later in this chapter).

EARLY

The incidence of proven early-onset neonatal infection is 1–2 per 1,000 live births. Up to 1 in 10 neonates may be treated with antibiotics for suspected early-onset neonatal infection. Most of these courses of antibiotics are stopped early, within 48 hours. Early-onset neonatal infection is caused by a limited range of bacteria. A baby may be well at birth and gradually deteriorate in the hours after birth. Sometimes the baby is acutely unwell at birth and the course is fulminant, requiring multi-organ support in intensive care.

The most common Gram-positive cause of early-onset neonatal infection in the UK is group B *Streptococcus* (GBS, *Streptococcus agalactiae*). Invasive GBS illness is severe. As described in **Chapter 11**, this bacterium is part of the intestinal flora for many people. About 20% of the population carries GBS in their stool at any one time, including pregnant women. Women colonized with GBS are at increased risk of having a baby with invasive GBS. For this reason, women are screened for GBS carriage, either universally or in a targeted manner. Evidence of GBS colonization triggers intra-partum antibiotic prophylaxis, which reduces the incidence of invasive GBS disease. GBS is susceptible to benzyl penicillin; therefore, benzyl penicillin is a useful agent for intra-partum antibiotic prophylaxis and treatment. A treatment course for proven GBS infection is at least 7 days.

Other Gram-positive causes of early-onset neonatal infection are *Staphylococcus aureus* and group A *Streptococcus*, but these are much less common.

A common cause of Gram-negative early-onset neonatal infection is *Escherichia coli*. As in other age groups, *E. coli* can cause a life-threatening systemic infection requiring full intensive care. Antimicrobial susceptibility varies with the local prevalence of antimicrobial resistance. Given the vertical pattern of infection, resistance patterns will vary with patterns of community resistance. A third-generation cephalosporin and gentamicin are used for the initial treatment of *E. coli* (and other Gram-negative bacteria). A lumbar puncture to rule out meningitis is essential in all proven culture positive infections and may be indicated if there are clinical concerns in the absence of a proven positive culture. *Haemophilus influenzae* is an occasional cause of early-onset neonatal infection due to vertical transmission. This is due to non-capsulate, non-serotypeable forms that are not covered by the routine immunization against *H. influenzae* type b. This is treated with cefotaxime.

LATE

Some late-onset neonatal infection occurs at home, in which case the babies will have community-acquired bacteria rather than hospital- acquired bacteria. Early or late neonatal infection can be associated with meningitis, which is often associated with a poor outcome in childhood. Meningitis may not have clinical signs, so neonatologists have a low threshold for performing a lumbar puncture.

OTHER INFECTIONS

Syphilis

Babies born to women with positive treponemal serology need clinical evaluation and syphilis serology testing unless there is definitive proof of maternal biological false-positive serology or cure. In the UK, congenital syphilis is rare. It affects around 10 babies a year, usually among women presenting to maternity services in the third trimester with backgrounds of socio-economic deprivation and chaotic lifestyles. The diagnosis of congenital syphilis is difficult, so maternity staff need to work closely with paediatricians, genitourinary medicine specialists and paediatric infectious disease specialists. Babies are treated if congenital syphilis is suspected or maternal treatment is within 4 weeks of birth or incomplete. The usual treatment is intravenous benzyl penicillin for 2 weeks or more. Guidance on treatment regimens by paediatric infectious disease specialists is essential.

Herpes simplex

Neonatal herpes simplex virus (HSV) infection is often fatal (20%) and leads to significant disability among survivors (>60%). Neonatal HSV is usually vertically transmitted. If an active, maternal primary infection is underway at the time of birth, the baby has a significant risk of developing systemic herpes. If a recurrence of genital herpes is underway at the time of birth, the risk of neonatal herpes is much lower (<3%). Thus, it is very important to notify the neonatal team if a mother has evidence of genital herpes and to provide as much information as possible about the clinical history and diagnosis. Caesarean section is an effective way to reduce the incidence of infection among women known to have primary genital herpes.

Neonatal HSV infection presents in three ways: localized, central nervous system (CNS) and disseminated. The localized form is relatively benign, but the neurological and disseminated manifestations of neonatal HSV are severe illnesses often requiring extensive intensive care. The treatment is intravenous acyclovir. Various treatment algorithms exist on the management of suspected HSV infection. Again, consultation with paediatric infectious disease specialists is essential.

Varicella zoster

Neonatal varicella occurs in the babies of mothers who develop chicken pox. If the baby is born more than 5 days after the mother develops the rash, then transplacental antibodies provide some protection and the illness is not severe. If the baby is born fewer than 5 days after the mother develops the rash, then the baby is not protected and can develop a severe infection complicated by pneumonitis. The severity of neonatal varicella can be reduced if the baby receives varicella zoster immunoglobulin (VZIG) as soon after birth as possible.

Babies born to women who develop chicken pox 7 days before or 7 days after birth should receive VZIG. If a woman has shingles, then the baby is protected from infection with varicella zoster virus by maternal antibodies; the mother and the baby can stay together, and routine observation should occur.

Human immunodeficiency virus

The management of babies born to mothers with human immunodeficiency virus (HIV) is well described in national guidelines. The principles are that each woman needs an individualized care plan that reflects her risk status and is drawn up by a multidisciplinary team.

UK guidance is that babies born to women with a low viral load (<50 HIV ribonucleic acid (RNA) copies/mL plasma) should receive monotherapy with zidovudine for 4 weeks. If a woman has >50 HIV RNA copies/mL plasma or maternal HIV is diagnosed within 3 days of birth, combination post-exposure prophylaxis with three agents should be started under expert supervision. With appropriate post-exposure prophylaxis, less than 1% of babies born to HIV-positive mothers will be infected. In the absence of post-exposure prophylaxis, 15% of babies born to HIV-positive mothers became infected in a UK cohort study.

Cytomegalovirus

Symptomatic congenital cytomegalovirus (CMV) causes learning disabilities or sensorineural hearing loss. Congenital CMV can be treated with ganciclovir intravenously for 6 weeks. This reduces the severity of CNS damage and hearing loss. As with the various infections listed previously, consultation with a paediatric disease specialist to determine risk and the need for intervention should always occur.

PULMONARY HYPERTENSION

Persistent pulmonary hypertension of the newborn (PPHN) is a relatively common condition occurring in 0.5 to 7 per 1,000 live births and results in a mortality ranging between 4% and 33% depending on the underlying pathology. Inhaled nitric oxide (iNO) and extracorporeal membrane oxygenation are the only current therapeutic options systematically evaluated in clinical trials. The vasodilatation induced by iNO is mediated by increasing concentrations of the second messengers: cyclic guanyl monophosphate and cyclic adenosine monophosphate in pulmonary vascular smooth muscle. The widespread use of iNO has resulted in a reduction in the need for extracorporeal membrane oxygenation. However, up to 40% of infants treated with iNO either have only a transient response or fail to demonstrate an improvement. Furthermore, the increasing cost of administering iNO to infants with PPHN may prohibit its use in developing countries. Alternative interventions continue to be trialled including sildenafil and bosantan.

The condition is clinically characterized by hypoxemic respiratory failure due to the lack of transition of the pulmonary vasculature from a high-resistance fetal to a low-resistance extrauterine circuit. Pulmonary vascular resistance remains high resulting in right to left shunting across the patent foramen ovale and the patent ductus arteriosus (PDA) resulting in hypoxemia. The key to successful management is lowering the pulmonary vascular resistance and increasing myocardial performance. One potential cause of pulmonary hypertension is meconium aspiration syndrome. Meconium staining of amniotic fluid (MSAF) occurs in approximately 10–15% of term deliveries. MSAF is thought to be a sign of fetal distress and is often associated with other conditions such as placental insufficiency and cord compression. The management of babies born through MSAF has changed significantly over the years. Previously, the head was suctioned on the perineum, but this practice changed following a trial highlighting a worse neonatal outcome when routine suctioning occurred. The Newborn Resuscitation Program (NRP) previously recommended endotracheal intubation and suctioning with a meconium aspirator in all infants born through MSAF for the prevention of meconium aspiration syndrome. This subsequently changed to only intubating when the baby was non-vigorous. In the more recent 2015 International Liaison Committee on Resuscitation recommendations, the emphasis has changed to initiating positive pressure ventilation during the first minute of life, even in non-vigorous infants. The indication for intubation for tracheal suctioning may be necessary if positive pressure ventilation does not allow for adequate ventilation and it is suspected that there is mechanical obstruction due to meconium.

> ## 🔑 KEY LEARNING POINTS
>
> - The more common reasons for admission to the special care unit include transient tachypnoea, jaundice and hypoglycaemia.
> - Early infection is rare, but can be devastating.
> - Management of congenital infections such as syphilis, CMV and HIV require multidisciplinary input.
> - The key to the management of pulmonary hypertension is lowering pulmonary pressures.

AN APPROACH TO THE DYSMORPHIC INFANT

Dysmorphic features are common in the general population. One or two dysmorphic features may not lead to a diagnosis or have any effect on the child. For example, 5% of the population may have a single palmar crease. It is important to adopt a standard approach to the examination and to document all of the features of concern. A constellation of features may represent an underlying condition. Always look at the parents, as they may have some similar features. A detailed family history is also important. If concerns remain, then the need to perform genetic testing should be discussed with the family, and karyotype, microarray or additional testing may need to be done. Discussion with a clinical geneticist may help guide appropriate investigations.

TRISOMY 21 IN NEONATES

The most common syndrome in the neonate is trisomy 21: Down syndrome. This can be expected based on sonographic or genetic analyses conducted during pregnancy or sometimes can be unexpected. Unexpected cases occur in people who decline antenatal screening for this condition and in people who have been screened as low risk. A risk of 1:2,000 means that 1 in 2,000 women will have a baby with Down syndrome. The older the mother, the greater the risk.

Honesty and transparency are important when dealing with a case of suspected Down syndrome. The ideal is to share suspicions with both parents in a calm, private setting. However, this is not always possible. If a parent raises concerns about Down syndrome, those concerns should be acknowledged and a paediatric opinion sought as soon as possible.

A paediatric assessment of suspected Down syndrome will usually take the form of a shared examination of the baby with the parents. All features of the baby are described and positives are shared. Features that are different from many children are pointed out (not abnormal features). A genetic test is always done, even if an experienced clinician can make a definitive diagnosis based on the examination alone. If there is a clinical suspicion of trisomy 21, but not all of the typical features are present, it is usually worth doing the genetic test, even if the likelihood is low. If one set of clinicians raise the concern, other groups are likely to raise the same concern. The genetic test is usually a fluorescent in situ hybridization (FISH) test that can give a result within 24–48 hours. A definitive karyotype is needed to report the type of trisomy and to indicate the value of genetic testing in parents and the future risk. Non-disjunction does not need testing of family members and is associated with a low risk of recurrence (1%).

The days after diagnosis are traumatic for the family. Some common problems can be present in the first day. These include an oxygen dependency secondary to pulmonary hypertension (which generally settles over a few days), hypoglycaemia, polycythaemia and jaundice. The dominant clinical problem is establishing feeds. Some babies with trisomy 21 can learn to feed on the postnatal wards with their mother, but some are admitted to the neonatal unit for a period of tube feeding. Breastfeeding should be encouraged. A cardiac defect is seen in about half of all cases of trisomy 21 and is sought using echocardiography. Ideally, an echocardiogram should be performed prior to discharge. Rarer conditions associated with trisomy 21 include duodenal atresia and Hirschsprung disease. The parents are given information about the condition overall. The family may wish to connect with various support groups. Input from early-intervention services in the community should be sought prior to discharge. Babies go home when they can feed. Appropriate clinical follow-up should be arranged, including cardiology follow-up if required.

NEUROLOGICAL CONCERNS

SEIZURES

Seizures are relatively common in the newborn period, affecting 1–2 per 1,000 livebirths. Hypoxic ischaemic encephalopathy (HIE) is the most common cause of neonatal seizures, causing about half of neonatal seizures. However, there is a broad differential. Other causes of neonatal seizures include cerebral infarction (stroke), intracranial haemorrhage (intraventricular haemorrhage (IVH) and subdural), meningitis, electrolyte disturbances (hypocalcaemia, hypomagnesemia), hypoglycaemia, and rarer metabolic disorders and structural brain disorders.

The assessment of neonatal seizures is based on description followed by interpretation. Neonates have specific patterns of seizures, including tonic, clonic, subtle and myoclonic. Tonic–clonic seizures are rare in neonates. Clinical observation is not reliable. Ideally, electroencephalography (EEG) or cerebral function monitoring is used, albeit the latter may have limited use in seizure detection. Other features such as autonomic changes (respiratory rate, blood pressure, oxygen saturations) are also important features of seizures. Jitters are not seizures. Jitters affect up to half of babies. Jitters involve repeated movements at 1–3 Hz, typically on stimulation. Jitters can be restrained, in contrast with seizures. Benign sleep myoclonus can mimic seizures and can be frightening for parents. Parents should be reassured that these are a normal phenomenon. Clear history taking is essential, and often parents will have recorded the event on their mobile phone, which can be very helpful on review.

Investigations are directed towards finding the cause of the seizures and looking for a prognosis. While cranial ultrasound may be useful, brain magnetic resonance imaging (MRI) is the first-line imaging modality.

The evidence base for the treatment of neonatal seizures is limited. Conventional therapy involves phenobarbital. Supplementary agents include midazolam, levetiracetam, phenytoin and sodium valproate.

The prognosis of neonatal seizures depends on the cause. Overall, about half of children with neonatal seizures will have neurodevelopmental abnormalities. The proportion is much higher if there is cerebral dysgenesis. Of children with neo-natal seizures, 10% to 20% have seizures in later life (this proportion will be higher if there is a brain malformation).

NEONATAL ENCEPHALOPATHY

Neonatal encephalopathy has a broad differential diagnosis. Neonatal encephalopathy is often, but not always, associated with events during and after labour. Thus, the neonatal approach is to evaluate the diagnosis with an open mind and assess the baby systematically before making a diagnosis and offering a prognosis. It may take some time to come to a definitive answer. In the meantime, the baby is treated aggressively for potential conditions. Causes of neonatal encephalopathy are wide and include HIE, infection (bacterial and viral, e.g. HSV), drugs (maternal therapeutic drugs, maternal abuse of drugs or neonatal therapeutic drugs), CNS malfor-mations and metabolic conditions (hypoglycaemia, aminoacidaemias, organic acidaemias, pyridoxine dependency, mitochondrial disorders, urea cycle dis-orders, etc.). The most common condition is HIE.

HYPOXIC ISCHAEMIC ENCEPHALOPATHY

Perinatal asphyxia accounts for approximately 6 per 1,000 live births. When the asphyxia is severe or prolonged, it can lead to HIE. This is the lead-ing cause of acquired brain injury in term infants, affecting 1–2 per 1,000 live births in the developed world. HIE is caused by a disruption in blood and/or oxygen supply to the brain. HIE can be caused by antenatal insults secondary to placental or cord problems or to peri-partum events such as placental abruption, shoulder dystocia, significant antepartum haemorrhage or cord accident. Postnatal events are a very rare cause. The severity of the condition and clinical features vary depending on the duration and severity of the original event. Following the original event, if circulation is restored, reperfusion occurs. Secondary energy failure occurs 6–48 hours after the initial insult. HIE is typically classified into three categories: mild, moderate and severe (described in **Table 16.1**). These categories are not necessarily independent of one another. Grading is currently assigned based on clinical assessment.

Mild HIE accounts for almost 40% of all HIE cases. Infants with mild HIE are noted to be hyper-alert or

Table 16.1 Modified Sarnat Scoring System for hypoxic ischaemic encephalopathy

Area	Stage 1 (mild)	Stage 2 (moderate)	Stage 3 (severe)
Level of consciousness	Hyperalert	Lethargic	Stuporous or comatose
Spontaneous activity	Active	Decreased	Absent
Posture	Mild distal flexion	Strong distal flexion, complete extension or 'frog-legged' position	Decerebrate
Tone	Hypertonic, jittery	Hypotonia (axial and/or limb)	Flaccid
Primitive reflexes			
Suck	Weak	Weak/absent	Absent
Moro	Strong, low threshold	Incomplete, high threshold	Absent
Autonomic function			
Pupils	Mydriasis	Miosis	Variable, fixed, dilated, unresponsive to light
Heart rate	Normal, tachycardia	Bradycardia	Variable, irregular
Respiratory rate	Regular, spontaneous breathing	Periodic, irregular breathing effort	Apnoeic
Seizures	None	Common: focal or multi-focal	Uncommon

irritable. They may demonstrate mild distal flexion of their limbs. They may have a weak suck and have mydriasis and tachycardia. They may have a strong Moro reflex, which is easy to elicit. Muscle tone can be normal with normal spontaneous activity and normal respirations. Although previously thought to have a normal outcome, studies now show that anywhere up to 25% of infants with mild HIE may have an abnormal motor or emotional/behavioural outcome, although this may not become apparent until school-going age or beyond.

Approximately 40% of infants with HIE will fall into the moderate HIE group. These infants are lethargic with decreased spontaneous activity. They have central hypotonia and demonstrate strong distal flexion. Their suck may be weak or absent and their Moro reflex may be weak or incomplete. They may have a low heart rate, have miosis and demonstrate periodic breathing. Seizures may occur in this group and, if present, they tend to occur between 12 and 72 hours of life. These infants meet current criteria for intervention with therapeutic hypothermia (TH) and have a 20–40% risk of significant adverse outcome.

Severe HIE is the least common but most devastating category of HIE. These infants are stuporous or in a coma. Their muscle tone is significantly decreased. They are flaccid and may demonstrate decerebrate posturing of their limbs. They have an absent suck and Moro. Their heart rate is variable, they tend to be apnoeic and their pupils can be unequal, fixed, dilated or show poor light reflex. Seizures are most common in this group. This group also display evidence of multi-organ dysfunction and may have signs of acute renal and liver failure. These infants tend to die in the neonatal period or, if they survive, have significant impairments, including cerebral palsy and significant learning difficulties.

TH has now become the standard of care for all infants with moderate to severe HIE. TH involves lowering an infant's core temperature to 33–34°C for 72 hours then slowly rewarming over 12 hours. To be effective, TH must be initiated early, within 6 hours of birth. In this short time frame, the infants who may benefit from TH must be resuscitated, stabilized and identified. To further complicate matters, HIE is an evolving and dynamic process. Clinical examination may remain the same, improve or

deteriorate over these 6 hours. The decision to initiate TH is currently based on the use of clinical and biochemical assessments.

ELECTROENCEPHALOGRAPHY

Neonatal EEG is extremely useful for the assessment of neurological function in infants with perinatal asphyxia and seizures. EEG is an electrophysiological technique for the recording of electrical activity arising from the brain. This is performed by placing electrodes on the scalp, which provides a recording of brain activity. Multichannel EEG, the gold standard for EEG monitoring, can be challenging in neonates, as electrode application can be difficult, it is complex and it requires expert interpretation. Personnel with the level of experience required to interpret neonatal multichannel EEG are usually not readily available in most NICUs.

A simpler EEG method is used in many NICUs across the world – amplitude integrated EEG (aEEG). aEEG is a compressed version of the traditional EEG that utilizes a limited number of channels. aEEG has some potential limitations. The recording is crude and non-experts still struggle in the interpretation of it. aEEG is also heavily affected by artefact, that is, any recorded electrical activity that was not created in the brain. This could be cardiac activity, neonatal movement or external factors such as a healthcare worker administering medications. Training in aEEG application and interpretation is essential.

MAGNETIC RESONANCE IMAGING

MRI is the radiological imaging method of choice for brain imaging in infants with HIE. MRI is highly correlated with long-term neurodevelopmental outcome and is therefore a good surrogate marker of outcome. It is superior to cranial ultrasound at detecting injury in the deep grey matter. MRI provides a detailed assessment of the infant's brain structure.

The most common sequences reported in neonatal imaging are T1- and T2-weighted images, diffusion weighted imaging (DWI) and magnetic resonance spectroscopy. T1 and T2 images are useful for assessing grey and white matter abnormalities and anatomical structure. DWI measures the diffusion of water molecules in a tissue and is the best modality to detect acute infarction. A combination of T1, T2 and DWI sequences of the brain are best for identifying hypoxic ischaemic injury. Numerous scoring systems exist, one of the most common being the Barkovich MRI Scoring System as outlined in **Table 16.2**.

Appropriate communication with the family at this time is essential, as this can be a very stressful time. The provision of information, including on the evolution of the clinical assessment, EEG and MRI data, is key to assessing long-term outcome risk. Appropriate multidisciplinary input from neurology, neurophysiology, radiology, physiotherapy, occupational therapy and speech and language are essential and individualized to the patient's needs.

Table 16.2 Barkovich MRI Scoring System

Score	Description
Basal ganglia (BG)	
0	Normal or isolated focal cortical infarct
1	Abnormal signal in thalamus
2	Abnormal signal in thalamus and lentiform nucleus
3	Abnormal signal in thalamus, lentiform nucleus and perirolandic cortex
4	More extensive involvement
Watershed (W)	
0	Normal
1	Single focal infarction
2	Abnormal signal in anterior or posterior watershed white matter
3	Abnormal signal in anterior or posterior watershed cortex and white matter
4	Abnormal signal in both anterior and posterior watershed zones
5	More extensive cortical involvement
Basal ganglia/watershed (BG/W)	
0	Normal
1	Abnormal signal in basal ganglia or thalamus
2	Abnormal signal in cortex
3	Abnormal signal in cortex and basal nuclei (basal ganglia or thalami)
4	Abnormal signal in entire cortex and basal nuclei
Summation (S)	
Arithmetic sum of BG and W	
Enhancement (E)	
0	No enhancement
1	Enhancement in white matter only
2	Enhancement in deep grey matter nuclei
3	Enhancement in cerebral cortex
4	Enhancement in cortex and deep grey matter or white matter

LOCALIZED NEUROLOGY

UPPER LIMB

Brachial plexus palsies are often noted after birth. These may be associated with difficult deliveries, but this does not explain all cases. Erb palsy affects the C5 and C6 nerve roots, giving rise to a distinctive posture with the arm held at the baby's side, internally rotated and pronated. Klumpke palsy affects C8 and T1 but is rare. Total recovery occurs in 75% of babies over a few weeks to months. Referrals to physiotherapy and orthopaedics are essential to minimize complications such as contracture and to assess for surgical intervention if there is no improvement.

FACE

Facial palsy is seen in neonates and is likely to be due to pressure from the mother's sacral promontory during labour. The use of forceps may exacerbate this in some cases. Recovery is usually complete within a few weeks. Asymmetric crying facies is often misinterpreted as a facial palsy. This entity is related to hypoplasia of the orbicularis oris muscle.

LUMBOSACRAL AREA

Small 'dimples' at the bottom of the back are common, affecting around 5% of babies. They can be associated with spinal lesions if the bottom of the dimple is not visible, if the area is high up or to the side or if there is a change to the skin nearby. Ultrasound of the lower spine is indicated if there is any suspicion of a worrying feature.

NEONATAL FRACTURES

The most common sites of neonatal fracture are clavicle, humeral shaft and femoral shaft. Less common sites are at the epiphyses of the humerus or femur. Some fractures are sustained during birth. Almost all neonatal fractures heal without sequelae. Immobilization is difficult in this age group and may not help. Analgesia is important (e.g. with paracetamol).

🔑 KEY LEARNING POINTS

- Seizures are common in newborn infants, affecting 1–2 per 1,000 live births.
- HIE is the leading cause of acquired brain injury in newborns.
- HIE accounts for approximately 50% of all seizures.
- EEG and MRI are essential investigations in the care of infants with HIE.
- Communication with the family is key.

PREMATURITY

Preterm infants are at a greater risk of morbidity than term infants. The moderate to late preterm infant group represents approximately 75–80% of all preterm births. UK data show that babies born between 32 and 36 weeks' gestation represent approximately 6–7% of all births and approximately 75% of all preterm births, equating to approximately 40,000 babies born each year in England and Wales. Mortality for this group of infants is very low, but there are many short- and longer term morbidities associated with late preterm birth. Typically, all babies delivered at <35 weeks are admitted to the SCBU, with variable admission rates above 35 weeks. Often, the reasons for admission include poor feeding, hypoglycaemia or jaundice.

Very preterm birth refers to infants delivered at less than 32 weeks, and extreme preterm infants are those delivered at less than 28 weeks. With continuing advances in technology, pharmacology and medical innovation, the boundaries for survival continue to be lowered. The gestational age at which a live born neonate has a 50% chance of survival has decreased from approximately 32 weeks' gestation in the 1960s to 23/24 weeks' gestation today.

Decision-making at the limit of viability (22–24 weeks), in particular whether resuscitation should occur or not and whether one should continue with intensive care or withdraw support, remains a very challenging process for all involved. There are a number of key players, namely the parents and the healthcare providers, all of whom have the baby's best interest as their primary concern. To help make complex decisions at the borderline of viability, it is important that the most up-to-date outcome data are available. Numerous sources of data are available, including large single-unit cohort studies and national and international studies.

The most important data when counselling expectant parents at the borderline of viability are one's own institutional data, and it is important that those involved in the antenatal discussions are aware of the most up-to-date data to inform families. The original EPICure data from 1995 were very informative for families and healthcare staff caring for extremely preterm infants. Those data equally highlighted some of the challenges around delivery of care at this time, including the high proportion of infants that were cared for in units that had small numbers of babies in this gestation category. Today, we see significant differences in outcomes across countries, some of this related to the approach to care. Survival is higher in regions where there is a much more proactive approach to management. A more centralized approach to care is now taken, along with more active neonatal management. Caring for extreme preterm infants in tertiary centres is perhaps one of the most important elements in managing peri-viable birth.

One of the principle concerns is that, as survival improves at lower gestational ages, so too will the number of babies with significant problems, resulting in lifelong issues for the parents and family. Long-term neurodevelopmental outcome is essential when expectant parents are being counselled. The original EPICure study reported on long-term outcomes at a median of 6 years and found rates of severe, moderate and mild disability to be 22%, 24% and 34%, respectively, in all survivors of delivery at less than 26 weeks. The American Academy of Paediatrics reported in 2002 that 30–50% of surviving children born at less than 25 weeks had moderate to severe impairment. Prevalence studies of the rate of cerebral palsy over different time periods have produced different results, with some seeming to support better longer-term outcomes. There are undoubtedly many methodological issues with each of these studies, but it is fair to surmise that, the lower the gestational age, the greater the risk of mortality and the higher incidence of significant problems (however these are defined) in the survivors.

The recent British Association of Perinatal Medicine (BAPM) publication entitled *Perinatal Management of Extreme Preterm Birth Before 27 Weeks of Gestation* provides an excellent and timely overview of the challenges faced by caregivers and families and provides a new risk-based framework for management. This is an updated framework from the previous 2008 version and an important point to note is that survival at 23 weeks in 2008 is more similar to survival at 22 weeks today (2022). One of the key concerns highlighted previously is the risk of severe impairment in survivors. This is estimated to be approximately one in four survivors with delivery at 23 weeks and one in seven with delivery at 24 weeks. The number of babies surviving delivery at 22 weeks with severe impairment is difficult to quantify; such data would have wide confidence intervals due to the relatively small numbers. However, it would, at best, be the same as that at 23 weeks, although one would have to assume that the rate of severe impairment was higher at 22 weeks (**Table 16.3**).

There are a number of key factors that influence outcome. These include gestational age, birthweight, sex, multiplicity and antenatal steroid administration. The BAPM framework describes a predominantly gestation-based risk assessment, refined by other factors including fetal factors (male sex, multiple pregnancy, congenital anomaly and poor fetal growth), clinical conditions (prolonged pre labour rupture of membranes before 24 weeks), therapeutic interventions (antenatal steroids and magnesium sulphate) and the clinical setting in which infants are cared for. Based on these risk factors, patients are categorized as extremely high risk (>90%), high risk (50–90%) or moderate risk (<50%) based on their chance of either dying or surviving with severe impairment.

Counselling of parents is critical. The information should be provided in a caring and empathetic way. The information needs to be communicated clearly and concisely and needs to be up to date. Ideally, senior members of staff should lead the discussion and, following the consultation, a clear treatment plan should be documented in the maternal notes. This may reflect an active management plan or a palliative approach to care. For example, for a male infant delivered at 22 weeks with a history of chorioamnionitis, no antenatal steroids administered and weighing less than 400 g, a palliative approach may be the most appropriate approach to take.

Some of the key obstetrical components to be addressed include the administration of antenatal steroids, the use of tocolysis, magnesium sulphate administration, the mode of delivery and delayed cord clamping. When there are concerns around infection or significant haemorrhage, tocolysis may not be appropriate. The main aim of tocolysis may be to achieve the maximum benefit from antenatal corticosteroids and allow timely transfer to a tertiary-level unit that cares for babies delivered at the cusp of viability. Perhaps one of the greatest areas of debate relates to the mode of delivery, especially when the fetus is in breech presentation and may require a classical incision. Extremely preterm caesarean delivery can be difficult and carries additional risks for the mother. These include haemorrhage, infection, bowel injury and risks for future pregnancies. Senior obstetrical decision-making in conjunction with the mother and the neonatal team is warranted. This highlights the importance of communication between the various specialities and the

Table 16.3 Outcome for babies born alive at 22–26 weeks*

Gestation	22 weeks	23 weeks	24 weeks	25 weeks	26 weeks
Survival	30% (21–49%)	40% (32–44%)	60% (55–65%)	70% (70–78%)	80% (70–85%)
Significant developmental problems	1 in 3	1 in 4	1 in 7	1 in 7	1 in 10

Source: Adapted from BAPM (2019). *Perinatal Management of Extreme Preterm Birth Before 27 Weeks of Gestation. A BAPM Framework for Practice.*
* Some babies born this prematurely cannot survive labour and birth. The figures in brackets indicate how certain we are of the true survival rate. Up to a quarter of children without severe disability may nonetheless have milder forms of disability such as learning difficulty, mild cerebral palsy or behavioural problems.

family. The antenatal consultation allows open and frank discussion. Parental views are explored, balanced information is provided to the family and outcome data are discussed. The consultation provides the family with an opportunity to discuss potential options and treatment plans.

Neonatal management plans are discussed in advance. It is important that exactly what these terms (active and palliative) mean is discussed during the antenatal consultation with the neonatology team. It is important to inform the families of how the infant might appear and that, in situations in which palliation may be chosen, some infants may cry at birth. There also has to be the caveat that, in certain circumstances (albeit rarely), plans may need to be revised (e.g. in situations in which the baby is born in unexpectedly good condition and the weight is significantly different from what had been determined previously).

When an active approach is taken, it is essential that a consultant neonatologist is present to guide the stabilization process. Delayed cord clamping for at least 60 seconds should occur, and stabilization should follow one of the standardized newborn resuscitation programmes being delivered in that institution (e.g. NLS, NRP). Prevention of hypothermia with the use of a plastic bag and the provision of CPAP with a face mask via a T-piece device to ensure lung inflation is central to newborn stabilization. A rising heart rate is a reflection of effective stabilization. Some centres will intubate and administer surfactant, others may try to avoid the placement of an endotracheal tube and instead insert a fine bore catheter to provide surfactant while the baby is spontaneously breathing and in receipt of CPAP. The stabilization process should typically occur in the same room as the parents who should be provided with the opportunity to touch their baby prior to subsequent transfer to the neonatal unit where hopefully a long journey will begin.

PREMATURITY AND COMPLICATIONS

A general understanding of some of the common morbidities associated with preterm birth is important for the obstetrician. These include morbidities such as respiratory distress syndrome (RDS), bronchopulmonary dysplasia (BPD), necrotizing enterocolitis (NEC), IVH and periventricular leukomalacia.

The importance of the antenatal consultation, detailing the journey and stressing the importance of breast milk provision cannot be overstated. We will begin this section by discussing the benefits of breast milk and then review the various morbidities associated with preterm birth.

BREAST MILK

Breastfeeding is the gold standard for newborn infants and has substantial health, growth and development benefits. The World Health Organization (WHO) recommends that infants should be exclusively breastfed for the first 6 months (WHO 2017). Formula feeding attempts to mimic breast milk, but it does not contain all of the nutritional and non-nutritional components. Breast milk has multiple bioactive and immune factors such as antibodies, immunoglobulins, lactoferrin, lysozyme, growth factors, white blood cells, microRNAs, stem cells and human milk oligosaccharides (HMOs). Each of these have direct health benefits and are critical for the developing infant immune system. Breast milk contains probiotics such as *Bifidobacterium* and *Lactobacillus* and HMOs encourage the proliferation of these probiotic microorganisms in the infant gut. Feeding preterm infants breast milk results in a significant reduction in the incidence of NEC and sepsis. It is easy to see how this may be the case when one considers the non-nutritional components outlined previously. Encouraging breast milk for the preterm infant is essential, and efforts should be made during antenatal visits to encourage mothers to consider breastfeeding.

Breastfeeding is also associated with longer term benefits such as a reduction in the risk of immune-mediated diseases including asthma, inflammatory bowel disease, type 1 diabetes and metabolic diseases later in life and it is probable that the infant gut microbiota plays a role here.

The intestinal microbiota in early life plays a major role in infant health and development, having an impact on maturation of the immune system, protection against pathogens and influencing the long-term metabolic welfare of the host. Breast milk provides the optimal active ingredients for the growth of beneficial microbial species. Our understanding of the intestinal microbiome is only in its infancy.

It must also be remembered that breastfeeding also confers health benefits to the mother. One must not forget the potential psychological benefits it gives to mothers to know that their milk has significant health benefits for their baby and that they are contributing to their infant's well-being. In situations in which breast milk is not available, there are donor milk banks available that can be used to supply breast milk for the very preterm population.

COMMON MORBIDITIES

Respiratory distress syndrome

RDS is caused by primary surfactant deficiency combined with structural immaturity of the lung. Antenatal corticosteroids significantly decrease the incidence of RDS. The more immature the infant, the greater the incidence of RDS, the greater the likelihood that they will receive mechanical ventilation and other modalities such as high-frequency oscillation and thus the greater chance of longer term pulmonary morbidity. Management has evolved over the last 20 years and the mainstay of therapy is now aimed at trying to avoid mechanical ventilation with CPAP and early surfactant replacement therapy. Advances in surfactant administration have included the intubation surfactant extubation (INSURE) technique, the less invasive surfactant administration (LISA) technique with a fine bore catheter and, more recently, nebulized surfactant therapy. When babies are intubated and mechanically ventilated for whatever reason (RDS, infection, apnoea), the goal must be to try and safely remove the endotracheal tube as quickly as possible to avoid all of the adverse effects of mechanical ventilation and the increased risk of BPD.

Bronchopulmonary dysplasia

BPD is one of the most common complications of prematurity, affecting up to 40% of infants delivered at less than 28 weeks' gestation. It is a complex multifactorial disorder. BPD occurs preterm when the lungs are evolving from the canalicular to the saccular stage of development. Exposure to air, oxygen, adverse effects of mechanical ventilation, infection and inflammation lead to a derangement of this normal process. Intrauterine growth failure, infection and chorioamnionitis can also have an

impact on this process and contribute to the development of deranged lung growth and abnormal vascular development.

The definition has continued to evolve from the original Northway classification through to more recent definitions such as the US National Institute of Child Health and Human Development definition from 2018, which classifies the condition as a continuum rather than a 'yes or no' phenomenon. The most recent suggested classification attempts to categorize babies as mild, moderate or severe based on the need for various levels of respiratory support and oxygen need.

Prevention is always better than cure. Strategies aimed at reducing BPD are aimed at avoiding some of the key factors associated with the development of the disorder. In the delivery suite, this means avoiding/minimizing oxygen toxicity, avoiding mechanical ventilation if possible, less invasive means of providing surfactant and, if ventilation is required, avoiding volutrauma and barotrauma. Reducing the number of days with an endotracheal tube in situ is important and the use of non-invasive ventilation such as CPAP is key. Infection often results in an increase in respiratory support and often an increase in the number of ventilator days. PDA has been associated with the development of BPD. Centres using prophylactic indomethacin as a therapy have lower rates of PDA and BPD than centres that do not. The next few years will provide more evidence around ductal management and adverse outcome in the extreme preterm infant group.

Medical therapies aimed at prevention include the use of caffeine, intramuscular vitamin A and postnatal corticosteroid administration. Caffeine was found to be associated with a lower incidence of BPD in the 'caffeine for apnoea of prematurity' trial and vitamin A decreased BPD rates. The issue with vitamin A administration is the frequent intramuscular injections that are required. Recent trials of steroid use have demonstrated some benefit.

Management of established cases of BPD should include input from multiple disciplines including neonatology, cardiology, pulmonology and dietetics. Therapies often include diuretics and bronchodilators but their efficacy is not well studied. Corticosteroids remain the mainstay of treatment. Controversy still remains around the optimal drug, timing and duration of therapy. Pulmonary hypertension is common in the setting of BPD. Additional therapies such as nitric oxide, sildenafil and bosentan are now being used, but there is currently little evidence to support their use.

Circulatory challenges

Circulatory instability is a common occurrence in the extreme preterm infant. It is often characterized by a low blood pressure. Hypotension is commonly diagnosed and treated in the very preterm infant, but there is enormous variation in practice, largely due to a lack of good evidence. It has been associated with adverse short-term and long-term outcomes. The evidence to support current management strategies is minimal and mostly dependent on small studies with short-term physiological end points. Preterm infants with blood pressure lower than average often have no biochemical or clinical signs of shock. Careful observation of such infants without intervention may well be appropriate.

Excessive intervention in preterm infants may be unnecessary or even harmful. The most common approach to treatment is to give one or more fluid boluses followed by dopamine. Fluctuations in blood pressure following commencement of inotropes are well recognized and could also trigger IVH. Furthermore, dopamine, the most used inotrope, has effects on many physiological functions, including pituitary effects, which lead to secondary hypothyroidism, a known risk factor for poor long-term neurodevelopmental outcome in the preterm infant.

Many clinicians rely on absolute blood pressure values to guide intervention. Blood pressure reference ranges are often based on birthweight, gestational age and postnatal age criteria. These statistically determined values vary considerably. The Joint Working Group of the BAPM has recommended that the mean arterial blood pressure in mmHg should be maintained above the gestational age in weeks. Despite little published evidence to support this 'rule', it remains the most common criteria used to define hypotension. Evidence is lacking in this area of newborn care and the next few years may bring clarity to a more individualized approach. The use of neonatal echocardiography has increased, and this should help provide greater clarity on the underlying pathophysiology. The hope then is that a more tailored approach may lead to an improved outcome.

Patent ductus arteriosus

The ductus arteriosus connects the pulmonary artery to the descending aorta. During the first days of the feto-neonatal transition, the ductus should close. Patency of the ductus arteriosus is the most common cardiovascular abnormality of the newborn and affects up to 60% of babies born at less than 28 weeks' gestation. PDA is associated with multiple morbidities (BPD, IVH, NEC, poor neurodevelopmental outcome) and death. Early identification and treatment of a haemodynamically significant duct may be important to ameliorate these associations.

Clinical signs can increase a clinician's suspicion of the presence of PDA, but they are not useful in identifying a haemodynamically significant duct without a bedside echocardiogram. Clinical signs most often present beyond the first few days of age at which stage the risk of morbidity is higher. Clinical effects of the ductus can be divided into those caused by excessive pulmonary blood flow and those due to reduced systemic blood flow, which occur in the setting of left to right flow at the level of the ductus (**Table 16.4**).

Despite multiple studies – some aimed at prophylaxis and others at treating a symptomatic ductus, with others advocating the complete opposite and adopting a conservative approach – the best approach remains elusive at present. Further trials in this area are warranted. When medical therapy fails, surgical treatment is warranted. Previously, this involved a thoracotomy, but today the duct can be closed percutaneously.

Necrotizing enterocolitis

NEC is a serious gastrointestinal complication that occurs primarily in preterm neonates and causes significant morbidity and mortality. Its incidence is approximately 5–10% in babies delivered at less than 32 weeks and is more likely with decreasing gestational age. It is a multifactorial problem characterized by by intestinal immaturity and bacterial overgrowth in association with altered blood flow. It is more common in the more immature and growth-restricted infants. Prolonged early courses of postnatal antibiotics are also associated with an increased incidence of NEC. It can be devastating when it occurs.

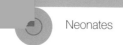

Table 16.4 Physiological and clinical effects of a haemodynamically significant patent ductus arteriosus

Excessive pulmonary flow	Reduced systemic flow
Physiological effects	
Reduced lung compliance	Fall in aortic end diastolic flow velocity
Pulmonary oedema	PDA steal phenomenon: reduction of cerebral/renal/mesenteric perfusion
Reduced gas exchange	Lactic acidosis
Increased pulmonary vascular resistance	
Clinical effects	
Tachypnoea	Low diastolic blood pressure
Increased oxygen requirements	Wide pulse pressure
Increased carbon dioxide retention	Bounding pulses
Ventilator dependence	Hepatomegaly (right heart failure)
Apnoea and bradycardia	Feeding intolerance
	Low urine output

PDA, patent ductus arteriosus.

The provision of the mother's own breast milk is the most effective way to decrease an infant's risk of acquiring NEC as outlined previously. The evidence base for the use of probiotics remains contentious. Studies are limited by low power and a lack of consistency between probiotic strains, treatment regimens and study design. However, meta-analyses have shown benefit, particularly when administered in conjunction with maternal-expressed breast milk, and is associated with a reduction in the incidence of NEC. A 2020 Cochrane review by Sharif *et al.* assessed 56 trials with over 10,000 infants; it found that the use of probiotics was associated with a 46% reduction in risk of NEC (relative risk (RR) 0.54, 95% confidence interval (CI) 0.45–0.65) with a number needed to treat of 33 (95% CI 25–50). Furthermore, probiotics were associated with an overall reduction in mortality (RR 0.76, 95% CI 0.65–0.89) with a number needed to treat of 50 (95% CI 50–100).

Intraventricular haemorrhage/periventricular leukomalacia

Acquired brain injury in very preterm infants usually results from haemodynamic instability and cerebral dysautoregulation. IVH in preterm neonates occurs in up to 60% of those weighing 500–750 g and in 10–20% of those weighing 1,000–1,500 g. The potential sequelae can be devastating, including death and significant long-term neurodevelopmental delay. Germinal matrix IVH and periventricular leukomalacia account for most of the cerebral brain injury in very preterm infants. The subependymal germinal matrix is rich in immature vessels, which are poorly supported by connective tissue. Fluctuations in cerebral blood flow with pressure changes promote a cycle of ischemia followed by reperfusion and this plays an important role in the pathogennesis of IVH. Most neonates with IVH are asymptomatic.

The Papile classification system of IVH is based on the degree of bleeding and is described as grades I to IV. Grades I and II represent mild IVH. Grades III and IV represent moderate-to-severe IVH – these neonates are at an increased risk of more significant outcomes including post-haemorrhagic hydrocephalus and shunt insertion, cerebral palsy and learning difficulties. Risk factors include prematurity (particularly in neonates <32 weeks' gestational age), low birthweight, hypotension, RDS, pneumothorax, PDA and hypoxia.

Periventricular leukomalacia is the most common form of white matter injury in preterm infants and results in cerebral palsy and learning difficulties in a large percentage of survivors. This area of the brain is particularly sensitive to low perfusion-related injury. Often this occurs in the setting of chorioamnionitis and premature rupture of membranes.

Retinopathy of prematurity

Babies born before 32 weeks' gestation or weighing less than 1,500 g are at risk of retinopathy of prematurity (ROP). Untreated, this condition leads to vascular proliferation in the retina and potentially retinal detachment and blindness. Treatment is effective and a screening programme is well established. The first successful treatment was cryotherapy, which has been superseded by laser treatment. Laser treatment may be superseded by other treatments such as intraocular injection with antibodies that block the actions of vascular endothelial growth factor (VEGF). In the past, ROP was thought to be due to administration of excessive amounts of oxygen. More recently, it has become clear that oxygen is only part of the problem. Other factors such as low birthweight, poor growth, low levels of insulin-like growth factor and excessive activity of VEGF are now thought to contribute to the development of ROP. The interventions listed here have significantly reduced the risk of significant visual impairment.

> ## 🔑 KEY LEARNING POINTS
>
> - Clear communication between caregivers and expectant parents is critical when extreme preterm birth is imminent.
> - An awareness of major outcome data is key.
> - An understanding of the key morbidities of preterm birth is essential.

PALLIATIVE CARE

While neonatal mortality remains very low, when newborns die, it is often in the immediate neonatal period. The perinatal team needs to develop a shared approach to this distressing circumstance. Fetal medicine services frequently identify the fetuses likely to die shortly after birth. When the families of babies with a potentially life-limiting condition choose to continue the pregnancy, a series of discussions is convened to discuss the options. Sometimes, it is possible to give a firm estimate that the baby will die within minutes of birth. More commonly, it may not be possible to be sure whether the baby will live

for minutes, hours or days. The neonatal contribution is to identify the possible scenarios and outline what is likely to happen in each scenario. Short-term survival for minutes or hours is often managed on the labour suite, preferably in a dedicated area that is designed to enhance family comfort. If the baby survives for 2–3 days, management in a sensitively selected area of the postnatal or neonatal ward may be optimal. If survival for more than 2–3 days is possible, then contact can be made with a local hospice so that families can consider that option.

Parallel planning is undertaken for several scenarios because of the uncertainty and variability between babies. Thus, a plan is made for each of the likely scenarios. These plans provide a framework for discussion and are often changed in the light of events. Parents should be given a range of options and should be supported to identify the course of action that meets their preferences. Paediatric palliative care team involvement is very helpful, even if the baby is not expected to travel to a hospice. The birth plan takes account of the neonatal options and the mother's obstetric needs and wishes. The trade-offs between type of birth (e.g. vaginal birth versus caesarean section) and the condition of the baby will be specific to each family. The team may need to account for the need for postnatal investigations if there is any uncertainty about the diagnosis or prognosis.

Families may wish to take a dying baby or a baby's body home and this should be facilitated. Organ transplant of some organs is technically possible in some cases but requires considerable planning and organization to ensure that an efficient system is in place before an opportunity to discuss transplantation arises.

The secret to the 'perinatal hospice' is shared working, advance planning and prospective mapping of the relevant services. Once a plan (or a set of parallel plans) has been agreed for a family, then all members of the team need to be aware of the plan and to follow it. This requires very clear, comprehensive documentation that is immediately available to all caregivers. Unexpected events need to be escalated rapidly to the most experienced member of the team so that appropriate adaptations to the plan can be made. Palliative care services can facilitate

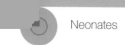

follow-up for the family. Supporting a family before and after the death of a baby is demanding work and staff should be offered debrief sessions and other support as appropriate.

IMPORTANCE OF CLINICAL TRIALS IN NEONATAL CARE

Research-active centres generally have better outcomes overall for patients than non-research-active centres. It is important that obstetricians and neonatologists are aware of ongoing studies within both fields. These studies have contributed significantly to the evidence base upon which many interventions now occur (e.g. antenatal steroids, antenatal magnesium sulphate, surfactant administration, probiotics and TH). Obtaining informed consent in newborn trials presents many challenges that are not necessarily encountered in other areas of medicine. The process of informed consent requires several pre-specified criteria to be met. These include adequate disclosure and comprehension of the information provided, voluntariness and that the patient (in this case the parent) is deemed to be competent. The provision of information involves both disclosure of adequate information and comprehension of the information provided. The wording of information booklets and consent forms is critical to the parents' understanding of what is being asked of them. A summary of the intervention in non-medical terms is essential, and information on the risks and benefits of the treatment addressed, confidentiality, refusal to participate or withdrawal at any point is also provided.

Therapeutic research in neonatal care is essential. Most parents are happy for their children to participate in clinical research. There are challenges with the current informed consent process. Some of these relate to the inherent difficulties associated with having a sick newborn in the NICU. It is important that parents are given sufficient time to comprehend this information. It is important that parents are approached at an appropriate time and do not in any way feel coerced into participating. Listening to parents and getting their opinions on the consent process is critical to our ability to conduct trials in this

area. Their involvement in aspects of study design is important. Through a collaborative approach, we will be able to conduct important future trials to help address many of the unanswered questions in perinatal and neonatal care.

CONCLUSION

This chapter addresses some of the key areas of perinatal care. Normal adaptation is described, along with many of the transient transitional problems that arise during the first days of life. Many of the challenges in caring for newborn infants born extremely preterm, babies born with suspected neonatal encephalopathy and babies with significant adaptation challenges such as pulmonary hypertension are highlighted. An understanding of these conditions will facilitate effective communication between healthcare providers, but most importantly with families at what can be a very challenging time.

FURTHER READING

BAPM (2019). *Perinatal Management of Extreme Preterm Birth Before 27 Weeks of Gestation. A BAPM Framework for Practice*. https://www.bapm.org/resources/80-perinatal-management-of-extreme-preterm-birth-before-27-weeks-of-gestation-2019.

Martinello K, Hart AR, Yap S, *et al.* (2017). Management and investigation of neonatal encephalopathy: 2017 update. *Archives of Disease in Childhood – Fetal and Neonatal Edition*, 102: F346–F358.

Moore T, Hennessy EM, Myles J, *et al.* (2012). Neurological and developmental outcome in extremely preterm children born in England in 1995 and 2006: the EPICure studies. *BMJ*, 345: e7961. https://doi.org/10.1136/bmj.e7961.

Morton SU, Brodsky D (2016). Fetal physiology and the transition to extrauterine life. *Clinics in Perinatology*, 43(3): 395-407. https://doi.org/10.1016/j.clp.2016.04.001.

Resuscitation Council UK. NLS (Newborn Life Support) Course. https://www.resus.org.uk/training-courses/newborn-life-support/nls-newborn-life-support.

SELF-ASSESSMENT

For interactive SBAs and EMQs relating to this chapter, visit www.routledge.com/cw/mccarthy.

CASE HISTORY 1

A 34-year-old primigravid woman is found to have anhydramnios at an 18-week scan. No kidneys can be seen on the scan and a follow-up MRI scan also failed to identify renal tissue. A diagnosis of renal aplasia is made. The couple elect to continue the pregnancy. A follow-up scan 4 weeks later confirms anhydramnios. An antenatal discussion takes place at 28 weeks. Please discuss the key factors that need to be addressed.

A **Input from the multidisciplinary team:** fetal medicine specialists, neonatologists, nephrologists and the paediatric palliative care team.

B **The diagnosis and prognosis:** the baby will most likely die due to severe pulmonary hypoplasia. Extensive resuscitation is not in the baby's best interests.

C **The implications for the baby:** the baby may die in utero or during labour; the baby may die within minutes of birth – if this is likely, the baby will stay with the mother immediately after birth; rarely, the baby survives for a longer period if full intensive care support is provided. However, the outcome will be the same: the baby will die within the first days of life. The sequence of events may turn out to be different but an initial good response after birth does not change the ultimate prognosis. Anhydramnios from 18 weeks in the presence of bilateral multicystic kidneys is not compatible with life.

D **The range of options for the family:** the family can ask the professionals to do what they think best; the family can be part of joint decision-making. The family can stay together at all times. Careful planning needs to take place around end-of-life care and the family need to be involved. Some families may have requested a trial of breathing support and the extent of this support should be addressed well in advance. Clear communication is key.

E **The extent and nature of resuscitation that is offered immediately after birth:** a senior neonatologist should be present to direct the management. Clear plans need to be developed. The goal should be to ensure that the baby is comfortable.

CASE HISTORY 2

A 28-year-old dentist presents in preterm labour at 26 weeks' gestation. You have been asked to have an antenatal discussion with the couple. Please discuss the key points you would like to address.

A Survival overall at 26 weeks is over 80–85%.

B The duration of stay in the neonatal unit is approximately 3 months, but can be longer if significant problems are encountered along the way. These include breathing difficulties, the risk of bleeding into the immature brain, the risk of infection and the risk of inflammation/infection in the abdomen.

C The family should be reassured that the neonatal team will be present at the delivery and will communicate fully with them in the delivery suite.

D Many babies will need ventilatory support at birth and for some time period thereafter.

E The importance of breast milk and its benefits should be stressed.

F The majority of survivors will go to mainstream school. Some will need additional support with reading or paying attention.

G 10% of survivors are at risk of significant disability.

Index